RADIATION
PROTECTION
in Medical Radiography

RADIATION PROTECTION
in Medical Radiography

Mary Alice Statkiewicz-Sherer,
A.S., R.T.(R), F.A.S.R.T.

Paul J. Visconti, Ph.D.

E. Russell Ritenour, Ph.D.

SECOND EDITION

with 128 *illustrations*

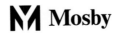 Mosby

St. Louis Baltimore Boston Chicago London Philadelphia Sydney Toronto

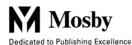

Publisher: David T. Culverwell
Editorial Project Supervisor: Cecilia Reilly
Developmental Editor: Christi Mangold
Production Editor: Allan S. Kleinberg
Designer: Julie Taugner
Manufacturing Supervisor: Theresa Fuchs

Cover photograph: © Jamie Barnett/Custom Medical Stock Photo

SECOND EDITION

Printed in the United States of America

Mosby–Year Book, Inc.
11830 Westline Industrial Drive
St. Louis, Missouri 63146

Library of Congress Cataloging in Publication Data
Sherer, Mary Alice, 1945-
    Radiation protection in medical radiography / Mary Alice
Statkiewicz-Sherer, Paul J. Visconti, E. Russell Ritenour.—2nd
ed.
       p.   cm.
    Rev. ed. of: Radiation protection for student radiographers / Mary
Alice Statkiewicz, E. Russell Ritenour, c1983.
    Includes bibliographical references and index.
    ISBN 0-8016-5750-4
    1. Radiography, Medical—Safety measures. I. Visconti, Paul J.
II. Ritenour, E. Russell, 1953- . III. Sherer, Mary Alice, 1945-
Radiation protection for student radiographers. IV. Title.
    [DNLM: 1. Radiography—adverse effects. 2. Radiation Protection.
WN 200 S551n 1993]
RC78.3.S54   1993
616.07'57'0289—dc20
DNLM/DLC
for Library of Congress
                                             93-16166
                                              CIP

96 97 CL/MV 9 8 7 6 5 4 3

To dad,
and in memory of mom,

To my sons,
Joseph, Christopher, and Terry, with love,

and

To all with whom I may share my knowledge.

About the Authors

Mary Alice Statkiewicz-Sherer, A.S., R.T.(R), F.A.S.R.T., the primary author of this text, is a private radiography education and medical publishing consultant. She also performs radiographic procedures for HCA Donelson Hospital in Nashville, Tennessee. Mrs. Statkiewicz-Sherer was previously employed at Memorial Hospital of Burlington County in Mount Holly, New Jersey, where she served for over 16 years as Program Director for the institution's Radiography Program and then as Educational Administrative Assistant for the Department of Radiology for over a year.

After earning an A.R.R.T. certification in 1965, Mrs. Statkiewicz-Sherer filled several technical and teaching positions in the New Jersey Area and graduated with an Associate in Science degree from the College of Allied Health Professions, Hahnemann Medical College and Hospital of Philadelphia (now Hahnemann University) in 1980. She has been an active and leading member of several professional organizations, having served on American Society of Radiologic Technologists committees and task forces, as President of the 28th Mid-Eastern Conference of Radiologic Technologists, and as President and Chairman of the Board of Directors of the New Jersey Society of Radiologic Technologists. Most recent services to the A.S.R.T. include functioning as Chairman of the Editorial Review Board for the membership year 1989-91 and serving as a member of the Committee on Memorial Lectures for the membership year 1989-91 and for 1991-93. In June 1990 Mrs. Statkiewicz-Sherer was elevated to Fellow of the American Society of Radiologic Technologists for her services and contributions to the profession.

In addition to being the primary author of the first edition, *Radiation Protection for Student Radiographers,* and also of this second edition, Mrs. Statkiewicz-Sherer co-authored the textbook, *Radiation Protection for Dental Radiographers,* which was published by Multi-Media Publishing, Denver, in 1984. Articles written by Mrs. Statkiewicz-Sherer have been published in

Radiologic Technology, the *Journal of the American Society of Radiologic Technologists,* and *ADVANCE for Radiologic Science Professionals,* a weekly newspaper published by Merion Publications, King of Prussia, Pennsylvania. She also serves as a consultant to ADVANCE.

Paul J. Visconti, Ph.D., since 1982 has been Director of Medical Physics and Radiation Safety Officer at Memorial Hospital of Burlington County in Mount Holly, New Jersey. Dr. Visconti received a Ph.D. in physics from the City University of New York in 1971. He was a full-time instructor in the Physics Department at the City College of New York for several years therafter. Dr. Visconti began his career in medical physics at Montefiore Hospital and Medical Center in New York City, where he remained for five years as an Associate Physicist. During that time he lectured extensively in radiological physics both to diagnostic radiology residents and to student radiographers. Dr. Visconti is a member of the Society of the Sigma Xi, the American Association of Physicists in Medicine, the American College of Medical Physics, the American College of Radiology, and is certified in Therapeutic Radiological Physics by the American Board of Radiology.

E. Russell Ritenour, Ph.D. is Associate Professor and Director of the Physics Section, Department of Radiology, University of Minnesota School of Medicine. He is also a member of the graduate faculty of Biophysical Sciences at the University of Minnesota. Dr. Ritenour received his Ph.D. in physics from the University of Virginia, completed a post-doctoral fellowship in medical physics sponsored by the National Institutes of Health, and was a member of the faculty of the University of Colorado School of Medicine for ten years, serving as director of the graduate medical physics training program until moving to Minnesota. He has served as radiation safety officer for several hospitals and research foundations, served as consultant to the Army for resident training programs, and written a number of audiovisual training programs for radiologic technologists, radiology residents, and medical physicists. He has been active on committees of the American College of Radiology, the American Board of Radiology, the American Association of Physicists in Medicine, and is a past president of the Rocky Mountain Chapter of the Health Physics Society.

Foreword

This textbook, originally conceived as an updated version of *Radiation Protection for Student Radiographers,* which was published in 1983, has advanced well beyond that concept. The same fundamental principles and goals employed in the initial text have been vastly expanded. New concepts and data have been incorporated into the second edition.

The authors have included information in radiation protection and radiation biology that will meet not only the needs of current student and graduate radiographers but also will be very germane for both radiology residents and practicing radiologists. Hence, the new title, *Radiation Protection in Medical Radiography,* is justified and appropriate.

Each chapter of this text clearly states its objectives, teaches the material in a concise, simple format using multidisciplinary techniques, and summarizes all salient concepts in a precise manner.

While the knowledge in this text is essential to understanding the biological effects of ionizing radiation and radiation protection at a basic scientific level, clinically this same information will serve as a standard to radiographers and physicians alike to promote the safe use of medical ionizing radiation. It is an important text that can be used either as a learning tool or reference guide by all radiography personnel.

Howard Scott Berinson, M.D.
Memorial Hospital of Burlington County,
Mount Holly, New Jersey
Diagnostic Radiologist
Member of the American College of Radiology

Preface to the Second Edition

When *Radiation Protection for Student Radiographers* was published in 1983, it was intended only as a fundamental text for instructional use in extablished medical radiography programs. Since that time, in addition to being widely accepted in that role, the book has also become a popular resource and reference guide to the safe use of x-rays by practicing radiographers, radiology residents, medical physicists, and physicians internationally. Hence, to reflect the wide range acceptance and use of the text, the title of the second edition has been changed to *Radiation Protection in Medical Radiography*. To facilitate a working knowledge of the principles of radiation protection, study materials presented in the second edition remain sophisticated enough to be true to the complexity of the subject yet simple and concise enough to permit adequate and efficient comprehension by all readers.

The format of the book remains unchanged. Each chapter begins with a list of learning objectives and ends with a set of multiple-choice review questions with which the reader can measure the knowledge acquired. Several new questions have been added to each chapter, and answers to all test questions are given in Appendix A. Appendix B gives the metric system equivalents for length, and Appendix C reprints the Consumer-Patient Radiation Health and Safety Act of 1981. The Glossary has had numerous terms added. Each chapter has had its Bibliography updated and expanded.

While there has been little change in most of the concepts of radiation protection and radiation biology, some new ideas and some significant modifications considered to be important to diagnostic radiology personnel have been incorporated in the second edition. Many radiation protection and radiation biology principles have been expanded on to increase the overall knowledge of the reader. Tables have been updated to reflect the most current information. Additional photographs and illustrations have been inserted to enhance the visual impact of the text and to promote retention of the study material.

For student radiographers and radiology residents this text is not intended as a complete self-teaching tool; rather, it should be used in conjunction with lectures presented by a qualified instructor. The practicing radiographer, medical physicist, and physician may use this book as a self-teaching instrument to broaden and reinforce existing knowledge of the subject matter.

By mastering the material covered in this monograph and by applying this knowledge in the performance of radiologic procedures, the reader will help to ensure the safety of the patient and all diagnostic radiology personnel.

Mary Alice Statkiewicz-Sherer

Acknowledgments

The greatest treasure a person can have is the love and support of family and good friends. To my family, who are my greatest treasure, and to my many caring friends, I wish to express my sincerest thanks for your support, encouragement, and understanding during the preparation of this second edition. I also extend special thanks to the radiologists, radiographers, and Radiology Department ancillary personnel at HCA Donelson Hospital, Nashville, Tennessee, who have provided inspiration and encouragement. Their friendship and support helped to make possible the completion of this manuscript.

A most sincere expression of gratitude is extended to my collaborator, Paul J. Visconti, Ph.D., for numerous technical recommendations, contribution of materials, encouragement, and valuable advice. Dr. Visconti has greatly contributed to enhancing the technical and scientific value of this publication. Sincere appreciation is also expressed to my other collaborating author, E. Russell Ritenour, Ph.D., for contribution of materials, technical recommendations, and valuable advice for the second edition and also for his significant contribution to the first edition. Both Dr. Visconti and Dr. Ritenour have contributed to making this publication a valuable resource for radiation protection and radiation biology.

Thanks is given to the professional staff of Mosby, with special acknowledgement to Cecilla F. Reilly, Editorial Project Supervisor and Christi Mangold, Developmental Editor, for assistance in the preparation and publication of this text. A special note of thanks is also extended to Publisher David Culverwell for granting me the additional time I needed to complete this edition following an automobile accident in which I sustained injury.

Radiography students and radiology residents are the hope of the medical imaging profession. They are the radiologic technologists and radiologists of the future. To my former radiography students from Memorial Hospital of Burlington County in Mount Holly, New Jersey, I extend a special thanks for inspiring me to prepare both the first and second editions. To those who will use this text, it is my hope that the materials contained in this second edition will greatly contribute to enhancing your knowledge of radiation protection and radiation biology.

Appreciation is extended to those who have given permission to reproduce illustrations, diagrams, quotations, and pictures from their work. Their material enhances this manuscript. In particular, special thanks for use of materials is given to Stewart C. Bushong, Sc.D, Philip W. Ballinger, M.S., R.T.(R), and Professor Elizabeth LaTorre Travis.

Acknowledgments and thanks for permission to reproduce photographic materials are also given to the National Council on Radiation Protection and Measurements (Bethesda, Maryland); the U.S. Department of Energy, Office of LWR Safety and Technology and the Office of Nuclear Energy (Washington, D.C.); and the U.S. Department of Energy, Nevada Operations Office (Las Vegas, Nevada). Many manufacturers of products and commercial suppliers have provided technical information about their products and have given permission for the reproduction of photographs and other illustrations. Thanks for the use of these materials is given to the following companies: Baird Corporation (Bedford, Massachusetts); Dosimetry Corporation of America (Cincinnati, Ohio); Eberline Instruments (Santa Fe, New Mexico); Landauer, Inc. (Glenwood, Illinois); Machlett Labs, Inc. (Stamford, Connecticut); Nuclear Associates (Carle Place, New York); Solon Technologies, Inc. (Solon, Ohio); Victoreen, Inc. (Solon, Ohio); and X-Rite, Inc. (Grandville, Michigan). Sincere gratitude is also expressed to Ramanik Patel, M.S., for discussions in radiation biology.

As acknowledged in the first edition of the text, a very special rememberance is noted to my parents, Felix and the late Elizabeth (Markovitch) Krohn, for all they have done for me. The education they made possible helped me to gain the knowledge necessary to prepare this monograph.

Finally, to my sons, Joseph F. Statkiewicz, Christopher R. Statkiewicz, and Terry Richard Sherer, Jr., a special thanks for the many times each of you has said, "I love you, mom. You can do it." You always provided love and encouragement when it was most needed. Your support gave me the necessary incentive to complete this edition.

Mary Alice Statkiewicz-Sherer

Contents

9
Radiation Monitoring, 242

Appendix A

Appendix B

Appendix C

Introduction to Radiation Protection

OBJECTIVES

Upon completion of this chapter, the reader will be able to:

- explain the need for radiation protection procedures
- define ionizing radiation
- describe the potential for ionizing radiation to cause biological damage
- define *sievert* and *rem* and explain their functions
- identify the various sources of natural background ionizing radiation and the different sources of man-made, or artificial, ionizing radiation
- describe the magnitude of medical radiation exposure
- explain the responsibility for radiation protection in the field of radiology

Since the early 1900s, scientists have been aware of the beneficial as well as the destructive potential of ionizing radiation. By using the knowledge of radiation hazards that has been gained over the years and by employing effective methods to limit or eliminate those hazards, humans can exercise greater control over the use of "radiant energy." Various methods of radiation protection can be applied to ensure safety for persons employed in radiation industries, including the healing arts, and for the population at large. This discussion focuses on radiation protection for the patient, all diagnostic radiology personnel, and the general public.

JUSTIFICATION AND RESPONSIBILITY FOR RADIOLOGIC PROCEDURES

For persons in good health, radiation exposure should *always* be kept to the *lowest* possible level. In certain cases of illness or injury, however, it is accepted medical practice to expose the patient to ionizing radiation for the purpose of obtaining valuable diagnostic information. Ionizing radiation possesses a beneficial as well as a destructive potential, and, when employed in the healing arts for the welfare of the patient, the potential benefits of exposing the patient to ionizing radiation outweigh the risk involved (Fig. 1-1).

Physicians who order radiologic examinations must accept basic responsibility for patient safety from radiation exposure. Relying on competent technical personnel is one way they can exercise this responsibility. As qualified professionals, radiographers accept a portion of the responsibility by providing quality patient care and radiologic services. The radiologist and the radiographer share the responsibility for keeping medical radiation exposure to the lowest level possible. This can *best* be accomplished by using the smallest radiation exposure that will produce useful radiographs, and by producing high-quality radiographs with the *first* exposure; repeat examinations caused by technical error or carelessness must be avoided, because they significantly increase radiation exposure for both the patient and the radiation worker.

IONIZING RADIATION
Definition

In simple terms, *radiation* is a transfer of energy that results either because of a change occurring naturally within an atom (e.g., radioactive decay*) or a

---

*Refer to Glossary.

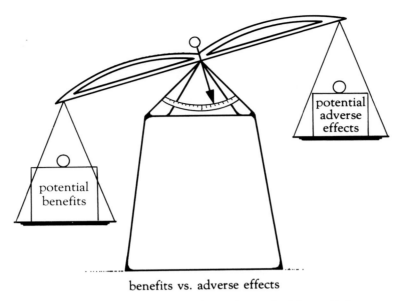

benefits vs. adverse effects

Fig. 1-1   The potential benefits of exposing the patient to ionizing radiation must outweigh the potential adverse effects.

process caused by the interaction of a particle with an atom. The latter occurs most commonly when a beam of high-energy electrons bombards the atoms composing the target of an x-ray tube (Fig. 1-2). When radiation as it passes through matter produces positively and negatively charged particles (ions), it is called *ionizing radiation*.

Not all forms of radiation, however, are capable of causing ionization. There exists, in fact, an entire spectrum of radiation that encompasses such familiar entities as the colors of the rainbow, microwaves, radio waves, and ultraviolet rays. X-radiation may be considered a special type of radiation because of its ability to create electrically charged particles by liberating orbital electrons from atoms with which it interacts. These electrically charged particles possess the potential to cause biological damage in humans by recombining disadvantageously; and the liberated, fast-moving electrons and x-ray photons that emerge from such interactions can cause further damage by producing further ionization.

Biological damage potential

While penetrating body tissues, ionizing radiation produces damage in the body primarily by ionizing the atoms of which the tissues are composed. De-

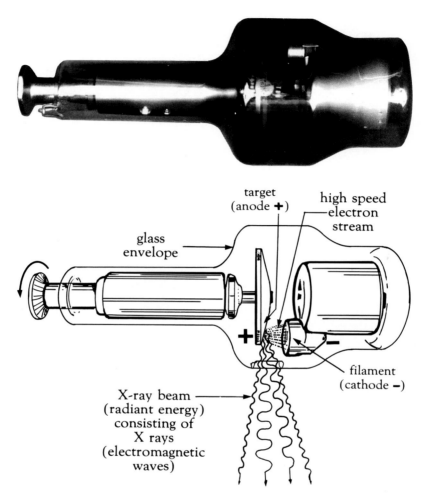

Fig. 1-2   Radiant energy is emitted from the x-ray tube in the form of waves (or particles).

structive radiation interaction at the atomic level results in molecular change, and this, in turn, can cause cellular damage which, in turn, may cause abnormal cell function or loss of cell function. When sufficient cellular damage results from destructive radiation interaction, the living organism may exhibit signs of organic damage (genetic or somatic changes in the organism such as mutations, cataracts, and leukemia). Changes in the blood count are a classic example of organic damage resulting from ionizing radiation exposure. An absorbed dose of x-radiation as low as 0.25 sievert (25 rem) can, within a few days, cause a decrease in the number of lymphocytes in circulating blood. Table 1-1 provides some basic information on the known biological effects of different radiation absorbed doses. Because this potential to cause biological damage exists, the use of radiant energy needs to be limited whenever possible.

Sievert (Sv) is the System International radiation quantity unit for absorbed dose equivalent, and the rem is the traditional radiation quantity unit for absorbed dose equivalent. These units consider the biological effects of various types of radiation in man. Both occupational and nonoccupational absorbed dose equivalents may be stated in sievert (rem). Radiation quantities and units are discussed further in Chapter 3.

Sources

Ionizing radiation has two kinds of sources: (1) natural and (2) man-made or artificial.

Natural sources of ionizing radiation have always been a part of the human environment. Ionizing radiation from natural sources is called natural background radiation and has three components: radioactive materials in the earth, cosmic radiation from outer space, and radionuclides deposited in the human body via natural processes.

Long-lived radioactive elements such as uranium, radium, and thorium, which emit ionizing radiations, are present in variable quantities in the earth. These sources of ionizing radiation are classified as terrestrial radiation, meaning "of the earth." The quantity of terrestrial radiation present in any area of the United States depends on the composition of the soil or rocks in

Table 1-1 Absorbed Radiation Dose Equivalent and Subsequent Biological Effect

Absorbed radiation dose equivalent	Subsequent biological effect
0.25 Sv (25 rem)	Blood changes
1.5 Sv (150 rem)	Nausea, diarrhea
2.5 Sv (250 rem)	To gonads, temporary sterility
3.0 Sv (300 rem) (midline)	50% chance of death; LD 50/30 (lethal dose for 50% of population over 30 days)
6.0 Sv (600 rem)	Death

Modified from *Radiologic health*. Unit #4, Slide #17, Denver, Multi-Media Publishing, Inc.

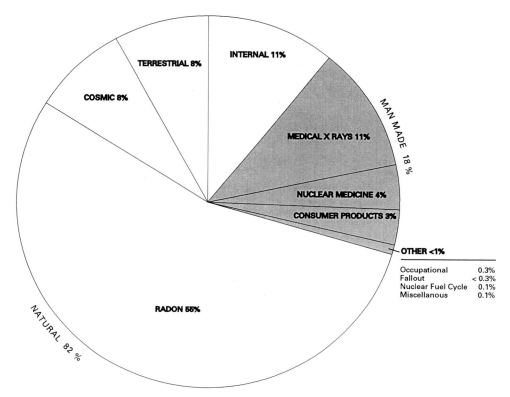

Fig. 1-3   Various radiation sources contribute to the total average effective absorbed dose equivalent for inhabitants of the United States. This diagram demonstrates the percentage contribution of each natural and man-made radiation source.
(From NCRP Report #93, p 55, Figure 8-1.)

that geographic area. Approximately 55% of man's gross common exposure from natural background radiation comes from radon (Fig. 1-3). It is by far the largest contributor to background radiation. It is estimated that a typical U.S. citizen receives approximately 1.98 mSv* (198 mrem†) per year from the indoor and outdoor levels of radon they normally encounter. Radon, which is the first decay product of radium, is a colorless, odorless, and heavy, radioactive gas that along with its decay products is always present to some degree in the air. Because it is a gas, radon can penetrate soil. It enters build-

*The millisievert (mSv) is equal to 1/1,000 of a sievert. See Chapter 3 for further information.
†The millirem (mrem) is equal to 1/1,000 of a rem. See Chapter 3 for further information.

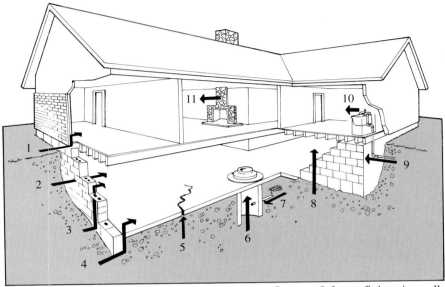

1. Spaces behind brick veneer on top of block foundation

2. Pores and cracks in concrete block foundation

3. Open top of block foundation walls

4. Floor to wall joints

5. Cracks in concrete floor

6. Exposed soil as in basement sump

7. Weeping drain tile draining into open sump

8. Mortar joints

9. Loose fitting pipe wall penetration

10. Well water from some wells

11. Some building materials such as stone

Fig. 1-4   Radon gas can penetrate through soil and enter a home through holes or cracks in its framework, crawlspaces under the living areas, floor drains, sump pumps, and porous cement block foundations. (Source: U.S. Environmental Protection Agency.)

ings through cracks or holes in their framework. In homes, it can gain access via crawlspaces under the living areas, through floor drains and sump pumps as well as through cement block foundations which are quite porous (Fig. 1-4). In many cases, there exists a pressure gradient between a house and the soil on which it rests so that, in effect, *the house draws on the ground like a vacuum cleaner.*

Radon concentrations in a particular structure vary from day to day and from one season to another. In the cooler months, when homes and buildings are tightly closed, radon levels are usually higher. This is the best time to perform tests for radon.

High indoor concentrations of radon have the potential to create serious health hazards for humans. When inhaled, this airborne, radioactive gas leaves alpha-emitting decay products, which remain in the lungs. As these products deteriorate, they give off radiation, which can injure lung tissue, thereby increasing the risk of lung cancer. Radon is considered by the Environmental Protection Agency (EPA) to be the second leading cause of lung cancer in the United States, responsible for approximately 20,000 cancer deaths per year. The EPA recommends that action be taken to reduce elevated levels of radon to below 4 picocuries* per liter (pCi/L) of air (a concentration that specifies the number of radioactive bursts per second that occur on average in 1 L of air). This level of radon presence is considered to be safe by the agency. The EPA estimates that 10% of the homes in the United States exceed the recommended limit of 4 pCi/L. Hence, accurate radon testing and appropriate structural repair, if required, are essential to the reduction of risk of lung cancer from radon.

Cosmic rays are of extraterrestrial origin and are the result of nuclear interactions that have taken place in the sun and other stars. The intensity of cosmic rays varies with altitude relative to the earth's surface. The greatest intensity occurs at high altitudes, and the lowest intensity occurs at sea level. The earth's atmosphere and magnetic field provide shielding from cosmic rays. The shielding is diminished at higher elevations, where there is less atmosphere. The average U.S. inhabitant receives an absorbed dose equivalent of approximately 0.3 mSv (30 mrem) per year from this extraterrestrial radiation. Cosmic radiations consist predominantly of high-energy protons but, because of interactions with molecules in the earth's atmosphere, are accompanied by alpha particles, atomic nuclei, mesons, gamma rays, and high-energy electrons. These other radiations are collectively referred to as a secondary cosmic radiation. The gamma rays among them are energetic enough to penetrate several meters of lead. Although the airplane is a man-made transportation vehicle, its normal use at high elevations brings many humans in closer contact with high-energy extraterrestrial radiation and consequently increases exposure. A flight in a typical commercial airliner results in a dose equivalent rate of 0.5 to 1 mrem/hr.

The human body contains many naturally existing radioactive nuclides within its tissues. Potassium-40 (^{40}K), carbon-14 (^{14}C), hydrogen-3 (^{3}H; tritium), and strontium-90 (^{90}Sr) are examples of radionuclides that exist in small quantities within the body. Radionuclides in the soil and the air also add to human internal radiation dose equivalent. The average member of the general population receives more than 0.67 mSv (67 mrem) per year from

---

*1 picocurie = 10^{-12} curie.

combined exposure to radiations from the earth's surface and radiation from within the human body. In total, including radon (1.98 mSv [198 mrem]), cosmic ray radiations (0.3 mSv [30 mrem]), and the internally deposited radionuclides (0.67 mSv [67 mrem]), the natural background radiation in the United States results in an estimated average annual individual absorbed dose equivalent of approximately 2.95 mSv (295 mrem). The quantity of natural radiation that humans are exposed to *cannot* be controlled.

Ionizing radiation created by humans for various uses is classified as man-made, or artificial, radiation. Sources of artificial ionizing radiation include airport surveillance systems, consumer products such as video display terminals and television receivers, medical procedures, nuclear reactors and the nuclear fuel cycle, and radioactive fallout from nuclear weapons tests where detonations have occurred above ground (Fig. 1-5). Man-made radiation contributes about 0.65 mSv (65 mrem) to the average annual radiation exposure of the U.S. population. Of this absorbed dose equivalent, 0.4 mSv

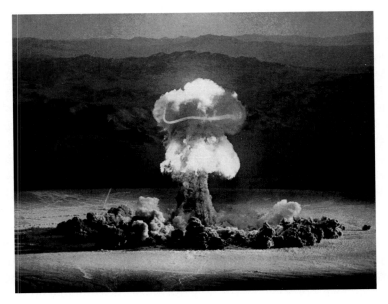

Fig. 1-5   The United States performed above ground nuclear weapons tests prior to 1963. During the Priscilla Test, this atomic cloud resulted from an explosion of a 37 kiloton testing device exploded from a balloon at the Nevada test site on June 24, 1957. The atomic cloud top which contains man-made ionizing radiation ascended approximately 43,000 feet above ground. (Courtesy U.S. Department of Energy (DOE), Nevada Operations Office, Las Vegas, NV.)

(40 mrem) results from medical diagnostic x-ray procedures, 0.14 mSv (14 mrem) results from nuclear imaging, and 0.11 mSv (11 mrem) results from consumer products.

When color TV monitors were first made available to consumers, radiation exposure levels from these devices were substantial. As a result of technological advances over the last two decades and the strict regulations imposed within the United States by the Food and Drug Administration (FDA) regarding such devices, the radiation exposure to the general public can be considered *negligible*.

When spread over the inhabitants of the United States, fallout from nuclear weapons tests and other environmental sources contributes less than 0.011 mSv (1.1 mrem) annually to the absorbed dose equivalent of each person. This annual absorbed dose equivalent is considered to have a *negligible* impact on the U.S. population.

Table 1-2 provides a quick reference for average annual radiation exposure of Americans from both natural background and man-made sources of radiation.

Although nuclear power benefits humans by creating a needed supply of electricity, unfortunate accidents involving nuclear reactors can occur. This can lead to additional, unplanned radiation exposure of humans and the environment. For example, on March 28, 1979, the Three Mile Island-2 (TMI-2) pressurized water reactor, located near Harrisburg, Pennsylvania, suffered a loss of coolant, which resulted in severe overheating (at a temperature of above 5,000° F) of the radioactive reactor core. Consequently, a significant melting of the core occurred.* The U.S. Department of Energy estimated that about 40% of the material in the TMI-2 nuclear reactor core reached a molten state. Approximately 15% of the melted uranium dioxide fuel of the core actually flowed through the undamaged portions of the core and settled on the bottom of the reactor vessel. This melted material in the nuclear reactor core and bottom of the reactor vessel formed crusts on its outside surfaces and in time cooled to form resolidified debris (Fig. 1-6, *A* to *C*). To remedy the hazardous condition, TMI has initiated a program to clean up the radioactive waste. It is important to note that although there was significant melting of the core and flowing of the molten radioactive material into intact portions of the reactor vessel, fortunately, there was no "melt-through" of the reactor vessel.

Although there was the potential for release of significant amounts of radioactive material, according to the General Public Utilities Nuclear Cor-

---

*Actual melting of the uranium dioxide fuel of the reactor core requires a temperature in excess of 5,000° F; melting of the metal alloys in the core structure that houses the uranium fuel would require a temperature of only about 2,000° F.

Table 1-2 Average Annual Radiation Exposure of Americans (NCRP 93)

Overall = 360 mrem (100%) All percentages listed below are percentages of 360 mrem.
~ 1 mrem/day

Natural = 295 mrem (82%)

~200		Radon	198 mrem	(55%)
~100		Cosmic, terrestrial, internal	97 mrem	(27%)
			295 mrem	(82%)

~65	Man-made = 65 mrem (18%)	Medical x-rays	40 mrem	(11%)
		Nuclear medicine	14 mrem	(4%)
		Consumer products	11 mrem	(3%)
			65 mrem	(18%)

"Other"		
Occupational	1.1 mrem	(0.3%)
Fallout	<1.1 mrem	(<0.3%)
Nuclear fuel cycle	0.4 mrem	(0.1%)
Miscellaneous	0.4 mrem	(0.1%)

NOTE—360 mrem = 0.36 rem = 3.6 mSv

$$\text{These are } \frac{\text{(effective dose equivalents)} \times \text{(number of persons exposed)}}{\text{total U.S. population (230 million in 1980)}}$$

EDE uses weighting factors to be able to adjust for internal versus external dose and distribution of dose among organs.

Adapted from data found in National Council on Radiation Protection and Measurements Report No. 93.

poration (GPU), the company that owns and operates TMI, the quantity of radiation that actually escaped during the accident was *not* sufficient to cause health problems.

An explosion at a nuclear power plant in Chernobyl (near Kiev in the Soviet Union) in April 1986 resulted in the release of a number of radioactive nuclides, including 17 million Curies of iodine-131 (^{131}I) and 2 million Curies of cesium-137 (^{137}Cs) or approximately one million times the amount of radioactive material released at TMI. More than two dozen workers died as a result of explosion-related injuries and the effects of receiving exposures exceeding 4 Sv (400 rem). The average dose to the

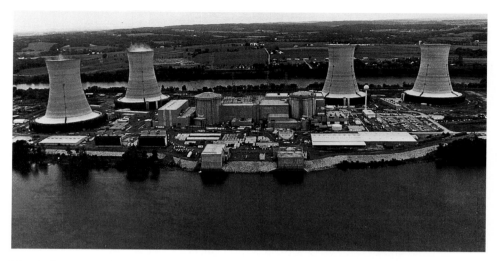

Fig. 1-6   *A,* Nuclear power stations such as that located on Three Mile Island (TMI) near Harrisburg, Pennsylvania, house nuclear reactors. The large, round containment buildings holding the reactors retain radioactive liquids and gases even in a high pressure environment.
(Courtesy U.S. Department of Energy, Washington, DC.)

approximately quarter of a million individuals living within 200 miles of the reactor was 0.2 Sv (20 rem), with thyroid doses (from drinking milk containing radioactive iodine) in some individuals possibly exceeding several hundred rem. Adverse health effects from radiation exposure are expected to occur for many years.

Because humans are unable to control natural background radiation, exposure from artificial sources *must* be limited to protect the general population from further biological damage.

MAGNITUDE OF MEDICAL RADIATION EXPOSURE

The two largest sources of artificial radiation are diagnostic x-ray and nuclear medicine procedures. These account for about 0.54 mSv (54 mrem) of the average annual individual absorbed dose equivalent of ionizing radiation. The average effective total absorbed dose equivalent from man-made plus natural radiation, including radon, is 3.6 mSv (360 mrem). Although the amount of natural background radiation remains fairly constant from year to year, the frequency of exposure to man-made radiation in the healing arts is rapidly increasing among all age groups in the United States. The reason for

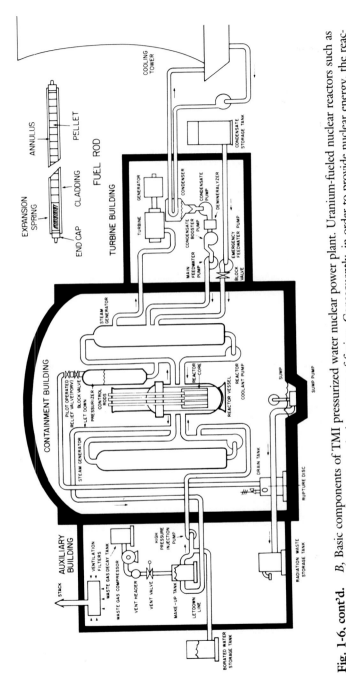

Fig. 1-6, cont'd.   *B,* Basic components of TMI pressurized water nuclear power plant. Uranium-fueled nuclear reactors such as this provide a source of nuclear power through the process of fission. Consequently, in order to provide nuclear energy, the reactor also produces man-made ionizing radiation. (From Shapiro, J: *Radiation protection: A guide for scientists and physicians,* 3rd ed, Cambridge: Harvard University Press, 1990, Figure 6.7, p 404.) *(Continued.)*

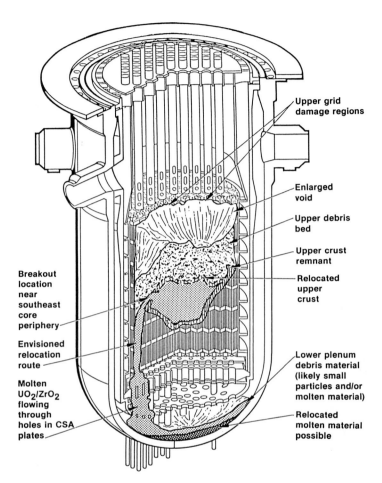

Upper grid damage regions

Enlarged void

Upper debris bed

Upper crust remnant

Relocated upper crust

Breakout location near southeast core periphery

Envisioned relocation route

Molten UO₂/ZrO₂ flowing through holes in CSA plates

Lower plenum debris material (likely small particles and/or molten material)

Relocated molten material possible

Fig. 1-6, cont'd.   *C,* TMI-2 end-state core conditions illustrating the damage to the radioactive nuclear reactor core after the loss of coolant accident on March 28, 1979. Some of the original core mass formed an upper layer of debris. A hard crust supports this material. Zones of prior-molten material and standing fuel rod segments account for some of the core mass lying beneath the upper debris bed. The lower reactor vessel head contains some of the core material that is melted. Closed-circuit television, mechanical probing, and core-boring operations contributed to assessing the TMI-2 end-state core conditions. (Courtesy U.S. Department of Energy, Washington, DC.)

this is that physicians are relying more and more on radiologic diagnosis to assist them in patient care. Greater accuracy in radiologic diagnosis resulting from educational and technological improvements makes this increased usage understandable. Yet to reduce the possibility of the occurrence of genetic damage in future generations, this increase in frequency of exposure in the healing arts must be counterbalanced by limiting the amount of patient exposure in individual procedures. This can *best* be accomplished through application of appropriate radiation protection measures and techniques.

Owing to the large variety of radiologic equipment and the differences in radiologic procedures and individual radiologist and/or radiographer technical skills, patient dose for each examination varies from one institution to another. Patient dose can be indicated in terms of skin dose, organ dose, or fetal dose. Tables 1-3 through 1-7 indicate permissible patient skin entrance exposure and typical patient skin, organ, and fetal exposures or absorbed doses for several different radiologic exams.

Table 1-3 Permissible Skin Entrance Exposures for Various Radiographic Examinations

Examination	Skin exposure (mR per projection)
Chest (PA)	12-26
Skull (lateral)	105-240
Abdomen (AP)	375-698
Retrograde pyelogram	475-829
Cervical spine (AP)	35-165
Thoracic spine (AP)	295-485
Extremity	8-327
Dental (bitewing and periapical)	227-425

These ranges are liberal and reflect the accessing devices, equipment, and techniques used in state-of-the-art technology.

Modified from Ballinger PW: *Merrill's atlas of radiographic positions and radiologic procedures,* ed 7, vol 1, St Louis, 1991, Mosby–Year Book, p 26.

Table 1-4 Typical Skin Exposure and Mean Tissue Glandular Dose for the Three Classifications of Mammography Examinations

Examination	Skin exposure per projection (mR)	Approximate glandular dose per projection (mrad)*
Direct exposure	6000-15,000	2500
Xeromammography	500-1500	400
Screen/film	200-1000	100

*The millirad (mrad) is equal to 1/1,000 of a rad. The rad is the traditional unit of the quantity, absorbed dose. See Chapter 3 for further information.

Modified from Ballinger PW: *Merrill's atlas of radiographic positions and radiologic procedures,* ed 7, vol 1, St Louis, 1991, Mosby–Year Book, p 27.

Table 1-5 Typical Bone Marrow Doses for Various Radiographic Examinations

X-ray examination	Mean marrow dose (mrad)
Skull	50
Cervical spine	20
Full-mouth dental	25
Chest	10
Stomach and upper gastrointestinal	400
Gallbladder	300
Lumbar spine	400
Intravenous urography	400
Abdomen	80
Pelvis	100
Extremity	10

From Ballinger PW: *Merrill's atlas of radiographic positions and radiologic procedures,* ed 7, vol 1, St Louis, 1991, Mosby–Year Book, p 27.

Table 1-6 Typical Gonad Doses from Various Radiographic Examinations

X-ray examination	Gonad dose (mrad) Male	Female
Skull	<1	<1
Cervical spine	<1	<1
Full-mouth dental	<1	<1
Chest	<1	<1
Stomach and upper gastrointestinal	2	40
Gallbladder	1	20
Lumbar spine	175	400
Intravenous pyelography	150	300
Abdomen	100	200
Pelvis	300	150
Upper extremity	<1	<1
Lower extremity	<1	<1

From Ballinger PW: *Merrill's atlas of radiographic positions and radiologic procedures,* ed 7, vol 1, St Louis, 1991, Mosby–Year Book, p 27.

Table 1-7 **Typical Fetal Dose as a Function of Skin Entrance Exposure**

X-ray examination	Fetal dose (mrad/R)
Skull	<0.01
Cervical spine	<0.01
Full-mouth dental	<0.01
Chest	2
Stomach and upper gastrointestinal	25
Gallbladder	3
Lumbar spine	250
Intravenous pyelography	265
Abdomen	265
Pelvis	295
Extremity	0.01

From Ballinger PW: *Merrill's atlas of radiographic positions and radiologic procedures,* ed 7, vol 1, St Louis, 1991, Mosby–Year Book, p 27.

SUMMARY

In this chapter, the reasons why humans must be protected from unnecessary exposure to ionizing radiation have been identified. The responsibility of professional radiation workers for providing radiation protection has also been explained.

REVIEW QUESTIONS

1. Which of the following is an acceptable reason for a person to undergo a radiologic procedure?
   a. the individual feels routine radiologic procedures should be performed each year
   b. people should have some exposure to ionizing radiation each year because it kills cancer cells that normally exist in the human body
   c. the physician ordering the radiologic procedure feels that the potential benefits of the procedure in terms of knowledge gained outweigh the risks of exposure to ionizing radiation
   d. there is no acceptable reason for an individual to be exposed to ionizing radiation

2. Which of the following persons has/have the responsibility for ordering a radiologic examination?
   a. radiographer
   b. referring physician and the radiologist
   c. radiographer and the radiologist
   d. radiographer and the referring physician

3. Radiation exposure to the patient and the radiographer is increased by:
   a. producing a high-quality diagnostic radiograph with the first radiographic exposure
   b. using appropriate radiation protection safety principles
   c. repeat radiographic exposures caused by technical error or carelessness
   d. the radiologist ordering a limited radiographic examination

4. A special form of radiation that is capable of creating electrically charged particles by removing orbital electrons from atoms with which it interacts is classified as:
   a. ionizing radiation
   b. non-ionizing radiation
   c. subatomic radiation
   d. ultrasonic radiation

5. Through which of the following routes can radon enter houses?
   1. crawl spaces under living areas
   2. floor drains
   3. porous cement block foundations
   a. 1 and 2 only
   b. 1 and 3 only
   c. 2 and 3 only
   d. 1, 2, and 3

6. If the circulating blood in the human body is exposed to an absorbed dose of ionizing radiation as low as 0.25 Sv (25 rem), the result can be:
   a. a noticeable increase in the number of lymphocytes
   b. a noticeable decrease in the number of lymphocytes
   c. the lymphocyte count would immediately drop to zero
   d. platelets would greatly increase in number

7. Which of the following are natural sources of ionizing radiation?
   a. medical x-radiation and cosmic radiation
   b. radioactive elements in the earth and in the human body
   c. radioactive elements in the human body and a diagnostic x-ray machine
   d. radioactive fallout and environs of atomic energy plants

8. Which of the following ionizing radiations are humans *unable* to control?
   a. radiation produced by an x-ray machine
   b. that existing in environs of nuclear reactors
   c. radioactive fallout from atomic weapons
   d. all natural background radiation

9. From which of the following sources do humans receive the *largest* dose of ionizing radiation?
   a. radioactive fallout from atomic weapons
   b. medical and dental radiation procedures
   c. the earth, outer space, and the human body
   d. environs of nuclear reactors

10. Why is radiologic diagnosis more accurate today than in previous years?
    1. improvements in education of medical personnel
    2. improvements in education of technical personnel
    3. greater sophistication in the design of diagnostic imaging equipment
    a. 1 only
    b. 2 only
    c. 3 only
    d. 1, 2, and 3

11. What do airport surveillance systems, video display terminals, television receivers, and nuclear reactors have in common?
    a. they are all sources of natural background radiation
    b. they are all sources of man-made radiation
    c. each member of the U.S. population receives 5 mrem per year from each of these radiation sources
    d. none of the items listed as choices are a source of radiation

12. The average effective total absorbed dose equivalent from man-made plus natural radiation is:
    a. 0.3 mSv (30 mrem) per year
    b. 0.6 mSv (60 mrem) per year
    c. 1.8 mSv (180 mrem) per year
    d. 3.6 mSv (360 mrem) per year

13. Terrestrial radiations include sources such as:
    a. radioactive elements such as uranium, radium, and thorium, which are present in variable quantities in the earth
    b. radioactive fallout from nuclear weapons tests where detonation occurred above ground
    c. the sun and other stars
    d. video display terminals and television receivers

14. How many millisievert (millirem) per year does the U.S. population receive as a consequence of nuclear weapons testing and other environmental sources?
    a. less than 0.01 mSv (1.1 mrem)
    b. 0.3 mSv (30 mrem)
    c. 0.6 mSv (60 mrem)
    d. 0.9 mSv (90 mrem)

15. Which of the following protects the world's population from exposure to essentially all high energetic, bombarding cosmic rays?
    a. clouds
    b. fog
    c. earth's atmosphere
    d. smog

16. Radon accounts for approximately _____ percent of humans' gross common exposure from natural background radiation.
    a. 15
    b. 25
    c. 55
    d. 75

17. According to the Environmental Protection Agency (EPA), radon levels in homes should *not* exceed a level of:
    a. 200 pCi/L
    b. 135 pCi/L
    c. 47 pCi/L
    d. 4 pCi/L

18. Which of the following is considered by the EPA to be the second leading cause of lung cancer in the United States?
    a. an annual chest x-ray
    b. cosmic rays
    c. radon
    d. a fluoroscopic examination of the esophagus

19. It is estimated that a typical U.S. citizen receives approximately _____ mSv (_____ mrem) per year from the indoor and outdoor levels of radon they encounter.
    a. 0.01, 1
    b. 0.1, 10
    c. 1, 100
    d. 1.98, 198

20. Man-made radiation contributes about _____ mSv (_____ mrem) to the annual exposure of the U.S. population.
    a. 0.3, 30
    b. 0.65, 65
    c. 1.2, 120
    d. 3.6, 360

Bibliography

Arena V: *Ionizing radiation and life,* St Louis, 1971, Mosby–Year Book.

Ballinger PW: *Merrill's atlas of radiographic positions and radiologic procedures,* ed 7, vol 1, St Louis, 1991, Mosby–Year Book.

Bushong S: *Radiologic science for technologists: physics, biology and protection,* ed 5, St Louis, 1993, Mosby–Year Book.

Fried S: Fear itself, *Philadelphia Magazine,* 77(9):126, 1986.

Herlitz Publications: Ionizing radiation exposure levels show less than estimated, *Oncology Times* 10(2):4, 1988.

Hildreth R: *From x-ray martyrs to low level radiation,* Kalamazoo, 1981, Industrial Graphics Services.

International Commission of Radiation Units and Measurements (ICRU): Radiation quantities and units, ICRU Report #33, Washington, DC, 1980.

Merion Publications: Radon returns to prominence on agency's list of dangers, *Advances for Radiologic Technologists,* 3(12):17, March 19, 1990.

Miller PE: Biological effects of diagnostic irradiation, *Radiologic Technology,* 48:11, 1976.

National Council on Radiation Protection and Measurements (NCRP) Reports, Bethesda, MD, NCRP Publications. #91, Recommendations on limits for exposure to ionizing radiation, 1987; #93, Ionizing radiation exposure of the population of the United States, 1987.

National Council on Radiation Protection and Measurements (NCRP) Reports, Washington, DC, NCRP Publications. #39, Basic radiation protection criteria, 1971; #43, Review of the current state of radiation protection philosophy, 1975.

New Jersey Department of Health, Division of Occupational and Environmental Health: Facts and Recommendations on Exposure to Radon, January 1987, p 1.

Ritenour ER: Radiation protection and biology: a self-instructional multimedia learning series, instructor manual, Denver, 1985, Multi-Media Publishing.

Scheele RV, Wakley, J: *Elements of radiation protection,* Springfield, IL, 1975, Charles C. Thomas.

Selman J: *Elements of radiobiology,* Springfield, IL, 1983, Charles C. Thomas.

Selman J: *The fundamentals of x-ray and radium physics,* ed 7, Springfield, IL, 1985, Charles C. Thomas.

Shapiro J: *Radiation protection: a guide for scientists and physicians,* ed 3, Cambridge, 1990, Harvard University Press.

Standard Education Society: *New standard encyclopedia,* vols Q-R, Chicago, 1960, Standard Education Society, p R-17.

Travis EL: *Primer of medical radiobiology,* ed 2, Chicago, 1989, Mosby–Year Book.

US Department of Defense: The effects of nuclear weapons, revised edition, Glasstone S, editor, reprinted Feb. 1964, US Atomic Energy Commission.

US Department of Health and Human Services, Public Health Service, Food and Drug Administration, Bureau of Radiological Health: The correlated lecture laboratory series in diagnostic radiological physics, HHS Publication FDA81-8150, Rockville, MD, 1981, HHS.

Vann JM: Radiation effects of Three Mile Island, Lecture, New Jersey Society of Radiologic Technologists, Nov. 28, 1979, State of NJ Nuclear Engineer, Bureau of Radiation Protection.

Basic Interactions of X-Radiation with Matter

OBJECTIVES

Upon completion of this chapter, the reader will be able to:

- define the terms *primary radiation, remnant radiation,* and *attenuation*
- identify four events that can occur when x-radiation passes through matter
- identify the events that result in the impingement of scattered radiation upon the patient, the radiographic film, and the radiographer
- identify the x-ray photon interactions with matter that are important in diagnostic radiology and differentiate between them
- describe the effect of kVp upon radiographic image quality and patient absorbed dose

X-rays are a form of energy. When x-rays enter a material such as human tissue, they may interact with the atoms of the material or they may pass through the material without interacting. If they interact, energy is transferred from the x-rays to the atoms of the material. This transference of energy is called *absorption* (Fig. 2-1), and the amount of energy absorbed per unit mass is referred to as the *absorbed dose*. The more energy transferred to or absorbed by the atoms of the patient's body, the greater the chance of the occurrence of biological damage in the patient. So, for the safety of the patient, the amount of energy transferred should be kept as small as possible. However, without the phenomenon of absorption and differences in the ab-

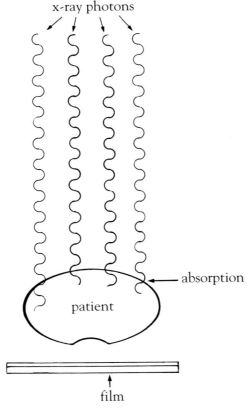

Fig. 2-1   X-ray photons can interact with atoms of the patient's body and transfer energy to the tissue. This transference of energy is called *absorption*.

sorption properties of different body structures, diagnostically useful radiographs, radiographs in which different structures can be perceived and distinguished, would not be possible. As we shall see, the radiographer also benefits when patient dose is kept low, because less radiation is scattered from the patient. The mechanisms by which radiation is absorbed and scattered by atoms help to explain many important concepts in radiography and radiation protection. The basic interactions of x-rays with matter are discussed in this chapter.

X-RAY BEAM PRODUCTION AND ENERGY

A diagnostic x-ray beam is produced by bombarding a positively charged target (the anode, which is usually made of tungsten, a metal with a high melting point and high atomic number) with a stream of high-speed electrons in a highly evacuated glass tube. As the electrons interact with the atoms of the target, x-ray photons of various energies, referred to collectively as *primary radiation,* emerge from the target (Fig. 2-2).

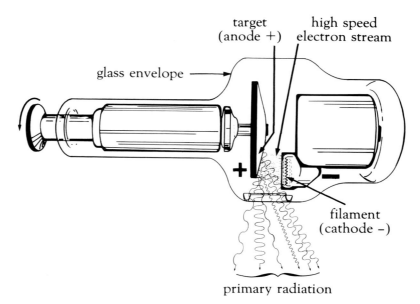

Fig. 2-2   Primary radiation emerges from the x-ray tube target and consists of x-ray photons of various energies. It is produced when the positively charged target is bombarded with a stream of high speed electrons and these electrons interact with the atoms of the target.

Although all photons* in a diagnostic x-ray beam do not have the same energy, we can say that the most energetic photon in the beam can have no more energy than the electrons that bombarded the target. The energy of the electrons inside the x-ray tube is expressed in terms of the electrical voltage applied across the tube. For diagnostic radiology this is expressed in thousands of volts or kilovolts (kV). Moreover, since the voltage across the tube fluctuates, it is usually expressed in kilovolts "at peak value," or kVp. When an electron is drawn across an electrical potential difference of one volt we say that it has acquired an energy of one "electron volt" or "eV". Thus, when a technique factor of 100 kVp is selected, it means that the electrons that bombard the target have an energy of 100 keV. X-rays of various energies will be produced, but the most energetic x-ray photon can have no more energy than 100 keV. For a typical diagnostic x-ray unit, the energy of the average photon in the beam is about one third of the energy of the most energetic photon. Therefore, a 100 kVp beam contains photons having energies of 100 keV or less with an average energy of about 33 keV.

ATTENUATION

Figure 2-3 illustrates the passage of four x-ray photons through an object. Before the four photons produced by the x-ray source enter the object, they are referred to as *primary* photons. Only two photons emerge from the object and strike the film below it. They are referred to as *remnant* photons because they remain in the beam after the beam has passed through the object. The two that do not strike the film are said to have been attenuated. The term *attenuation* is rather broad and with respect to x-rays is used to refer to any process that decreases the intensity of the primary photon beam that was directed toward some destination. The destination of the photons in Fig. 2-3 is the film. So, photon #3, which has deviated from its path (has been "scattered") to the extent that it will not strike the film, is said to have been attenuated. Photon #4 seems to disappear. It has transferred all of its energy to the atoms of the object and has therefore ceased to exist. Because a photon has no mass, no charge, and no attribute other than energy, when it gives up its energy it ceases to exist.

The term *attenuation,* then, refers to both absorption and scatter that prevent photons from reaching some predefined destination. Referring back to Fig. 2-3, we see that the path of photon #2 was bent but not so much that the photon missed the film. Insofar as photon #2 reached the film it is

---

*Refer to Glossary.

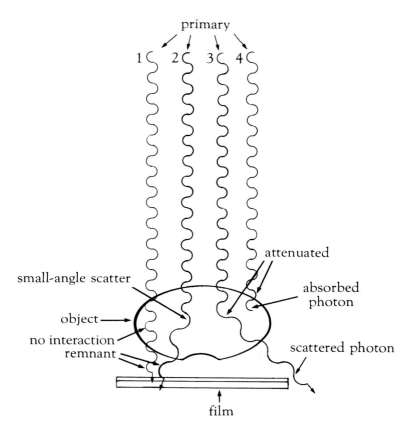

primary

PRIMARY − REMNANT = ATTENUATION

Fig. 2-3   Primary, remnant, and attenuated photons. Primary photons (photons #1, 2, 3, and 4) are those photons which emerge from the x-ray source. Remnant photons (photons #1 and 2) are those photons which pass through the object being radiographed and reach the film. Attenuated photons (photons #3 and 4) are those photons which have interacted with atoms of the object and been scattered or absorbed such that they do not reach the film.

part of the remnant radiation, but the bending of its path represents what is called *small-angle scatter* (forward scatter). Small-angle scatter will degrade the appearance of a radiograph. Sharp outlines of dense objects will be smeared out by the effects of such scatter. Moreover, because there will be millions of such small-angle scatter events, the film will acquire an overall darkening that interferes with the radiologist's ability to distinguish different structures in the image. This overall darkening is called radiographic *fog*. Reducing the amount of tissue irradiated reduces the amount of fog produced by small-angle scatter. Therefore adequately collimating the x-ray beam is one way to reduce fog (Fig. 2-4, A and B). Other methods used to reduce the image-degrading effects of scatter are discussed later.

PROBABILITY OF PHOTON INTERACTION WITH MATTER

There is some chance, some randomness involved in the interaction of photons with matter. We cannot predict exactly what will happen to a single photon when it enters matter. We can predict what will happen "on the average," however, and this is more than enough to determine the characteristics of the radiograph that results from such interactions. For example, it can be shown that a 50 keV photon has a 66% likelihood of interacting with the atoms of the tissue when it travels through 5 cm of soft tissue; 34% of the

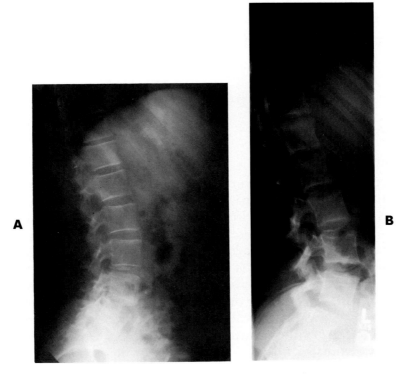

Fig. 2-4 *A,* Lateral view of the lumbar vertebrae evidencing improper collimation, which results in the production of radiographic fog and a consequent lack of radiographic clarity. *B,* Lateral view of the lumbar vertebrae evidencing proper collimation, which eliminates radiographic fog and, consequently, increases radiographic clarity.

time the photon will simply pass through. Another way to say this is that if 100 photons travel through 5 cm of soft tissue, we would expect 66 interactions to occur. Of the 66 interactions, 11% should be of a type called *photoelectric absorption;* thus about 7 out of 100 (11% of 66) interactions would be of the photoelectric type. In the photoelectric interaction, a photon is completely absorbed by the atoms of the tissue (i.e., removed from the beam). If this were the only interaction possible, then irradiating 5 cm of soft tissue with 50 keV photons would cast a "shadow" (create a light area) on a radiographic film, which would be the result of 7% fewer photons reaching that portion of the film. In reality the process is much more complicated, because there are several effects to take into account and a typical x-ray beam is composed of photons of various energies. In the remainder of this chapter, we will look more closely at the different interactions of photons with individual atoms and discuss the effect of the probability of occurrence of a particular type of interaction on the radiograph.

PROCESSES OF INTERACTION

There are four basic types of interaction between x-radiation and matter:
1. Coherent scattering.
2. Photoelectric absorption.
3. Compton scattering.
4. Pair production.

Coherent scattering

If a low-energy photon (less than 100 keV) interacts with an atom, the electrons of the atom as a whole may be caused momentarily to vibrate. This is analogous to the behavior of electrons in the antenna of a receiver when it intercepts a radio signal. Because they are charged particles, each of the atom's vibrating electrons will radiate energy in the form of electromagnetic waves. These waves coherently (i.e., cooperatively) combine with each other to form a resultant scattered wave. This represents the scattered photon. Its wavelength is the same as that of the incident photon. Thus no net energy has been absorbed by the atom. It is very likely, however, that there will be a change in direction of the emitted photon. In general, this change in direction will be less than 20 degrees with respect to the initial direction of the original photon. This is the net effect of *coherent scattering,* also known as *Rayleigh scattering,* in honor of the scientist who first explained it. Although coherent scatter is most likely to occur below 30 kV, some occurs throughout the diagnostic range and can result in a small amount of radiographic fog (Fig. 2-5).

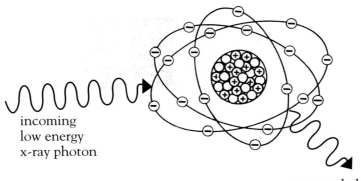

incoming
low energy
x-ray photon

scattered photon
posessing the same
wavelength and energy
or penetrating power
as that of the incident
x-ray photon

Fig. 2-5   Coherent scattering. The incoming low energy x-ray photon interacts with an atom, causing the electrons of the atom momentarily to vibrate. The electrons then radiate energy in the form of electromagnetic waves. These waves coherently combine with each other to form a resultant scattered wave. This represents the scattered photon. Its wavelength and energy or penetrating power is the same as that of the incident photon. Generally, the emitted photon may change in direction less than 20° with respect to the direction of the original photon.

Photoelectric absorption

Within the energy range of diagnostic radiology (30 to 150 kVp), photoelectric absorption is the *most important* mode of interaction between x-ray photons and atoms of the patient's body.

Photoelectric absorption is an interaction between an x-ray photon and an inner shell electron (usually in the K shell) tightly bound to an atom of the absorbing medium (Fig. 2-6, *A* to *C*). To dislodge an inner shell electron from its atomic orbit, the incoming x-ray photon *must* possess a quantity of kinetic energy as large as or larger than the amount of energy that binds the electron in orbit. Upon encountering an inner shell electron, such an incoming x-ray photon surrenders all of its energy to the orbital electron and ceases to exist. The electron will be ejected from its inner shell, creating a vacancy in that shell. The ejected orbital electron, called a *photoelectron,* possesses kinetic energy equal to the energy of the incoming photon less the binding energy of the electron shell. The photoelectron can interact with other atoms, causing excitation or ionization, until all of its kinetic energy has been expended. It is usually absorbed within a few micrometers of the me-

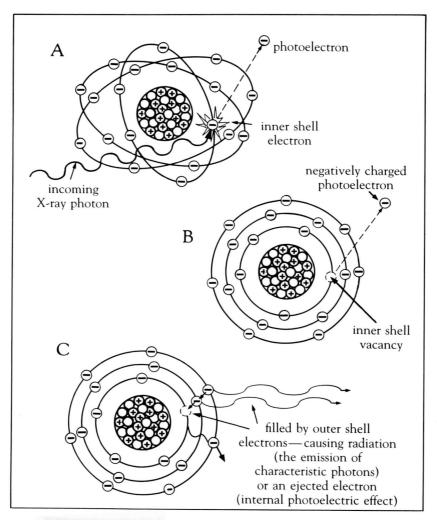

Fig. 2-6 Photoelectric absorption. *A,* The incoming x-ray photon, upon encountering an inner shell electron, surrenders all of its energy to the electron and the photon ceases to exist. *B,* The atom responds by ejecting the electron, called a *photoelectron,* generally from its inner shell, creating a vacancy in the shell. *C,* To fill the opening, an electron from an outer shell drops down to the vacated inner shell by releasing energy in the form of a characteristic photon. Then, to fill the new vacancy in the outer shell, another electron from the shell next furthest out drops down and another characteristic photon is emitted, and so on until the atom regains electrical equilibrium. A K shell vacancy characteristic photon may also interact with an outer shell electron, ejecting it from the atom.

The byproducts of photoelectric absorption are:

1. Photoelectrons (those induced by interaction with external radiation as well as the internally generated Auger electrons)
2. Characteristic x-ray photons (fluorescent radiation)

When their energy is locally absorbed in human tissue, patient dose and the biological damage potential both increase.

Fig. 2-7 Byproducts of photoelectric absorption.

dium through which it travels. In the human body this energy transfer results in increased patient dose and contributes to biological damage of tissues.

As a result of the photoelectric effect, in general, a vacancy will exist in the inner shell of the parent atom. To fill this opening, an electron from an outer shell drops down to the vacated inner shell opening, by releasing energy (equivalent to the difference in energy level between the two shells) in the form of a photon. This photon is termed a *characteristic photon*. It possesses relatively low energy in human tissue and is locally absorbed in the irradiated object. Ensuing vacancies in successive shells are filled and photons emitted in a like fashion until the atom regains electrical equilibrium (Fig. 2-7). It is also possible that a characteristic photon created as a result of a K-shell vacancy may not escape the confines of the atom but rather produce its own photoelectric effect by giving its energy to an electron of low binding energy, thereby ejecting that electron from the atom. Unbound electrons generated in this manner are known as Auger electrons. This *internal* photoelectric effect reduces the intensity of characteristic radiation (also called *fluorescent radiation*) emitted from atoms as a result of photoelectric interactions. The term *fluorescent yield* refers to the number of characteristic x-rays emitted per K-shell vacancy. The fluorescent yield per photoelectric interaction in general is lower in materials composed of higher atomic number atoms (Fig. 2-6, *C*).

The probability of occurrence of photoelectric absorption depends upon the energy of the incident x-ray photons and the atomic number of the atoms comprising the irradiated object; it increases in a pronounced fashion as the energy of the incident photons decreases and the atomic number of

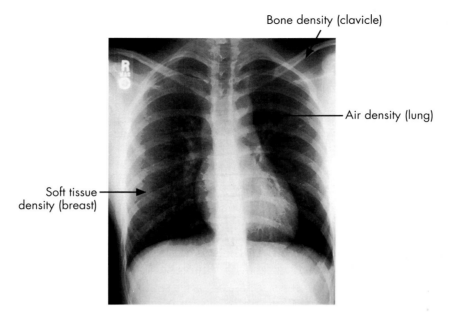

Bone density (clavicle)

Air density (lung)

Soft tissue density (breast)

Fig. 2-8   The less a given structure attenuates radiation, the darker (i.e., of greater density) will be its images on the finished radiograph and vice versa. Thus, bone, with a higher effective atomic number than either soft tissue or air cavities, absorbs more radiation and appears white on a diagnostic radiograph, whereas soft tissue presents a gray image and air-containing structures such as the lungs appear black.

the irradiated atoms increases.* Thus, in the radiographic kilovoltage range, bone (effective atomic number 13.8) undergoes much more photoelectric absorption† than an equal mass of soft tissue (effective atomic number approximately 7.4) and air (effective atomic number 7.6).

Such differences in absorption properties between different body structures make diagnostically useful radiographs possible. In other words, the ability to perceive and distinguish between different body structures in a radiograph depends upon there being differences in the amount of x-radiation these structures will permit to pass through them to reach the x-ray film.

The less a given structure attenuates radiation, the darker (i.e., of greater density) will be its image on the finished radiograph and vice versa. Thus bone, with a higher effective atomic number than either soft tissue or air cavities, absorbs more radiation and appears white on a diagnostic radio-

---

*Approximately Z^4/E^3 per atom, Z^3/E^3 per gram or per electron.
†Approximately 12 times per atom more likely.

graph, whereas soft tissue presents a gray image and air-containing structures (e.g., lungs, stomach) appear black (Fig. 2-8).

Within the energy range of diagnostic radiology, the greater the difference in the amount of photoelectric absorption, the greater will be the contrast in the radiographic image between adjacent structures. Yet, as absorption increases, so does the potential for biological damage. Thus, to ensure both radiographic image quality and patient safety, the radiologist or radiographer should choose the highest energy x-ray beam that permits adequate radiographic film contrast.

Compton scattering

Compton scattering, also known as *incoherent* or *modified scattering,* is responsible for *most* of the scattered radiation produced during radiologic procedures. This scatter is isotropic, meaning it can be directed onward as forward or small-angle scatter, backward as backscatter, and to the side as sidescatter. The direction of travel of the scatter is a major factor in planning protection for members of the medical radiography team during a radiologic examination (Fig. 2-9).

In the Compton process, an incoming x-ray photon interacts with a loosely bound outer shell electron of an atom of the irradiated object (Fig. 2-10). Upon encountering the electron, the incoming x-ray photon surrenders a portion of its kinetic energy to dislodge the electron from its outer shell orbit. The freed electron, called a *Compton scattered electron,* possesses kinetic energy and is capable of ionizing atoms. It loses its kinetic energy by interacting with atoms and finally recombines with an atom that needs another electron. This usually occurs within a few micrometers of the site of the original Compton interaction.

The weakened x-ray photon that surrendered some of its energy to free the electron from its orbit continues on its way but in a new direction. It possesses the potential to interact with other atoms it may encounter either by the process of photoelectric absorption or again by Compton scattering. It may also emerge from the patient, in which case it may contribute to degradation of the radiographic image (see "small-angle scatter," p. 26) or present a health hazard to the radiographer or radiologist (Fig. 2-11).

In diagnostic radiology, the probability of occurrence of Compton scattering relative to that of the photoelectric interaction increases as the energy of the x-ray photons increases. Compton scattering and photoelectric absorption in tissue are equally probable at about 35 keV. Therefore, in a 100 kVp x-ray beam, a significant number of Compton events occur.

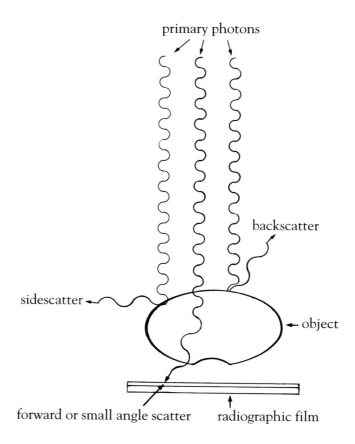

Fig. 2-9   Compton scattering results in all directional scatter. The scatter created can be directed onward as forward or small angle scatter, backward as backscatter, and to the side as sidescatter. The direction of travel of the scatter is a major factor in planning protection for members of the medical radiography team during a radiologic examination.

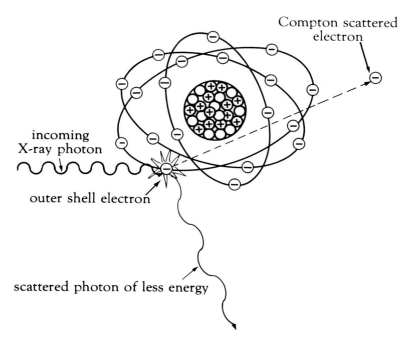

Fig. 2-10   Compton scattering. The incoming x-ray photon, upon encountering a loosely bound outer shell electron, surrenders a portion of its kinetic energy to dislodge the electron from its orbit. The weakened x-ray photon then continues on its way but in a new direction. The high speed electron ejected from its orbit is called a *Compton scattered electron.*

The two byproducts of Compton scattering are the:

1. Compton scattered electron
2. Scattered x-ray photon of lower energy

The weakened, scattered x-ray photon can emerge from the patient and contribute to degradation of the radiographic image as "fog" or it can scatter and present a health hazard for the radiographer or radiologist.

Fig. 2-11   Byproducts of Compton scattering.

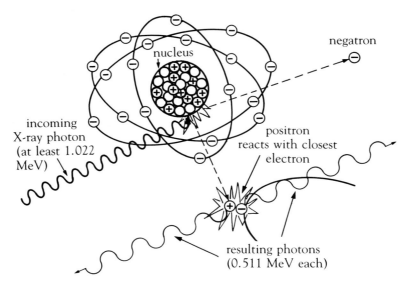

Fig. 2-12   Pair production. The incoming photon (equivalent in energy to at least 1.022 MeV) strongly interacts with the nucleus of an atom of the irradiated object and disappears. In the process the energy of the photon is transformed into two new particles, a negatron and a positron. The negatron eventually recombines with any atom which needs another electron. The positron interacts destructively with a nearby electron. During the interaction, the positron and the electron annihilate one another and in their place energy appears in the form of two 0.511 MeV photons, each moving in opposite directions.

Pair production

Pair production does not occur unless the energy of the incident photon is *at least* 1.022 million electron volts (MeV). Although this energy range is far above that used in diagnostic radiology, a brief description of pair production is included in this chapter for the purpose of furnishing the reader with a broader understanding of the basic interactions of x-radiation with matter.

In pair production (Fig. 2-12) the incoming photon strongly interacts with the nucleus of an atom of the irradiated object and disappears. In the process the energy of the photon is transformed into two new particles, a negatron (an ordinary electron) and a positron (a positively charged electron). The negatron and the positron have the *same* mass and magnitude of charge; the only difference is in the "sign" of their electrical charges. The incoming photon *must* have enough energy to produce the combined mass of these two particles. It is found that 1.022 MeV is the *minimum* energy required to produce an electron-positron pair.* This is why pair production does *not* occur at lower energies. The electron will lose its kinetic energy by exciting and ionizing atoms in its path. Eventually, the electron will have lost enough energy so that it can be captured by an atom in need of another electron.

As far as is known, there are no large quantities of positrons freely existing in the universe. The positron is classified as a form of antimatter. It interacts destructively with a nearby electron. During the interaction, the positron and the electron annihilate one another, and, in their place, energy appears that is carried off by two 0.511 MeV photons moving in opposite directions. Here, mass has been transformed into energy.

Annihilation radiation

Although pair production does not have any direct use in diagnostic radiology, annihilation radiation is made use of in positron emission tomography (PET).† In PET scanning, the source of the positrons are atomic nuclei that are unstable because they contain too many protons relative to their number of neutrons. To relieve this instability, the surplus proton is replaced in the nucleus by a neutron while a positron and another particle called a *neutrino*‡ are ejected from that nucleus. Some examples of atomic nuclei used in PET scanning are fluorine-18 (^{18}F), carbon-11 (^{11}C), and nitrogen-13 (^{13}N). The annihilation photons produced by the decay of such unstable nuclei are intercepted by a ring of detectors surrounding the patient and are used to build a cross-sectional image of the radioactivity within the patient.

SUMMARY

The number of photons absorbed or scattered from a beam of x-rays depends upon the energy of the photons and the composition of the material in the path of the beam. The photoelectric effect is the basis of radiographic imagery, whereas the Compton effect is its bane. When the kVp is decreased, the number of photoelectric interactions increases and the number of Compton interactions decreases. Therefore, one would say that radiogra-

---

*Mass (electron or positron) = 9.1×10^{-31} kg
  $c = 3 \times 10^8$ m/s
  $E\text{(total)} = E\text{(electron)} + E\text{(positron)} = mc^2 \text{(electron)} + mc^2 \text{(positron)} = 16.38 \times 10^{-14}$ J
  1 MeV = 1.6×10^{-13} J
Therefore $E = 16.38 \times 10^{-14} \div 1.6 \times 10^{-13} = 1.022$ MeV.
†Hendee WR, Ritenour ER: *Medical imaging physics,* ed 3, St Louis, 1992, Mosby–Year Book, p 332.
‡A neutrino is an electrically neutral particle that, according to present theory, possesses almost but not quite negligible mass. As a result, the neutrino demonstrates an exceedingly small tendency to interact with any type of matter.

phy should be done at low kVp. However, when kVp is decreased, more energy is absorbed by the patient (the entire energy of the photon is absorbed when a photoelectric interaction occurs, whereas only part of the photon's energy is absorbed when a Compton interaction occurs); consequently, patient dose is increased. Clearly, there must be a compromise between the needs for image quality and patient safety. For a given exam, there is an optimum technique (kVp and mAs combination) that minimizes the dose to the patient while providing a radiograph of acceptable quality. The kVp selections are usually based on the type of procedure and body part being radiographed. Other factors such as film/screen type, patient thickness, degree of muscle tissue, and so forth, affect the technique selected and cannot always be determined by referring to standard charts. It is the task of the radiographer to balance these variables to arrive at the technique which will provide an acceptable image in keeping with the standards of radiation protection.

REVIEW QUESTIONS

1. What is remnant radiation composed of?
   a. primary photons and Compton scattered electrons
   b. noninteracting and small-angle scattered photons
   c. attenuated photons
   d. absorbed photons

2. When a technique factor of 90 kVp is selected:
   a. the highest energy photon in the beam has an energy of 30 keV
   b. the electrons are accelerated from the cathode to the anode with an energy of 30 keV
   c. the energy of the average photon in the beam is 90 keV
   d. the energy of the average photon in the beam is 30 keV

3. Which of the following contributes *significantly* to the exposure of the diagnostic radiographer?
   a. positrons
   b. electrons
   c. Compton scattered photons
   d. Compton scattered electrons

4. Which of these defines *attenuation*?
   a. absorption and scatter
   b. absorption only
   c. scatter only
   d. Compton electrons

5. Which one of the following is *not* a type of interaction between x-radiation and matter?
   a. Compton scattering
   b. bremsstrahlung
   c. pair production
   d. photoelectric effect
   e. none of the above

6. In which of the following x-ray interactions with matter is the energy of the incident photon *completely* absorbed?
   a. Compton scattering
   b. photoelectric absorption
   c. bremsstrahlung
   d. pair production

7. In which of the following x-ray interactions with matter is the energy of the incident photon *partially* absorbed?
   a. Compton scattering
   b. photoelectric effect
   c. coherent scattering
   d. pair production

8. What is the result of coherent scattering?
   a. simply a change in direction of the incident x-ray photon
   b. a transfer of all the energy of the incident x-ray photon to the atoms of the irradiated object
   c. the production of a negatron and a positron
   d. a transfer of only some of the energy of the incident x-ray photon to the atoms of the irradiated object

9. A Compton scattered electron:
   a. annihilates another electron
   b. is absorbed within a few microns of the Compton interaction
   c. causes photoelectric interactions
   d. is a remnant photon

10. In photoelectric absorption, the kinetic energy of the incoming x-ray photon must be _____ in order to be able to dislodge an inner shell electron from its orbit.
   a. less than the energy that binds the atom together
   b. ten times as great as the energy that binds the atom together
   c. the same as or slightly greater than the energy that binds the electron in its orbit
   d. the incoming x-ray photon does not require kinetic energy to dislodge an inner shell electron from its orbit

11. Which of the following interactions between photons and matter involves a matter-antimatter annihilation reaction?
   a. Compton scattering
   b. coherent scattering
   c. pair production
   d. photoelectric absorption

12. The probability of the occurrence of photoelectric absorption _____ as the atomic number of the irradiated material _____ .
   a. increases, decreases
   b. decreases, increases
   c. increases, increases
   d. stays the same, increases

13. The radiation that occurs when an electron moves from an outer orbit to fill a vacancy in an inner orbit is called:
   a. characteristic radiation
   b. bremsstrahlung
   c. photoelectric radiation
   d. primary radiation

14. Most of the scattered radiation produced during radiographic procedures is the direct result of:
   a. photoelectric effect
   b. nuclear decay
   c. remnant electrons
   d. Compton interactions

15. Which one of the following is *not* another term for coherent scattering?
   a. characteristic
   b. classical
   c. Rayleigh
   d. unmodified

16. What is the effective atomic number of bone?
   a. 13.8
   b. 7.6
   c. 7.4
   d. 5.9

17. Before interaction with matter, what may an incoming x-ray photon be referred to as?
   a. attenuated photon
   b. primary photon
   c. remnant photon
   d. scattered photon

18. Which of the following are byproducts of photoelectric absorption?
    a. photoelectron and Compton scattered electron
    b. low-energy scattered x-ray photon and characteristic photon
    c. low-energy scattered x-ray photon and Compton scattered electron
    d. photoelectron and characteristic x-ray photon

19. Which two interactions between x-radiation and matter can result in the production of small-angle scatter?
    a. photoelectric absorption and Compton scattering
    b. coherent scattering and Compton scattering
    c. photoelectric absorption and pair production
    d. coherent scattering and pair production

20. Which of the following particles is considered to be a form of antimatter?
    a. electron
    b. positron
    c. x-ray photon
    d. scattered x-ray photon

21. Which of the following interactions results in the conversion of mass into energy?
    a. classical scattering
    b. photoelectric absorption
    c. modified scattering
    d. annihilation reaction

22. What is Compton scattering synonymous with?
    a. coherent scattering
    b. incoherent scattering
    c. photoelectric absorption
    d. pair production

23. What does the radiation permeability of a structure refer to?
    a. ionizing properties
    b. penetrability by radiation
    c. radiosensitivity
    d. radioinsensitivity

24. During the process of coherent scattering, what does the incident x-ray photon interact with?
    a. a single inner shell electron, ejecting it from its orbit
    b. a single outer shell electron, ejecting it from its orbit
    c. an atom's electrons, causing them to vibrate and emit radiation
    d. a scattered photon of lesser energy, annihilating it

25. What characteristic primarily differentiates the probability of occurrence of the various interactions of x-radiation with human tissue?
    a. energy of the incoming photon
    b. direction of the incident photon
    c. x-ray beam intensity
    d. difference in the binding energy of the atom's electron shells

Bibliography

Ball JL, Moore AD: *Essential physics for radiographers,* London, 1980, Blackwell Scientific.

Bushong S: *Radiologic science for technologists: physics, biology, and protection,* ed 5, St Louis, 1993, Mosby–Year Book.

Bushong S: *Radiologic science for technologists: physics, biology, and protection,* ed 2, St Louis, 1980, Mosby–Year Book.

Christensen EE, Curry III TS, Dowdey JE: *An introduction to the physics of diagnostic radiology,* ed 2, Philadelphia, 1978, Lea & Febiger.

Curry III TS, Dowdey JE, Murry Jr RC: *Christensen's introduction to the physics of diagnostic radiology,* ed 3, Philadelphia, 1984, Lea & Febiger.

Donohue DP: *An analysis of radiographic quality: lab manual and workbook,* ed 2, Rockville, MD, 1984, Aspen.

Frankel R: *Radiation protection for radiologic technologists,* New York, 1976, McGraw-Hill.

Graham BJ, Thomas WN: *An introduction to physics for radiologic technologists,* Philadelphia, 1975, Saunders.

Hewitt PG: *Conceptual physics. A new introduction to your environment,* ed 4, Boston, 1981, Little, Brown, p 612, Appendix 1.

Malott JC, Fodor III J: *The art and science of medical radiography,* ed 7, St Louis, 1993, Mosby–Year Book.

Noz ME, Maguire Jr GQ: *Radiation protection in the radiologic and health sciences,* ed 2, Philadelphia, 1985, Lea & Febiger.

Pizzarello DJ, Witcofski RL: *Basic radiation biology,* ed 2, Philadelphia, 1975, Lea & Febiger.

Ritenour ER: *Radiation protection and biology: a self-instructional multimedia learning series, instructor manual,* Denver, 1985, Multi-Media Publishing.

Scheele RV, Wakley J: *Elements of radiation protection,* Springfield, IL, 1975, Charles C Thomas.

Selman J: *The fundamentals of x-ray and radium physics,* ed 7, Springfield, IL, 1985, Charles C Thomas.

Stanton L: *Basic medical radiation physics,* New York, 1969, Appleton-Century-Crofts, Educational Division, Meredith Corporation.

US Department of Health and Human Services, Public Health Service, Food and Drug Administration, Bureau of Radiological Health: The correlated lecture laboratory series in diagnostic radiological physics, HHS Publication FDA81-8150. Rockville, MD, 1981, HHS.

3

Radiation Quantities and Units

OBJECTIVES

Upon completion of this chapter, the reader will be able to:

- describe the historical evolution of radiation quantities and units
- define the radiation units of exposure, absorbed dose, and absorbed dose equivalent
- identify and explain the traditional and System International (SI) units for radiation exposure, absorbed dose, and absorbed dose equivalent
- explain the importance of linear energy transfer (LET) as it applies to biological damage resulting from irradiation of human tissue
- define the term *quality factor* and identify this factor for each of the different ionizing radiations
- state the formula for determining absorbed dose equivalent
- determine the absorbed dose equivalent in terms of traditional and SI units when given the quality factor and absorbed dose for different ionizing radiations

As the potential harmful effects of ionizing radiation became known, the medical community decided it was necessary to reduce radiation exposure throughout the world by developing standards for measuring and limiting this exposure. Diagnostic radiology personnel should be familiar with the standardized radiation quantities and units discussed in this chapter to be able to measure patient and personnel exposure in a consistent and uniform manner. Chapter 4 will familiarize you with the standardized limits on radiation exposure expressed in these units and designed to minimize the potential harmful effects of such exposure.

HISTORICAL EVOLUTION OF RADIATION QUANTITIES AND UNITS

Wilhelm C. Roentgen announced the discovery of x-rays in December 1895. In the months that followed, experimentation with this new "wonder ray" resulted in acute biological damage for some patients and radiation workers. Cases of somatic damage (biological damage to the body of the exposed individual) caused by exposure to ionizing radiation were reported in Europe as early as 1896. In the United States, Clarence Dally, glassblower, tube maker, and assistant to Thomas A. Edison, became the first American radiation fatality. Dally died of radiation-induced cancer in 1904 at age 39. Cancer deaths among physicians, presumably attributable to x-ray exposure, were reported as early as 1910. Many other radiologists and dentists developed cancerous skin lesions on the hands as a result of their occupational exposure (Fig. 3-1). Blood disorders, such as aplastic anemia and leukemia, were more common among early radiologists than among nonradiologists.

Alarmed by the increasing number of radiation injuries reported, the medical community decided to investigate methods for reducing radiation exposure. In 1921 the British X-Ray and Radium Protection Committee was

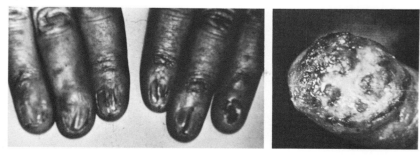

Fig. 3-1   Lesions of the fingers induced by ionizing radiation.

formed to perform this task. Unfortunately, because a workable unit of radiation exposure had not been generally agreed upon, the committee was unable to fulfill its responsibility.

The unit in use at that time was called the *skin erythema dose* and was defined as the dose of radiation that causes diffused redness over an area of skin after irradiation. This amount of radiation corresponds roughly to a modern dose of a few hundred rad. Because the amount of radiation required to produce the erythema reaction varied from one person to another, it was a crude and inaccurate way to measure radiation exposure. Scientists felt it was necessary to continue searching for a more reliable unit. The new unit selected was to be based upon some exactly measurable effect produced by radiation, such as ionization of atoms or energy absorbed in the irradiated object.

The International Commission on Radiation Units and Measurements (ICRU) was formed in 1925. In 1928 this commission was charged by the Second International Congress of Radiology to define a unit of exposure. In 1937 the commission finished its assignment, and, although not accurately defined, the roentgen (R) became internationally accepted as the unit for measurement of exposure to x-radiation and gamma* radiation. To increase accuracy and acceptability, the roentgen was redefined in 1962.

In 1948 the General Conference of Weights and Measures, which was responsible for the development and international unification of the metric system, assigned its International Committee for Weights and Measures the responsibility for developing guidelines for the units of measurement. To fulfill this responsibility, the committee developed the *International System of Units (SI)*. This system made possible an interchange of units among all branches of science. The roentgen, rad, and rem are special units that are to be used until a complete transition to the SI can be made. The ICRU adopted the SI units for use with ionizing radiation in 1980 and urges full implementation of these units as soon as possible.

The SI unit of absorbed dose (discussed later in this chapter) was named after L.H. Gray, who was instrumental in fashioning the Bragg-Gray theory, which is arguably the most important theory in all of radiation dosimetry. This theory relates the ionization produced in a small cavity within an irradiated medium or object to the energy absorbed in that medium as a result of its radiation exposure. Thus, with the use of appropriate correction factors it essentially links the determination of the absorbed radiation dose in a medium to a relatively simple measurement of ionization charge. Gray was also responsible for many pioneering papers in radiation biology. R.M.

---

*Refer to Glossary.

Sievert, for whom the SI unit of absorbed dose equivalent was named, is best known for his method* of determination of the exposure rates at various points near to linear radium sources (tubes).

RADIATION QUANTITIES
Exposure

When a volume of air is irradiated with x-rays or gamma rays, the interaction that occurs between the x-rays and the neutral air atoms results in some electrons being liberated from those atoms. Consequently, the ionized air can function as a conductor and carry electricity because of the negatively charged, free electrons and positively charged, associated ions that have been created. As the intensity of x-ray exposure of the air volume increases, the number of electron-ion pairs increases. Thus, by measuring the number of such pairs in a well-defined volume of air, the amount of radiation responsible for the ionization of that air can be determined. This radiation ionization in air is termed *exposure*.

Because it is essential for the reader to understand the concept of the radiation quantity, exposure, in order to differentiate it from other quantities used in medical radiography, exposure may be defined as the total electric charge per unit mass that x-ray and gamma ray photons with energies up to 3 MeV generate in air only. In a simplified sense, it may be viewed as the amount of ionizing radiation which may strike an object, such as the human body, when in the vicinity of a radiation source.

To obtain a precise measurement of radiation exposure in medical radiography, the total amount of ionization an x-ray beam produces in a known mass of air must be obtained. This type of direct measurement is accomplished in an accredited** calibration laboratory by using a standard or free-air ionization chamber (Fig. 3-2). A well-specified quantity of dry (i.e., non-humid) air under standard conditions of pressure and temperature (760 mmHg or 1 atm at sea level and 22° C) is contained in the chamber. If, in that specific volume of dry air, the total charge of all of the ions of one sign (either all pluses or all minuses) produced are collected and measured, the total amount of radiation exposure can be accurately determined.

Such an instrument, however, is not a practical device at locations other than a standardization laboratory. As a result, much smaller and less complicated instruments have been developed for use away from the laboratory. Although very convenient, these instruments must be periodically recalibrated in a standardization laboratory against a free-air chamber.

---

*Referred to as the Sievert Integral. Interested readers with some background in calculus may refer to Johns and Cunningham. The Physics of Radiology, 4th edition, Charles C. Thomas, 1983.
**By bodies such as the American Association of Physicists in Medicine, National Bureau of Standards, etc.

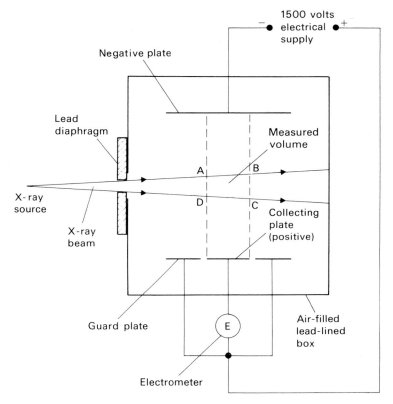

Fig. 3-2 This device determines radiation exposure by measuring the amount of ionization an x-ray beam produces within its air collection volume. The instrument consists of a box containing a known quantity of air, two oppositely charged metal plates, and an electrometer, an instrument that measures the total amount of charge collected on the positively charged metal plate. The chamber measures the total amount of electrical charge of all the electrons produced during the ionization of a specific volume of air at standard atmospheric pressure and temperature. The electrical charge is measured in units called coulombs (C) (charge of an electron = -1.6×10^{-19} C). A collected electrical charge of 2.58×10^{-4} C/kg of irradiated air constitutes an exposure of 1 roentgen (R). (From Ball JL, Moore AD: *Essential physics for radiographers,* London, 1980, Blackwell Scientific Publications, Fig. #18/I, p. 212.)

Absorbed dose

As ionizing radiation passes through an object, some of the energy of that radiation will be transferred to the object. Some of the radiation that is transferred to the object is absorbed (i.e., stays within the object). The quantity, "absorbed dose," is defined as the amount of energy per unit mass absorbed by the irradiated object. This absorbed energy is responsible for whatever biological damage occurs as a result of the tissues being exposed to radiation.

Anatomical structures in the body possess different absorption properties; some structures have the ability to absorb more radiant energy than others. The amount of energy absorbed by a structure depends on the atomic number of the tissue composing the structure and the energy of the incident photon; absorption increases as atomic number increases and photon energy decreases. That is, low-energy photons are, in general, more easily absorbed in a material than are high-energy photons.

The effective atomic number of a given tissue is a composite of the atomic numbers of the many different chemical elements composing the tissue. Bone has a higher effective atomic number (13.8) than does soft tissue (7.4) because bone contains calcium (atomic number = 20) and phosphorus (atomic number = 15), whereas soft tissue is composed mostly of fat (atomic number = 5.9) and structures with atomic numbers close to that of water (atomic number = 7.4). Bone absorbs more ionizing radiation than soft tissue in the diagnostic energy range of 30 to 150 kVp because the photoelectric process is the dominant mode of energy absorption within this range. The photoelectric interaction's probability of occurrence is strongly dependent upon the atomic number of the irradiated material. The higher the atomic number of a material, the greater will be the amount of energy absorbed by that material.

In the therapeutic radiology range of 100 keV and above, however, the difference in absorption between bone and soft tissue gradually decreases (Fig. 3-3). This is because the amount of photoelectric absorption decreases and the amount of Compton scattering relative to the photoelectric interaction increases as the energy of the x-ray beam increases; the amount of Compton scattering in a material does not depend on the atomic number of the material. Hence, as energy increases, the difference in amount of absorption between any two tissues of different atomic number decreases. Since it is the process of absorption that is responsible for biological damage and absorption properties vary with the quality of the radiation and the type of tissue irradiated, tissue dosage in therapeutic radiology is generally specified in terms of absorbed dose rather than in terms of exposure.

Absorbed dose equivalent

Absorbed dose equivalent provides a method with which to calculate the effective absorbed dose for all types of ionizing radiation, including protons* and neutrons* as well as x-rays. It has been found that equal absorbed doses

---

*Refer to Glossary.

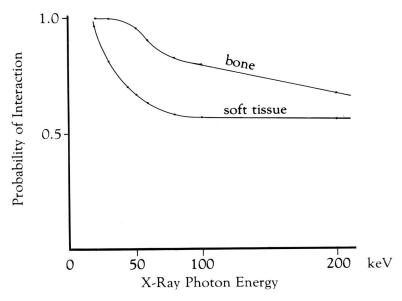

Fig. 3-3   Probability of interaction of x-rays when a 5 cm thick layer of soft tissue or bone is encountered. The probability is greater at lower energies and is greater for bone than soft tissue, particularly at low energies.

of different types of radiation produce different amounts of biological damage in body tissue. For example, a 50-rad absorbed dose of fast neutrons would cause more biological damage than a 50-rad absorbed dose of x-rays. The absorbed dose equivalent takes this into consideration by using a modifying or quality factor (QF) to adjust the absorbed dose value. This is accomplished by multiplying the absorbed dose by the quality factor and any other applicable modifying factor. The product obtained is called the absorbed dose equivalent. The following formula may be used to make the calculation:

ADE (absorbed dose equivalent) = AD (absorbed dose) × QF (quality factor)

X-rays, beta particles (high-speed electrons), and gamma rays are known to produce virtually the same biological effects in body tissue for equal absorbed doses. In terms of quality factor, these radiations have been given a value of 1 and are the base or standard against which to compare the effectiveness of other types of ionizing radiation in producing biological damage. The quality factors of different kinds of ionizing radiations are listed in Table 3-1. The concept of linear energy transfer (LET) helps to explain the need for a quality factor. LET is the amount of energy transferred on average by incident radiation to an object per unit length of travel through the object.

Table 3-1 **Quality Factors for Different Types of Ionizing Radiations**

Type of ionizing radiation	Quality factor*
X-ray photons	1
Beta particles	1
Gamma photons	1
Thermal neutrons	5
Fast neutrons	20
High-energy external protons	1
Low-energy internal protons†	20
Alpha particles	20
Multiple charged particles of unknown energy	20

*Data from National Council of Radiation Protection and Measurements (NCRP) Reports: #91, Recommendation on limits for exposure to ionizing radiation, Bethesda, MD, 1987, NCRP Publications, p 13.
†Protons produced as a result of neutrons interacting with the nuclei of tissue molecules.

Radiation having a high LET transfers a large amount of energy into a small area and can therefore do more biological damage than radiation having a low LET. Thus a high LET radiation has a quality factor that is greater than the quality factor for a low LET radiation. LET and its relationship to biological damage will be discussed again in Chapter 6.

RADIATION UNITS
Roentgen (traditional unit of exposure)—coulomb per kilogram (SI unit)

The roentgen (R) equals the amount of charge released by x-ray or gamma-ray photons as they pass through a specific quantity of dry air. It is precisely defined as the photon exposure that produces under standard conditions of pressure and temperature a total positive or negative ion charge of 2.58×10^{-4} C/kg of dry air. The coulomb (C) is a unit of electric charge that equals 1 ampere-second.* In the International System (SI) the exposure unit is simply the coulomb per kilogram (C/kg) produced in dry air by ionizing radiation. Thus one roentgen (traditional) equals 2.58×10^{-4} C/kg (SI). It may also be stated that an exposure of 1 C/kg of dry air equals $1/2.58 \times 10^{-4}$ R, or 3.88×10^3 R. Conversion of the roentgen (R), the traditional unit of exposure, to coulombs per kilogram (C/kg), the SI unit, may be accomplished by multiplying by 2.58×10^{-4} (C/kg)/R.

*The ampere is the SI unit of electric current. One ampere represents the flow of electrons amounting to a charge of one coulomb crossing unit area per second.

EXAMPLE: To convert 100 R to C/kg:

1. Set up the equation: $100 \text{ R} \times 2.58 \, (10)^{-4} \dfrac{\text{C/kg}}{\text{R}}$

2. Cancel R: $100 \text{ R} \times 2.58 \, (10)^{-4} \dfrac{\text{C/kg}}{\text{R}}$

3. Obtain answer: $258 \times 10^{-4} \dfrac{\text{C}}{\text{kg}}$

4. Write answer as a scientific notation: 2.58×10^{-2} C/kg

Conversion of coulombs per kilogram (C/kg) to roentgen (R) may be accomplished by dividing by 2.58×10^{-4}.

EXAMPLE: To convert 100 C/kg to R:

1. Set up the equation: $100 \text{ C/kg} \div 2.58 \, (10)^{-4} \dfrac{\text{C/kg}}{\text{R}}$

2. Cancel C/kg: $100 \text{ C/kg} \div 2.58 \, (10)^{-4} \dfrac{\text{C/kg}}{\text{R}}$

3. Obtain answer: 39×10^{4} R

Rad (traditional unit of absorbed dose)—gray (SI unit)

Traditionally, the rad has been used as the unit of the quantity, absorbed dose. The letters r a d stand for "*r*adiation-*a*bsorbed-*d*ose." This unit indicates the amount of radiant energy transferred to an irradiated object by any type of ionizing radiation. The rad is equivalent to an energy transfer of 100 erg (a unit of energy and work) per gram of irradiated object. One rad may be expressed mathematically as follows:

$$1 \text{ rad} = 100 \text{ erg/g}$$

or

$$1 \text{ rad} = 1/100 \text{ J/Kg}$$

(A joule [a unit of energy] may be defined as the work done or energy expended when a force of one newton acts on an object along a distance of one meter.)

The SI unit of absorbed dose is called a *gray* (Gy) and is defined as an energy transfer of one joule (J) per kilogram (kg) of irradiated object. One gray is therefore given by the simple relation:

$$1 \text{ Gy} = 1 \text{ J/kg}$$

Gray and rad are easily translated to compare absorbed dose values. If the absorbed dose is stated in rads, the equivalent number of gray may be determined by dividing by 100.

EXAMPLE: number of rad divided by 100 = number of gray
5000 rads = 5000 divided by 100 rads per Gy = 50 Gy

If absorbed dose is stated in gray, the number of rads may be determined by multiplying by 100.

EXAMPLE: number of gray multiplied by 100 = number of rad
15 gray = 15 × 100 rads per gray = 1500 rads

SI subunits facilitate conversion from rad to gray. The milligray (mGy) equals 1/1000 gray. This is a concept similar to a millirad (mrad), which equals 1/1000 rad. In therapeutic radiology the centigray (cGy) will eventually replace the rad for recording of absorbed dose.

$$1 \text{ cGy } (1/100 \text{ gray}) = 1 \text{ rad } (1/100 \text{ Gy})$$

EXAMPLE: number of centigray = 1 × number of rad; therefore, if a patient receiving x-ray therapy treatment has received a total dosage of 5000 rad, the dosage can be recorded in SI subunits as 5000 × 1 cGy = 5000 cGy.

Rem (traditional unit of absorbed dose equivalent)—Sievert (SI unit)

Traditionally, the rem has been used as the unit of the quantity, absorbed dose equivalent and may be defined as the absorbed dose equivalent of any type of ionizing radiation that produces the "same biological effect" as one rad of x-radiation. One rem of neutrons will thus represent a different absorbed dose than does one rem of alpha particles. An absorbed dose in rad may be converted to a dose equivalent by use of the quality factor for the type of radiation being considered. The letters r e m mean "*rad-equivalent-man*." If a person is exposed to various types of ionizing radiation on the job, absorbed dose equivalent must be determined to measure the biological effect.

EXAMPLE: (using traditional units, rad and rem) An individual received the following absorbed doses: 10 rad of x-radiation, 5 rad of fast neutrons, and 20 rad of alpha particles; what is the total absorbed dose equivalent?
The formula for determining absorbed dose equivalent is:
ADE = absorbed dose × quality factor
(rem) = (rad) × (QF)
(The quality factor for each of the radiations in question may be obtained from Table 3-1.)

ANSWER:

Radiation type	Absorbed dose	×	QF	=	ADE
x-radiation	10 rad	×	1	=	10 rem
fast neutrons	5 rad	×	20	=	100 rem
alpha particles	20 rad	×	20	=	400 rem
	Total absorbed dose equivalent			=	510 rem

In the SI system the unit of absorbed dose equivalent is the sievert (Sv). One sievert equals one hundred rem. Sievert and rem are easily compared. If the absorbed dose equivalent is stated in rem, the number of sievert may be determined by dividing by 100, the number of rem.

EXAMPLE: 500 rem = 500 divided by 100 rem per Sv = 5 Sv

If the absorbed dose equivalent is stated in sievert, the number of rem may be determined simply by multiplying by 100.

EXAMPLE: 10 Sv = 10 × 100 rem per Sv = 1000 rem

If a person receives exposure from various types of ionizing radiation, the absorbed dose equivalent for measuring biological effects can be determined and expressed in sievert.

EXAMPLE: (using gray and sievert) An individual received the following absorbed doses: 0.1 Gy of x-radiation, 0.05 Gy of fast neutrons, and 0.2 Gy of alpha particles; what is the total absorbed dose equivalent?
The formula for determining absorbed dose equivalent is:
ADE = absorbed dose × quality factor
(sievert) = (gray) × (QF)
(The quality factor for each of the radiations in question may be obtained from Table 3-1.)

ANSWER:

Radiation type	Absorbed dose	×	QF	=	ADE
x-radiation	0.1 G	×	1	=	0.1 Sv
fast neutrons	0.05 G	×	20	=	1.0 Sv
alpha particles	0.2 G	×	20	=	4.0 Sv
	Total absorbed dose equivalent			=	5.1 Sv

Subunits may also be used to specify dose limits; e.g.:

1 rem = 10 millisievert (mSv)

Thus, if the dose limit is stated in rem, the number of millisievert may be obtained by multiplying by 10.

EXAMPLE: 15 rem = 15 × 10 millisievert (mSv) per rem = 150 mSv = 0.150 Sv

Tables 3-2 and 3-3 provide a summary of radiation quantities, units, and equivalents.

Table 3-2 Traditional and SI Unit Equivalents

1 roentgen (R) equals:	1. 2.58×10^{-4} C/kg of air 2. 86.9 erg/g of air
1 milliroentgen (mR) equals:	1. 1/1000 R (10^{-3} R)
1 rad equals:	1. 100 erg/g 2. 1/100 J/kg 3. 1/100 Gy 4. 1 cGy
1 millirad equals:	1. 1/1000 rad
1 rem equals:	1. 1/100 J/kg (for x-radiation, q.f. = 1) 2. 1/100 Sv 3. 1 centisievert (cSv) 4. 10 mSv
1 millirem equals:	1. 1/1000 rem
1 SI exposure unit equals:	1. 1 C/kg = $\dfrac{1}{2.58 \times 10^{-4}}$ R
1 coulomb equals:	1. 1 ampere-second
1 coulomb per kilogram of air equals:	1. 1 SI unit of exposure 2. $\dfrac{1}{2.58 \times 10^{-4}}$ R
1 gray equals:	1. 1 J/kg 2. 100 rad 3. 10 decigray 4. 100 cGy 5. 1000 mGy
1 sievert equals:	1. 1 J/kg (for x-radiation, QF = 1) 2. 100 rem 3. 10 dSv 4. 100 CSv 5. 1000 mSv
1 erg equals:	1. 10^{-7} J
1 joule equals:	1. 10^{7} erg 2. 1 newton-meter 3. 6.24×10^{18} eV

Table 3-3 **Summary of Radiation Quantities and Units**

Type of radiation	Quantity	Traditional unit	SI unit	Measuring media	Effect measured
X- or gamma	Exposure	roentgen (R)	coulomb per kilogram (C/kg)	Air	Ionization of air
All ionizing radiations	Absorbed dose	rad	gray (Gy)	Any object	Amount of energy per unit mass absorbed by object
All ionizing radiations	Absorbed dose equivalent	rem	sievert (Sv)	Body tissue	Biological effects

SUMMARY

Radiation quantities and units have been described in this chapter. The traditional and System International units for radiation exposure, absorbed dose, and absorbed dose equivalent have been identified and defined. The reader should now be able to determine the absorbed dose equivalent in terms of traditional and SI units when given the quality factor and absorbed dose for different ionizing radiations.

REVIEW QUESTIONS

1. Who was the first American to die from radiation-induced cancer (in 1904)?
   a. Thomas A. Edison
   b. Wilhelm C. Roentgen
   c. Clarence Dally
   d. Marie Curie

2. Which of the following served as the *first* unit used to measure exposure to ionizing radiations?
   a. roentgen
   b. skin erythema
   c. sievert
   d. rad

3. To determine the total amount of radiation exposure in a specific volume of dry air under standard conditions of pressure and temperature, the effect that must be measured is:
   a. energy absorption
   b. biological damage
   c. cellular activity
   d. quantity of ionization

4. Which of the following provides a method by which to calculate the effective absorbed dose for *all* types of ionizing radiations?
   a. absorbed dose
   b. absorbed dose equivalent
   c. exposure
   d. ionization of air

5. The ionizing radiations that produce virtually the *same* biological effects for equal absorbed doses in body tissue are:
   a. x-rays, beta particles, and gamma rays
   b. alpha particles, beta particles, and gamma rays
   c. x-rays, neutrons, and gamma rays
   d. x-rays, alpha particles, and fast neutrons

6. Which of the following is the SI unit of exposure?
   a. sievert
   b. roentgen
   c. gray
   d. coulomb per kilogram

7. Select the correct statement:
   a. 1 C/kg of dry air $= \dfrac{1}{2.58 \times 10^{-4}}$ gray
   b. 1 C/kg of dry air $= \dfrac{1}{2.58 \times 10^{-4}}$ roentgen
   c. 2.58×10^{-4} C/kg of dry air $= 10$ sievert
   d. 2.58×10^{-4} C/kg of dry air $= 50$ roentgen

8. If the absorbed dose is stated in rad, gray may be determined by:
   a. multiplying by 100
   b. adding by 100
   c. dividing by 100
   d. subtracting by 100

9. The amount of energy per unit mass transferred from an x-ray beam to an object is called the:
   a. exposure

b. absorbed dose equivalent
c. SI
d. absorbed dose

10. The measurement of ionization produced by x-ray or gamma ray photons in air defines *only*:
    a. exposure
    b. absorbed dose
    c. absorbed dose equivalent
    d. skin erythema dose

11. In the diagnostic radiology energy range from 30 to 150 kVp, which of the following tissues possesses the *greatest* ability to absorb radiant energy through the process of photoelectric absorption?
    a. muscle
    b. bone
    c. fat
    d. air

12. Which of the following factors can be multiplied to determine absorbed dose equivalent?
    a. rad × quality factor
    b. rem × roentgen
    c. gray × quality factor
    d. a and c only

13. In the SI, 1 J of energy absorbed from any type of ionizing radiation in 1 kg of any irradiated object equals:
    a. 10 Sv
    b. 5 C/kg
    c. 1 rad
    d. 1 Gy

14. If a patient receiving x-ray therapy treatment receives a total dosage of 6000 rad, the dosage may be recorded as _____ if SI is used.
    a. 12,000 Gy
    b. 6000 cGy
    c. 600 rad
    d. 60 R

15. 200 rem equal:
    a. 2 mSv
    b. 20 mSv
    c. 200 mSv
    d. 2000 mSv

16. Which of the following is used to adjust the absorbed dose value to measure biological effects of different types of ionizing radiation?
    a. exposure-absorbed dose ratio
    b. ionization factor
    c. quality factor
    d. rate of linear energy transfer

17. The *greatest* amount of biological damage in human tissue is produced by ionizing radiation with a:
    a. high LET and a high specific ionization
    b. low LET and a high specific ionization
    c. high LET and a low specific ionization
    d. low LET and a low specific ionization

18. A quality factor has been established for each of the following ionizing radiations: x-rays, fast neutrons, and alpha particles. Determine the total absorbed dose equivalent in sievert for a person who has received the following exposures: 5 rad of x-rays, 2 rad of fast neutrons, and 4 rad of alpha particles.
    a. 1.25 Sv
    b. 10.5 Sv
    c. 125 Sv
    d. 1250 Sv

19. Which of the following units are *not* SI units?
    a. roentgen
    b. coulomb per kilogram, gray, sievert
    c. rad and rem
    d. a and c only

20. Of the following equivalents, which equals 1 rad?
       1. 100 erg/g
       2. 1/100 J/kg
       3. 0.01 Gy
    a. 1 only
    b. 2 only
    c. 3 only
    d. 1, 2, and 3

21. To determine absorbed dose, the amount of energy absorbed by the irradiated object must be measured by:
    a. determining the quantity of ionization in a specific volume of dry air at atmospheric pressure
    b. calculating the absorbed dose equivalent
    c. calculating the skin-entrance exposure of the object
    d. determining the quantity of energy deposited per kilogram of the object

22. For x-ray and gamma ray photons with energies up to 3 MeV, one of the following quantities may be defined as the measure of the total electric charge per unit mass that these radiations generate in air only:
    a. absorbed dose
    b. absorbed dose equivalent
    c. exposure

23. As the intensity of x-ray exposure of air increases, the electrical resistance of the air will:
    a. decrease
    b. increase
    c. remain the same

24. 10 C/kg equal _____ roentgen.
    a. 2.58×10^{-4}
    b. 25.8×10^{-4}
    c. 3.9×10^{4}
    d. 39×10^{4}

25. 1 millirem equals _____ rem.
    a. 1/10
    b. 1/100
    c. 1/1000
    d. 1/10,000

Bibliography

American Association of Physicists in Medicine. Fullerton, GD et al, editors: Medical Physics Monograph No. 5., *Biological risks of medical irradiation,* New York, 1980, American Association of Physicists in Medicine.

Ball JL, Moore, AD: *Essential physics for radiographers,* England, 1980, Blackwell Scientific Publications.

Bushong S: *Radiologic science for technologists: physics, biology, and protection,* ed 5, St Louis, 1993, Mosby–Year Book.

Christensen EE, Curry III TS, Dowdey JE: *An introduction to the physics of diagnostic radiology,* ed 2, Philadelphia, 1978, Lea & Febiger.

Curry III TS, Dowdey JE, Murry Jr RC: *Christensen's introduction to the physics of diagnostic radiology,* ed 3, Philadelphia, 1984, Lea & Febiger.

Frankel R: *Radiation protection for radiologic technologists,* New York, 1976, McGraw-Hill.

Hildreth R: *From x-ray martyrs to low level radiation,* Kalamazoo, 1981, Industrial Graphics Services.

International Commission on Radiation Units and Measurements (ICRU): *Radiation quantities and units,* ICRU Report #33. Washington, DC, 1980, ICRU.

Malott JC, Fodor III J: *The art and science of medical radiography,* ed 7, St Louis, 1993, Mosby–Year Book.

National Council of Radiation Protection and Measurements (NCRP) Reports: *#91 Recommendations on limits for exposure to ionizing radiation,* Bethesda, MD, 1987, NCRP Publications.

Noz ME, Maguire Jr GQ: *Radiation protection in the radiologic and health sciences,* ed 2, Philadelphia, 1985, Lea & Febiger.

Ritenour ER: *Radiation protection and biology: a self-instructional multimedia learning series,* instructor manual, Denver, 1985, Multi-Media Publishing.

Scheele RV, Wakley J: *Elements of radiation protection,* Springfield, IL, 1975, Charles C Thomas.

Selman J: *The basic physics of radiation therapy,* ed 2, Springfield, IL, 1973, Charles C Thomas.

Selman J: *The fundamentals of x-ray and radium physics,* ed 7, Springfield, IL, 1985, Charles C Thomas.

Shapiro J: *Radiation protection: a guide for scientists and physicians,* ed 3, Cambridge, 1990, Harvard University Press.

Thomas CL, editor: *Taber's cyclopedic medical dictionary,* ed 13, Philadelphia, 1973, FA Davis.

US Department of Health, Education, and Welfare, Public Health Service, Food and Drug Administration, Bureau of Radiological Health: Barnett MH: *The biological effects of ionizing radiation: an overview,* HEW Publication FDA 77-8004. Rockville, MD, 1976, HEW.

Limits for Exposure to Ionizing Radiation

OBJECTIVES

Upon completion of this chapter, the reader will be able to:

- identify the various agencies in the United States that share the responsibility for evaluating the relationship between absorbed dose equivalent and subsequent biological effects of radiation exposure, and also for formulating risk estimates of subsequent somatic and genetic effects of irradiation
- identify the national agency that has the responsibility to enforce established radiation absorbed dose limiting standards
- define the term *effective absorbed dose equivalent limits*
- explain the purpose of the Radiation Control for Health and Safety Act of 1968
- explain the ALARA concept
- explain the purpose of the Consumer-Patient Radiation Health and Safety Act of 1981
- state the goal for radiation protection
- state the formula for determining the maximum permissible dose equivalent
- calculate the maximum permissible dose equivalent
- describe current radiation protection philosophy
- identify the risks to health from exposure to ionizing radiation at low absorbed doses

- explain the premise upon which the effective absorbed dose equivalent limits system is based
- describe recent changes in National Council on Radiation Protection and Measurements (NCRP) recommendations
- describe the radiation hormesis effect
- state in terms of traditional units and also in terms of System International (SI) units the:
  a. annual effective absorbed dose equivalent limit for whole-body occupational exposure* of persons during routine operations (stochastic effects)
  b. annual occupational absorbed dose equivalent limits for tissues and organs (nonstochastic effects) such as the crystalline lens of the eye, and all other tissues and organs (e.g., reproductive cells, red bone marrow, breast, lung, skin, and extremities)
  c. guidance for radiation protection programs: cumulative exposure
  d. annual effective absorbed dose equivalent limit for continuous or frequent exposure* of the public
  e. annual effective absorbed dose equivalent limit for infrequent exposure* of the public
  f. annual effective absorbed dose equivalent limit for education and training exposures* of radiation workers
  g. total absorbed dose equivalent limit for exposures* of the embryo-fetus
  h. absorbed dose equivalent limit in a month for embryo-fetus exposures*

Exposure of patients and radiation workers to ionizing radiation must be limited to minimize the likelihood of harmful biological effects. Occupational and nonoccupational effective absorbed dose equivalent limits have been developed by health physicists to this end. This effective absorbed dose equivalent-limiting system is the system in use at the time of publication of this text. It supersedes the maximum permissible dose system (MPD system) previously used.

The concept of radiation exposure and associated "risk" of possible radiation-induced malignancy is behind the establishment of the system currently in use. Information contained in NCRP Report #91† and ICRP Pub-

---

*Sum of external and internal exposure.
†National Council on Radiation Protection and Measurements: NCRP Report #91, *Recommendations on limits for exposure to ionizing radiation*, Bethesda, MD, 1987, NCRP Publications.

lication #26* serve as resources for the revised recommendations. Future radiation protection standards will, more likely, be based on risk rather than absorbed dose equivalent.

Because members of the medical radiography team share the responsibility for patient safety from radiation exposure and are themselves subject to such exposure in the performance of their professional duties, they must be familiar with previous, existing, and new guidelines.

REGULATORY AGENCIES

Various groups share the responsibility for evaluating the relationship between radiation absorbed dose equivalent and subsequent biological effects resulting from radiation exposure. They are also responsible for formulating risk estimates of somatic and genetic effects of irradiation.

These groups include:
1. International Commission on Radiological Protection (ICRP)
2. United Nations Scientific Committee on the Effects of Atomic Radiation (UNSCEAR)
3. National Academy of Sciences Advisory Committee on the Biological Effects of Ionizing Radiation (NAS-BEIR)
4. National Council on Radiation Protection and Measurements (NCRP)

Recommendations for effective absorbed dose equivalent limits are made by these different agencies. Based on these recommendations, limits on radiation exposure can be established by an act of Congress or other lawmaking body. National and state agencies have been charged with the responsibility of enforcing standards once they have been established. The Nuclear Regulatory Commission (NRC), formerly known as the Atomic Energy Commission (AEC), is the federal agency that has the power to enforce the standards.

The majority of states have entered into agreements with the NRC to assume the responsibility of enforcing radiation protection regulations through their respective health departments. These states are known as "agreement" states. In "nonagreement" states, both the state and the NRC enforce radiation protection regulations by sending their agents to facilities, such as hospitals, that use radiation and radioactive materials to determine if the facilities comply with existing radiation safety regulations. Individual

---

*International Commission on Radiological Protection: ICRP Publication #26, *Recommendations of the ICRP,* Elmsford, NY, 1977, Pergamon Press.

states may also draft their own regulations regarding radiation safety. Inspection of nuclear reactors and assurance of compliance with federal radiation safety regulations of such facilities in agreement or nonagreement states fall solely under the jurisdiction of the NRC.

TERMINOLOGY

Effective absorbed dose equivalent limit, conceptually, refers to the *upper boundary* dose of ionizing radiation that a person can absorb during the course of a year, or in a single exposure in any given year, with a *negligible risk* of sustaining bodily injury or genetic damage as a result of the exposure.

The previously used term, *maximum permissible dose (MPD),* was used to indicate the maximum absorbed dose (equivalent) of ionizing radiation that an occupationally exposed person could absorb without sustaining appreciable bodily injury as a result of the exposure. Nonoccupational or public radiation absorption limits, were previously described in terms of (absorbed) dose limits.*

RADIATION CONTROL FOR HEALTH AND SAFETY ACT OF 1968 (PUBLIC LAW 90-602)

In 1968, the U.S. Congress passed the Radiation Control for Health and Safety Act (Public Law 90-602) to protect the public from the hazards of unnecessary radiation exposure resulting from electronic products such as microwave ovens and color televisions. Diagnostic x-ray equipment was also included. The Act permitted the establishment of the Bureau of Radiological Health (BRH) under the Food and Drug Administration (FDA). In 1982 this Bureau became known as the Center for Devices and Radiological Health. Essentially, it is responsible for conducting an ongoing electronic products radiation control program. This includes setting up standards in the manufacture, installation, assembly, and maintenance of machines used for radiologic procedures, ensuring continued compliance of such devices with these standards, assessing the biologic effects of ionizing radiation, evaluating radiation emissions from electronic products in general, and conducting research to reduce radiation exposure.

The code of standards for diagnostic x-ray equipment went into effect on August 1, 1974. This code applies to complete systems and major components manufactured *after* that date (equipment in use before August 1,

---

*National Council on Radiation Protection and Measurements: NCRP Report #39, *Basic radiation protection criteria,* Washington, DC, 1971, NCRP Publications.

1974, does *not* need to be modified or discarded). Some of the important provisions of the standards for diagnostic x-ray equipment include:

1. Automatic limitation of the radiographic beam to the image receptor regardless of image receptor size (known as *positive beam limitation*).
2. Appropriate minimum permanent filtration to ensure an acceptable level of beam quality (i.e., a significant reduction in the intensity of very "soft" x-rays which contribute only to added patient absorbed dose).
3. Ability of the machines to duplicate certain radiation exposures for any given combinations of kilovolts at peak value (kVp), milliamperes (mA), and time to ensure both exposure reproducibility (consistency in output in radiation intensity from an individual exposure to other subsequent exposures) and exposure linearity (consistency in radiation intensity stated in milliroentgens per milliampere-seconds (mR/mAs) when changing from one milliampere station to another with a variance of not more than 10%).
4. Inclusion of beam limitation devices for spot films taken during fluoroscopy. Such devices should be located between the x-ray source and the patient.
5. Presence of "beam on" indicators to give visible warnings when x-ray exposures are in progress and audible signals when exposure has terminated.
6. Inclusion of manual backup timers for automatic (phototimed) exposure control to ensure the termination of the exposure if the automatic timer fails.

Public Law 90-602 does *not* regulate the diagnostic x-ray user. It is strictly an equipment performance standard.

ALARA CONCEPT

In 1954 the National Committee on Radiation Protection* put forth the principle that radiation exposures should be kept "As Low As Reasonably Achievable." This concept, known as the ALARA concept, is accepted by all regulatory agencies. Medical radiographers and radiologists share the responsibility to keep occupational and nonoccupational absorbed dose equivalents as *low* as is possible. In practice, this translates into absorbed dose equivalents *well below* maximum allowable levels. This can usually be achieved through the employment of proper safety procedures.

---

*Later to be known as the National Council on Radiation Protection and Measurements (NCRP).

CONSUMER-PATIENT RADIATION HEALTH AND SAFETY ACT OF 1981

The Consumer-Patient Radiation Health and Safety Act of 1981 (Appendix C), signed by then president of the United States, Ronald Reagan, in August of that year, provides federal legislation requiring the establishment of minimum standards for the accreditation of education programs for persons who administer radiologic procedures and for the certification of such persons. The purpose of this act is to ensure that medical and dental radiologic procedures are consistent with rigorous safety precautions and standards. The practices of radiologic technology (which encompasses radiography, radiation therapy, and nuclear medicine), dental hygiene, and dental assistants are covered by this legislation.

Federal enactment of this law under the directorship of the secretary of Health and Human Services occurred on October 1, 1981. Individual states are encouraged to enact similar statutes and to administer certification and accreditation programs based on the standards established therein. There is no legal penalty for noncompliance. Because of this, many states have not followed with appropriate legislation.

GOAL FOR RADIATION PROTECTION

NCRP Report #91, "Recommendations on Limits for Exposure to Ionizing Radiation," has put forth the goal of limiting "the probability of radiation induced diseases in persons exposed to radiation (somatic effects) and in their progeny (genetic effects) to a degree that is reasonable and acceptable in relation to the benefits from the activities that involve such exposure."* This goal defines the essence of radiation protection.

CURRENT RADIATION PROTECTION PHILOSOPHY

Both genetic and somatic responses to ionizing radiation were considered in developing the present effective absorbed dose equivalent-limiting recommendations. Current radiation protection philosophy is based on the assumption that there is a linear, nonthreshold relationship between radiation dose and biological response ("response" refers here to biological effects). This means that the chance of sustaining biological damage and the amount of damage sustained are directly proportional to the amount of radiation absorbed, and that there is no known level of radiation dose below which one has zero probability of sustaining biological damage. Consequently, even the most miniscule

---

*NCRP Report #91, p. 3.

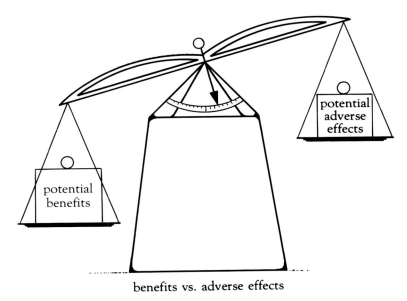

benefits vs. adverse effects

Fig. 4-1   The potential benefits of exposing the patient to ionizing radiation must outweigh the potential adverse effects.

dose of radiation has the potential to cause some damage. The current philosophy also accepts the premise that ionizing radiation possesses a beneficial as well as a destructive potential and proposes that, when employed in the healing arts for the welfare of the patient, the potential benefits of exposing the patient to ionizing radiation must outweigh the risks involved (Fig. 4-1).

RISK

The members of the medical profession and the general public share a common concern regarding the potential adverse biological effects of ionizing radiation from low levels of exposure. Predominantly associated with low levels are stochastic effects* (e.g., the random inducement of cancer or genetic effects). For higher radiation levels, nonstochastic effects† must be considered. There is as yet *no conclusive proof* that low-level ionizing radiation causes a statistically significant increase in the risk of malignancy. Although this *risk,* in fact, *may be negligible,* the subject is still highly controversial. A discussion

---

*Nonthreshold randomly occurring biological effects of ionizing radiation in which the probability of occurrence of the effects rather than the severity is proportional to the dose.

†Biological effects of ionizing radiation that demonstrate the existence of a threshold and the severity of the biological damage increases as a consequence of increased absorbed dose.

of risk estimates for causing cancer in humans, biological effects of ionizing radiation from low-level exposure, and stochastic and nonstochastic effects is presented in Chapter 6.

Revised concepts of radiation exposure and risk have brought about the recent NCRP changes in recommendations for limits on exposure to ionizing radiation. These changes are addressed later in this chapter. Because there are many conflicting views on assessing the risk of cancer inducement from low-level radiation exposure, the trend has been to create stricter radiation protection standards. A direct consequence of this conservatism has been the adoption of the effective absorbed dose equivalent limits system.

For the patient, as previously stated, the benefit obtained from any diagnostic radiologic procedure *must always* be weighed against the risk that must be taken. Methods for assessing risk estimates for cancer induction are discussed in Chapter 6.

For radiation workers such as medical imaging personnel, occupational risk due to radiation may be equated with occupational risk in other "safe" industries (i.e., the number of fatal injuries per 10,000 workers) (see Chapter 8 for further information). This numerical value, however, is difficult to equate with the effective absorbed dose equivalent limits. The NCRP wants the lifetime risk of fatal stochastic effects kept *below* one in a hundred.

To achieve this end, the NCRP proposes that radiation protection programs for radiation workers should be designed so that individual workers do not have cumulative (i.e., from external plus internal sources) absorbed dose equivalents in excess of their age in years times 10 mSv (1 rem).* As an example of this concept, consider the following situation. A worker of age 40 has been employed at a nuclear power plant for 10 years. Before this, he had been employed as a radiation worker in another industry during the course of which he received a cumulative absorbed dose equivalent of 100 mSv (10 rem). Thus the radiation protection program for his current position should be such that he has not accumulated a total absorbed dose equivalent greater than 300 mSv (30 rem) in his 10 years of employment.

PREMISE UPON WHICH THE EFFECTIVE ABSORBED DOSE EQUIVALENT LIMITS SYSTEM IS BASED

The essential concept is that any organ in the human body is vulnerable to damage from exposure to ionizing radiation and, therefore, every organ is

---

*NCRP Report #91, p 47.

essentially at risk because of the assumed stochastic (probabilistic) nature of incidence of radiation-induced effects (somatic or genetic).

Unlike its predecessor, the now abandoned Maximum Permissible Dose System (MPD),* the Effective Absorbed Dose Equivalent Limits System includes for the determination of effective absorbed dose equivalent (H_E) "all" radiation-vulnerable human organs that can contribute to potential risk rather than just using the human organs considered to be critical organs.†‡ The Effective Absorbed Dose Equivalent Limits System tries to equate the various risks of cancer and genetic effects to the tissue or organ that was exposed to radiation. Because various tissues and organs do not have the same degree of sensitivity to these effects, the system employed must compensate for the differences in risk from one organ to another. Hence, an organ weighting factor (W_T) is used. This factor "indicates the ratio of the risk of stochastic effects attributable to irradiation of a given organ or tissue *(T)* to the total risk when the whole body is uniformly irradiated."§ Weighting factors recommended by the ICRP in 1977 and adopted by the NCRP in 1987 are reproduced in Table 4-1. A more complete discussion of this important topic is on page 17 of NCRP Report #91.

RECENT CHANGES IN NCRP RECOMMENDATIONS

Since 1983, numerous changes have been made in radiation protection standards. Recommendations contained in NCRP Report #91 now supersede those contained in NCRP Report #39. A summary of some of the important changes follows.

The formula, MPD = 5 (N − 18) rem [MPD = 50 (N − 18) mSv], governing cumulative whole-body occupational exposure, was abandoned by the NCRP (NCRP Report #91), along with the Maximum Permissible Dose System. Therefore, the traditional age proration formula (where 50 mSv [5 rem] represents the absorbed dose equivalent of ionizing radiation allowed in any one year for persons employed in radiation industries [such as medical radiography], N represents the actual age [in years] of the individual concerned, and 18 specifies the legal age at which a person could become employed as a radiation worker) will be eliminated from radiation protection standards. It is instructive, however, to give an example demonstrating the proper usage of this formula.

---

*Absorbed dose limits that indicate the maximum absorbed dose which an individual may incur.
†Examples of critical organs identified in NCRP Report #39 are the gonads, blood-forming organs (specifically red bone marrow), and lung tissue.
‡NCRP Report #39, pp. 73, 74.
§NCRP Report #91, p. 51.

Table 4-1 **Weighting Factors for Calculating Effective Dose Equivalent (H_E)***

Tissue	Weighting factor (W_T)
Gonads	0.25
Breast	0.15
Red bone marrow	0.12
Lung	0.12
Thyroid	0.03
Bone surfaces	0.03
Remainder†	0.30

From ICRP: *Recommendations of the International Commission on Radiological Protection,* Publication #26, New York, 1977, Pergamon Press.

*$H_E = \sum_i (H_T)_i (W_T)_i$ where $(H_T)_i$ is the dose equivalent determined for a specific tissue and the summation is overall possible irradiated tissues.

†Remainder includes the five nonlisted tissues receiving the highest dose equivalents and are associated with the specific region being irradiated (e.g., for GI tract exposure, the Remainder tissues include stomach, small intestine, upper large intestine, and the lower large intestine). The Remainder group does not include extremities or the lens of the eye.

EXAMPLE: Determine the maximum accumulated whole-body absorbed dosage of x-radiation that a 33-year-old staff radiographer may receive.

ANSWER: In traditional terms:

MPD = 5 ($N - 18$) rem

= 5 (33 − 18) rem

= 5 (15) rem

= 75 rem

In SI units:

MPD = 50 ($N - 18$) mSv

= 50 (33 − 18) mSv

= 50 (15) mSv

= 750 mSv

This represents the total cumulative whole body absorbed dose equivalent that the radiographer was permitted to receive during the course of a 15 year employment. Should the radiographer have accumulated by age 33 an absorbed dose equivalent in excess of 75 rem (750 mSv), then that person could not be permitted to accumulate additional radiation dosage until compliance was reestablished with the ($N - 18$) rule.

Because the NCRP has recommended that this method of calculation be discontinued, members of the medical radiography team should check with their state health department concerning current regulations.

It should be noted that medical imaging personnel generally do *not* receive an annual absorbed dose equivalent of more than a few hundred millirem while performing their respective duties. Because occupational exposure should be maintained *well below* 50 mSv (5 rem) in any given year, the traditional MPD formula is simply not practical.

To replace the old MPD formula, the NCRP recommends limiting the cumulative absorbed dose equivalent in rem to the occupationally exposed person's age in years. Therefore, the cumulative absorbed dose equivalent should *not* exceed the age of the individual in years $\times$ 10 mSv (years $\times$ 1 rem).*

Other significant changes include the use of 50 mSv (5 rem) as the annual effective absorbed dose equivalent limit for whole-body occupational exposure of persons during routine operations. NCRP Report #91 emphasizes that this limit is an upper boundary.

The ICRP and NCRP are considering the possibility of reducing exposure standards because of (1) revised risk estimates derived from recent re-evaluations of dosimetric studies on the atomic bomb survivors of Hiroshima and Nagasaki† and (2) the appearance, due to longer follow-up time, of increased numbers of solid tumors in the survivor population. According to these studies, ionizing radiation was estimated to be three times more damaging than previously thought. This implies that both atomic bombs may well have emitted a smaller quantity of radiation than previously believed and, consequently, that radiation-induced cancers in the survivors were caused by lesser doses of radiation than originally projected. Because of this, levels of ionizing radiation formerly considered "acceptable" have been revised downward.

Perhaps in the future the annual effective absorbed dose equivalent limit for occupationally exposed persons may be limited to 10 or 20 mSv (1 or 2 rem) per year.‡ Of course, such a change will necessitate further evaluation of actual risk for persons employed in radiation industries. Lowering

---

*NCRP Report #91, p. 47.

†Committee on Biological Effects of Ionizing Radiations, National Research Council, Commission of Life Sciences. Board on Radiation Research: *Health effects of exposure to low levels of ionizing radiation* (BEIR V Report), National Academy Press, 1989.

‡In fact, contained within Manual #60 of the International Commission on Radiation Protection (ICRP 60), Pergamon Press, Oxford, 1991, is a recommendation for lowering the allowable occupational level of exposure to ionizing radiation from 50 mSv/yr (5 rem/yr) to 20 mSv/yr (2 rem/yr) averaged over defined periods of five years. This lower limit is not enforced in the United States.

of the current limits would be the responsibility of the NRC, individual states, and the FDA.

While an annual effective absorbed dose equivalent limit for whole-body occupational exposure has been set at 50 mSv (5 rem) by the NCRP, a limit has also been set for individual members of the general public *not* occupationally exposed. The NCRP recommended annual limit is 1 mSv (0.1 rem) for continuous or frequent exposures from man-made sources other than medical irradiation and 5 mSv (0.5 rem) for infrequent annual exposure. Chapter 8 contains further information pertaining to these limits.

To reduce exposure for pregnant female members of the medical radiography team, the NCRP now recommends that the effective absorbed dose equivalent limit for the unborn child (5 mSv [0.5 rem]) "*not* be received at a rate greater than 0.5 mSv (0.05 rem) per month."*

Radiography students are another important absorbed dose equivalent limiting consideration. Eighteen-year-old students, exposed as part of their educational experience, should *not* exceed 1 mSv (0.1 rem) annually.

Genetic and somatic general population dose limits (each limit being 0.17 rem per year) have been deemed unnecessary and have been abandoned because they are not likely to be exceeded if the occupational annual effective absorbed dose equivalent limit of 50 mSv (5 rem) and the maximum general population annual effective absorbed dose equivalent limit of 5 mSv (0.5 rem) are adhered to.

MPD quarterly dose equivalent limits have also been discarded as a consequence of the same school of thought that caused the deletion of the genetic and somatic population dose limits.

To provide a low-exposure cut-off level so that regulatory agencies could dismiss a level of individual risk as negligible, an annual effective absorbed dose equivalent of 0.01 mSv (0.001 rem) has been set. This means that below this absorbed dose equivalent level it is *not* necessary to try to reduce individual exposure.

RADIATION HORMESIS

In the BEIR V Report of the National Academy of Science in the Biological Effects of Ionizing Radiation, conclusions regarding the adverse effects on health from low levels of ionizing radiation are founded on extrapolations from radiation dose equivalents greater than 0.5 Sv (50 rem). (See Chapter 6 for more information.) Such radiation levels are significantly greater than ordinary background radiation levels (3.5 mSv or 350 mrem). BEIR V em-

*NCRP Report #91, p. 47.

braces the linear "no threshold" view of the Japanese atomic bomb lifetime survival study (LSS) data. However, recent studies from the Radiation Effects Research Council in Hiroshima indicate an apparent "threshold" dosage in the atomic bomb LSS data somewhere between 0.2 and 0.5 Sv (20 to 50 rem). This lower value corresponds to the amount of natural radiation that average U.S. residents receive in their lifetime. What is curious is that the lifetime survival data appear to indicate that Japanese A-bomb survivors with moderate radiation exposure (5 mSv to 50 mSv or 0.5 rem to 5 rem, about equivalent to 1.5 to 15 years of natural radiation) have a reduced cancer death rate compared with a normally exposed "control" population. This contradicts the cancer death increase predictions of the BEIR V Report and, *if substantiated,* would seem to cast doubt on the BEIR V conclusion that "any" amount of radiation is potentially harmful. The reverse might, in fact, be true, at least for moderate amounts of radiation exposure. As additional support of this conclusion, consider that, for seven Western states having background radiation levels higher than other states by about 1 mSv per year (100 mrem per year), the residents of those states experience about 15% fewer cancer deaths per 1000 individuals than the U.S. average. In addition, a study in China made in 1972 to 1975 of two stable populations of about 70,000 persons each of whose annual background radiation levels differed by about 2 mSv (200 mrem) disclosed a cancer rate in the more exposed population of only about 50% of that of the other group. Other intriguing studies exist. From these, one might conclude that there is a radiation hormesis effect (i.e., a beneficial consequence of radiation) for populations continuously exposed to moderately higher levels of radiation. It is possible that, during the course of humankind's long progress up the evolutionary ladder, advantageous genetic mutations with respect to radiation exposure would have occurred resembling those that allow lower animals today to demonstrate radiation hormesis. Thus, by predicting risk from even the smallest amounts of radiation exposure (e.g., two or three times normal background levels), the BEIR commission may be unduly alarming the general public.*

OCCUPATIONAL AND NONOCCUPATIONAL ABSORBED DOSE EQUIVALENT LIMITS

For the protection of radiation workers, as well as the population as a whole, absorbed dose equivalent limits (Table 4-2) have been established as guides. All medical imaging personnel should be familiar with new NCRP recom-

---

*For a more detailed discussion on the topic of radiation hormesis and references to the studies cited for China and seven U.S. Western states, see the letter by John Cameron, *Physics Today,* 45(3):13, 1992.

Table 4-2 Summary of NCRP Recommendations*†
(NCRP Report #91)

A. Occupational exposures (annual)‡
  1. Effective dose equivalent limit (stochastic effects) — 50 mSv — (5 rem)
  2. Dose equivalent limits for tissues and organs (nonstochastic effects)
     a. Lens of eye — 150 mSv — (15 rem)
     b. All others (e.g., red bone marrow, breast, lung, gonads, skin, and extremities) — 500 mSv — (50 rem)
  3. Guidance: Cumulative exposure — 10 mSv × age — (1 rem × age in years)
B. Planned special occupational exposure, effective dose equivalent limit‡
C. Guidance for emergency occupational exposure‡
D. Public exposures (annual)
  1. Effective dose equivalent limit, continuous or frequent exposure‡ — 1 mSv — (0.1 rem)
  2. Effective dose equivalent limit, infrequent exposure‡ — 5 mSv — (0.5 rem)
  3. Remedial action recommended when:
     a. Effective dose equivalent§ — >5 mSv — (>0.5 rem)
     b. Exposure to radon and its decay products‖ — >0.007 Jhm^{-3} — (>2 WLM)
  4. Dose equivalent limits for lens of eye, skin, and extremities‡ — 50 mSv — (5 rem)
E. Education and training exposures (annual)‡
  1. Effective dose equivalent limit — 1 mSv — (0.1 rem)
  2. Dose equivalent limit for lens of eye, skin, and extremities — 50 mSv — (5 rem)
F. Embryo-fetus exposures‡
  1. Total dose equivalent limit — 5 mSv — (0.5 rem)
  2. Dose equivalent limit in a month — 0.5 mSv — (0.05 rem)
G. Negligible individual risk level (annual)‡ Effective dose equivalent per source or practice — 0.01 mSv — (0.001 rem)

*Excluding medical exposures.
†See Table 4.1 in NCRP Report #91 for recommendations on Q.
‡Sum of external and internal exposures.
§Including background but excluding internal exposures.
‖WLM stands for working level month and refers to a cumulative exposure for a working month (170 hours). As applied to radon and its daughter products, 1 WLM represents the cumulative exposure experienced in a 170-hour period due to a radon concentration of 100 pCi/L. The occupational limit for miners is 4 WLM/yr, which results in an absorbed dose equivalent of approximately 0.15 Sv (15 rem) per year.

mendations. For this group, the most important item is the 50 mSv (5 rem) per year whole-body occupational effective absorbed dose equivalent limit. This upper boundary annual absorbed dose equivalent limit on the monitoring badge reading (to be discussed in Chapter 9) is designed to restrict "whole body" exposure levels, thereby limiting stochastic effects of radiation. It takes into account the absorbed dose equivalent in all radiation-sensitive organs that are found in the body. The absorbed dose equivalent limits for tissues and organs, such as lens of the eye, extremities, and skin, which are subject to nonstochastic effects, are higher than 50 mSv (5 rem) per year. When the effective absorbed dose equivalent for stochastic effects is maintained, protection from nonstochastic (threshold) effects also occurs.

SUMMARY

The concept of occupational and nonoccupational absorbed dose equivalent limits have been described in this chapter. The reader should be able to state current NCRP absorbed dose equivalent limits in terms of both traditional and System International units. The reader should also be able to discuss correct radiation protection philosophy and identify the risks to health from exposure to ionizing radiation at low absorbed doses.

REVIEW QUESTIONS

1. Which of the following agencies has the responsibility to enforce radiation safety standards that have been established by an act of Congress or other law-making body?
   a. ICRP
   b. NRC
   c. NCRP
   d. UNSCEAR

2. Which term was formerly used to indicate the absorbed dose of ionizing radiation to which a person in a radiation-related occupation could be exposed to over a given period of time without sustaining appreciable bodily injury?
   a. quality factor
   b. maximum absorbed dose
   c. maximum permissible dose
   d. exposure rate

3. Which of the following terms was previously used to specify nonoccupational radiation absorption limits, such as radiation absorption by the general public?
   a. dose limits
   b. maximum permissible dose

c. maximum absorbed dose

d. quality factor

4. Biological effects (e.g., cataracts) resulting from exposure to ionizing radiation appear to follow a:
   a. sigmoid dose-response nonthreshold relationship
   b. circular dose-response threshold relationship
   c. curvilinear threshold dose pattern
   d. linear, nonthreshold dose pattern

5. Conceptually, the upper boundary dose of ionizing radiation that a person can absorb per year, or in a single exposure in any given year, with a negligible risk of sustaining bodily injury or genetic damage as a result of the exposure defines:
   a. maximum permissible dose
   b. dose limits
   c. effective dose
   d. effective absorbed dose equivalent

6. Select the *former* maximum permissible dose equivalent formula.
   a. $MPD = 5 (N - 18)$ rem
   b. $MPD = 50 (N - 18)$ mSv
   c. $MPD = 18 (N - 5)$ rem/mSv
   d. a and b

7. Using the *former* MPD formula, determine the maximum accumulated dose of ionizing radiation that a 27-year-old radiographer's whole body is allowed to have absorbed over the course of his or her lifetime.
   a. 750 mSv (75 rem)
   b. 600 mSv (60 rem)
   c. 450 mSv (45 rem)
   d. 250 mSv (25 rem)

8. Which of the following annual whole-body occupational radiation annual effective absorbed dose equivalent limits applies to the radiographer during routine operations?
   a. 5 mSv (0.5 rem)
   b. 50 mSv (5 rem)
   c. 250 mSv (25 rem)
   d. 750 mSv (75 rem)

9. During the entire period of gestation, the fetus in utero may not receive more than _____ from occupational exposure of a pregnant woman with the rate of this absorbed dose equivalent limit not exceeding _____ per month.

a. 5 mSv (0.5 rem), 0.5 mSv (0.05 rem)
b. 50 mSv (5 rem), 5 mSv (0.5 rem)
c. 300 mSv (30 rem), 150 mSv (15 rem)
d. 500 mSv (50 rem), 250 mSv (250 rem)

10. For members of the general public *not* occupationally exposed, the NCRP recommends a limit of _____ for continuous (or frequent) exposures from artificial sources of ionizing radiation other than medical and _____ for infrequent annual exposure.
    a. 1 mSv (0.1 rem), 5 mSv (0.5 rem)
    b. 3 mSv (0.3 rem), 8 mSv (0.8 rem)
    c. 10 mSv (1 rem), 20 mSv (2 rem)
    d. 50 mSv (5 rem), 75 mSv (7.5 rem)

11. Eighteen-year-old radiography students, exposed as part of their educational experience, should *not* exceed an absorbed dose equivalent limit of _____ annually.
    a. 0.5 mSv (0.05 rem)
    b. 1 mSv (0.1 rem)
    c. 5 mSv (0.5 rem)
    d. 50 mSv (5 rem)

12. The NCRP recommends replacing the cumulative whole-body occupational exposure MPD formula (MPD = 5 (N − 18) rem) by limiting cumulative exposure to the age of the individual in years times _____ .
    a. 1 mSv (0.1 rem)
    b. 10 mSv (1 rem)
    c. 100 mSv (10 rem)
    d. 1000 mSv (100 rem)

13. When whole-body occupational exposure is controlled by keeping the effective absorbed dose equivalent *well below* the upper boundary limit, the *possibility* of inducing stochastic effects of radiation is:
    a. increased
    b. maintained at an acceptable level
    c. minimized
    d. none of the above

14. In 1968, the Radiation Control for Health and Safety Act (Public Law 90-602) was passed by the U.S. Congress to protect the public from the hazards of unnecessary radiation exposure resulting from:
    a. diagnostic x-ray equipment only
    b. therapeutic x-ray equipment only
    c. electronic products excluding diagnostic x-ray equipment
    d. electronic products including diagnostic x-ray equipment

15. For radiation workers such as medical imaging personnel, occupational risk may be equated with occupational risk in:
    a. other safe industries
    b. somewhat hazardous industries
    c. hazardous industries
    d. extremely hazardous industries

16. What is the term applied to a beneficial consequence of radiation for populations continuously exposed to low levels of radiation above background?
    a. nonoccupational absorbed dose equivalent effect
    b. radiation negligible risk level effect
    c. radiation hormesis effect
    d. radiation benevolent effect

Bibliography

Ballinger PW: *Merrill's atlas of radiographic positions and radiologic procedures,* ed 7, vol 1, St Louis, 1991, Mosby–Year Book, pp 18-33.

Bushong S: *Radiologic science for technologists: physics, biology and protection,* ed 2, St Louis, 1980, Mosby–Year Book.

Bushong SC: *Radiologic science for technologists: physics, biology and protection,* ed 4, St Louis, 1988, Mosby–Year Book.

Cameron JR: Radiation hormesis (letter), *Physics Today* 45(3):13, 1992.

Christensen EE, Curry III TS, Dowdey JE: *An introduction to the physics of diagnostic radiology,* ed 2, Philadelphia, 1978, Lea & Febiger.

Curry III TS, Dowdey JE, Murry Jr RC: *Christensen's introduction to the physics of diagnostic radiology,* ed 3, Philadelphia, 1984, Lea & Febiger.

Frankel R: *Radiation protection for radiologic technologists,* New York, 1976, McGraw-Hill.

Fullerton GD et al, editors: *Medical Physics Monograph No 5,* Published for the American Association of Physicists in Medicine by the American Institute of Physics, New York, 1980.

Hagler M: Radiation protection update, *RT Image* 3(20):10, 1990.

Hall EJ: *Radiobiology for the radiologist,* ed 3, Philadelphia, 1988, JB Lippincott.

Hendee WR, editor: *Health effects of low-level radiation,* Norwalk, CT, 1984, Appleton-Century-Crofts.

International Commission on Radiation Units and Measurements (ICRU): *Radiation quantities and units,* ICRU Report #33. Washington, DC, 1980, ICRU.

International Commission on Radiological Protection: *Recommendations of the ICRP,* ICRP Publication No. 26. Elmsford, NY, 1977, Pergamon Press.

Loudin A: The radiation debate continues, *RT Image* 3(51):10, 1990.

National Council on Radiation Protection and Measurements (NCRP): Report #39, *Basic radiation protection criteria,* Washington, DC, 1971, NCRP Publications.

National Council on Radiation Protection and Measurements (NCRP): Report #43, *Review of the current state of radiation protection philosophy,* Washington, DC, 1975, NCRP Publications.

National Council on Radiation Protection and Measurements (NCRP): Report #91, *Recommendations on limits for exposure to ionizing radiation,* Bethesda, MD, 1987, NCRP Publications.

Noz ME, Maguire Jr GQ: *Radiation protection in the radiologic and health sciences,* Philadelphia, 1979, Lea & Febiger.

Noz ME, Maguire Jr GQ: *Radiation protection in radiologic and health sciences,* ed 2, Philadelphia, 1985, Lea & Febiger.

Reimenschneider J: Rethinking radiation protection standards, *RT Image* 3(6):6, 1990.

Reimenschneider J: ICRP recommends lower maximum dose, *RT Image* 3(28):22, 1990.

Scheele RV, Wakley J: *Elements of radiation protection,* Springfield, IL, 1975, Charles C Thomas.

Selman J: *The fundamentals of x-ray and radium physics,* ed 6, Springfield, IL, 1978, Charles C Thomas.

Selman J: *The fundamentals of x-ray and radium physics,* ed 7, Springfield, IL, 1985, Charles C Thomas.

Sevcik J: Putting the radiation risk into perspective, *RT Image* 2(12):1, 1989.

Travis EL: *Primer of medical radiobiology,* ed 2, Chicago, 1989, Year Book Medical Publishers.

US Department of Health, Education, and Welfare (HEW), Public Health Service, Food and Drug Administration, Bureau of Radiological Health, Division of Compliance X-Ray Products Branch: *Assembler's guide to diagnostic x-ray equipment,* HEW Publication (FDA) 76-8002, Rockville, MD, 1975, HEW.

US Department of Health, Education, and Welfare (HEW), Public Health Service, Food and Drug Administration, Bureau of Radiological Health, Division of Compliance (HFX-400): *A practitioner's guide to the diagnostic x-ray equipment standard,* Publication (FDA) 78-8050, Rockville, MD, 1978, HEW.

Webster EW et al: American Association of Physicists in Medicine (AAPM) Report No. 18, *A primer on low-level ionizing radiation and its biological effects,* New York, 1986, American Institute of Physics (published for the AAPM).

5

Overview of Cell Biology

OBJECTIVES

Upon completion of this chapter, the reader will be able to:

- explain the need for having a basic knowledge of cell structure, composition, and function as a foundation for radiation biology
- identify and describe some important functions of the major classes of organic and inorganic compounds that exist in the cell
- describe the molecular structure of DNA and explain how it functions in the cell
- list the various cellular components and identify their physical characteristics and functions
- distinguish the two types of cell division, mitosis and meiosis, and describe each process

Biology is a science that explores living things and life processes. Cells are the basic units of all living matter and are essential for life. The cell is the fundamental component of structure, of development and growth, and of life processes. Before the reader can develop an understanding of the effects of ionizing radiation on a living system such as the human body, which is composed of large numbers of various types of cells, a basic knowledge of cell structure, composition, and function must be acquired. This chapter provides the reader with an overview of cell biology as a foundation for radiation biology.

THE CELL

Cells exist in many different forms and perform many different functions. Some cells function as free-moving, independent units, some belong to loosely organized communities that wander from one place to another, and some remain fixed in one position functioning as part of the tissue of a larger organism throughout their lifetime. Every mature human cell is highly specialized, having predetermined tasks to perform in support of the whole body. Cells move, grow, react, protect themselves, regulate life processes, and reproduce. To ensure efficient cell operation, the body must provide food as a source of raw material for the release of energy, oxygen to help break down the food, and water to transport inorganic substances* such as calcium and sodium into and out of the cell. In turn, normal cellular functioning enables the body to maintain homeostasis or equilibrium, to return to and maintain normal functioning despite the changes it has been forced to undergo as a result of the influences to which it has been subjected.

Cells are engaged in an ongoing process of obtaining energy and converting it to their own special purposes. They absorb molecular nutrients through the cell membrane and use these nutrients in the production of energy and the synthesis of molecules. If exposure to ionizing radiation damages the components involved in molecular synthesis beyond repair, cells will function abnormally or die.

CELL CHEMICAL COMPONENTS
Protoplasm

Cells are made of protoplasm, the building material for all living things. This substance carries on the complex process of metabolism,† the reception and

---

*See *inorganic compounds* in Glossary.
†See *cell metabolism* in Glossary.

processing of food and oxygen and the elimination of waste products, which enables the cell to perform the vital functions of synthesizing proteins and producing energy.

Protoplasm consists of organic* and inorganic materials, either dissolved or suspended in water. Twenty-four elements form the biomolecules that compose protoplasm, the four main elements involved being carbon, hydrogen, oxygen, and nitrogen. When combined with phosphorus and sulfur, they compose the essential major organic compounds: proteins,* carbohydrates,* lipids,* and nucleic acids.* The most important inorganic substances are water and mineral salts. Water aids in sustaining life and is the most abundant inorganic compound in the body. Depending on cell type, it normally accounts for 70% to 85% of protoplasm. Mineral salts exist in smaller quantities and are also of vital importance.

Organic compounds

The four major classes of organic compounds (proteins, carbohydrates, lipids (fats), and nucleic acids [Fig. 5-1]) all contain carbon. Carbon is the basic constituent of all organic matter. By combining with hydrogen, nitrogen, and oxygen, it makes life possible. Of all the organic compounds, protein contains the most carbon.

Proteins

Proteins make up about 15% of cell content. They are essential for growth, the construction of new body tissue, and the repair of injured or debilitated tissue. Proteins are formed by combining amino acids* (the structural units of protein) into a long chainlike molecular complex. In this complex, a chemical link called a *peptide bond* connects each amino acid to the other. Protein production or protein synthesis involves twenty-two different amino

---

*See Glossary.

MAJOR CLASSES OF ORGANIC COMPOUNDS
WHICH COMPOSE THE CELL:

PROTEINS

CARBOHYDRATES

LIPIDS (FATS)

NUCLEIC ACIDS

Fig. 5-1   Major classes of organic compounds composing the cell.

acids. The order of arrangement of these amino acids determines the precise function of each protein molecule, and the type of protein that any given cell contains determines the characteristics carried by that cell. Chromosomes* and genes* organize the amino acids into the proper sequences to form specific structural and enzymatic proteins (Fig. 5-2).

Structural proteins, such as those found in muscle, provide the body with its shape and form and a source of heat and energy. By functioning as catalysts,* enzymatic proteins (enzymes) control the cell's various physiological activities. Enzymes cause an increase in cellular activity, which, in turn, causes biochemical reactions to occur more rapidly to meet the needs of the cell. Hence, proper functioning of the cell depends on the enzymes.

---

*See Glossary.

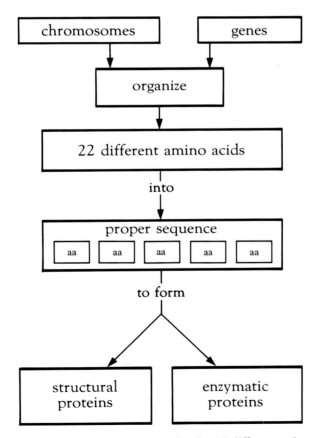

Fig. 5-2   Chromosomes and genes organize the 22 different amino acids into the proper sequences to form the different structural and enzymatic proteins.

Besides providing structure and support for the body, proteins can also function as hormones and antibodies. Hormones are chemical secretions manufactured by various endocrine glands and carried by the bloodstream to influence activities of other parts of the body. They regulate body functions such as growth and development. Antibodies are produced by the lymphocytes. They are materials developed by the body in response to the presence of foreign antigens such as bacteria or a flu virus. The antibodies provide a primary defense mechanism against such antigens. Hence, they defend the body against infection and disease.

Proteins also function as building blocks for numerous acellular tissues of the human body, such as hair and nails.

Carbohydrates

Carbohydrates, which may also be referred to as saccharides, make up about 1% of cell content. They include starches and various sugars. Carbohydrates range from simple to complex compounds even though they are composed of only carbon, hydrogen, and oxygen. The simple sugars such as glucose, fructose, and galactose have six carbon atoms and six molecules of water (e.g., glucose with the chemical formula $C_6H_{12}O_6$). Glucose is the primary energy source for the cell. Because it is a simple sugar, it is called a *monosaccharide*. *Disaccharides* are also sugars. These have two units of a simple sugar or two monosaccharides linked together. Sucrose (cane sugar) is an example of a disaccharide. Both monosaccharides and disaccharides have relatively small molecules. *Polysaccharides* contain several or many molecules of simple sugar. Plant starches and animal glycogen are the two most important polysaccharides.

Carbohydrates, simply described as long chains of sugar molecules, function as short-term energy storers for the body. Their primary purpose is to provide fuel for cell metabolism.* They are also important structural parts of cell walls and intercellular materials.

Lipids

Lipids, which are also referred to as fats or fatlike substances, constitute about 2% of cell content. They are made up of a molecule of glycerine* and three molecules of fatty acid.* Lipids are water-insoluble organic macromolecules that consist of carbon, hydrogen, and oxygen. They are the structural parts of cell membranes. Lipids are present in all body tissue and perform a variety of functions for the cell. They serve as a reservoir for the long-term storage of energy, insulate and protect the body against the environment,

---

*See Glossary.

support and protect organs such as the eyes and kidneys, provide essential fatty acids necessary for growth and development, and assist in the digestive process.

Nucleic acids (Fig. 5-3)

Nucleic acids, which compose about 1% of the cell, are large, complex macromolecules.* The small structures that make up nucleic acids are called *nucleotides*. Each nucleotide is a unit formed from a nitrogenous base such as adenine, guanine, cytosine, or thymine, a five-carbon sugar molecule (deoxyribose), and a phosphate molecule. Cells contain two types of nucleic acids that are important to human metabolism: deoxyribonucleic acid* (DNA) and ribonucleic acid* (RNA). The DNA macromolecule is composed of two long sugar-phosphate chains, which twist around each other in a double helix configuration and are linked by pairs of nitrogenous bases (organic bases that contain the element nitrogen) at the sugar molecules of the chains to form a tightly coiled structure resembling a twisted ladder or a spiral staircase. The sugar-phosphate chains are the rails, and the pairs of nitrogenous bases, which consist of complementary chemicals, are the steps or rungs of the DNA ladderlike structure (Fig. 5-4). Hydrogen bonds attach the bases to each other, joining the two side rails of the DNA ladder.

The four nitrogenous bases in DNA macromolecules are: adenine (A), guanine (G), cytosine (C), and thymine (T). Adenine and guanine are compounds called purines, whereas the compounds cytosine and thymine are classified as pyrimidines. A significant characteristic of the nitrogenous bases is that purines* always link only with pyrimidines* in certain specific combinations; more precisely, adenine always bonds only with thymine and cytosine bonds only with guanine. This characteristic is why the two strands of DNA are described as complementary.

DNA, the master chemical, contains all the information the cell needs to function. It carries the genetic information necessary for cell replication and regulates all cellular activity to direct protein synthesis (the building of new proteins). DNA determines the characteristics of a person by regulating the sequences of amino acids in the person's constituent proteins during the synthesization of these proteins; these sequences of amino acids are determined by the order of adenine-thymine and cytosine-guanine base pairs in the DNA macromolecules (which constitute the genetic "codes" of the macromolecules). Different sequences of amino acids produce different kinds of proteins with different functions. Protein characteristics determine cell characteristics, and cell characteristics, ultimately, determine the characteristics of

---

*See Glossary.

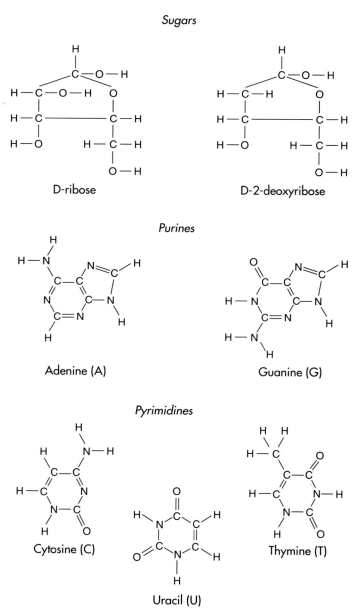

Fig. 5-3   The components of nucleic acids (H = hydrogen, C = carbon, N = nitrogen, O = oxygen). Sugars are strung together with phosphate groups, and a base is attached to each sugar. DNA uses D-2-deoxyribose sugar and RNA D-ribose. Both nucleic acids use the same two purines, but thymine in DNA is replaced by uracil in RNA.

(From Cherfas, J., *Man-made life*, Pantheon Books, New York, 1982; with permission.)

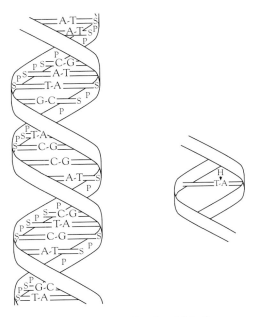

Fig. 5-4   Diagram of a DNA macromolecule which illustrates its twisted ladder-like or spiral-staircase–like configuration. Alternating sugar and phosphate molecules form the side-rails of the ladder, while the nitrogen bases, which consist of the complimentary chemicals adenine (A), thymine (T), guanine (G), and cytosine (C) form the rungs or steps. A hydrogen bond joins the bases together.

the entire individual. It is as if all of the information necessary to construct and maintain a living organism were written in a book (DNA) where the letters, words, and sentences are composed of the nitrogenous bases.

Because DNA is found mostly in the cell nucleus, it cannot directly influence cellular activity such as growth and differentiation, which occur in the cytoplasm (that part of the cell that lies outside of the nucleus). Instead, DNA regulates cellular activity *indirectly,* transmitting its genetic information outside of the cell nucleus by reproducing itself in the form of messenger RNA (mRNA), the substance responsible for making proteins out of amino acids.

DNA serves as a prototype for mRNA. mRNA is identical to DNA except that mRNA contains the five-carbon sugar molecule ribose rather than deoxyribose, and uracil* (U) replaces thymine as the nitrogenous base. An

*See Glossary.

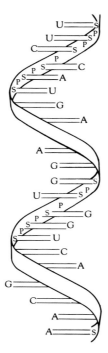

Fig. 5-5   Messenger RNA (mRNA) resembles one-half of a DNA macromolecule. It appears as a single strand (one side-rail) of the DNA ladder-like configuration, the ladder being severed in half lengthwise. Uracil (U) replaces thymine (T) as one of the nitrogenous bases in the mRNA molecule.

mRNA macromolecule resembles one half of a DNA macromolecule. It appears as a single strand of the DNA ladderlike configuration, the ladder being severed in half lengthwise (Fig. 5-5).

mRNA macromolecules carry their genetic codes (in the form of their sequences of nitrogenous bases—U, U, C, C, A, U, G, for example) from the cell nucleus through the endoplasmic reticulum (the network of sacs and canals that winds through the cytoplasm) to the ribosomes where proteins are manufactured. Here, the mRNAs transfer their genetic codes to another kind of RNA molecule called transfer RNA (tRNA). tRNAs combine with and transport individual amino acids from different areas of the cell to the ribosomes, where the amino acids are arranged and attached in specific orders to form chainlike protein molecules. Each tRNA molecule is coded for a particular amino acid; because each of the twenty-two different amino acids has a tRNA, there are at least twenty-two different types of tRNA. The cell's "protein factories," the ribosomes, travel along the mRNAs linking tRNAs

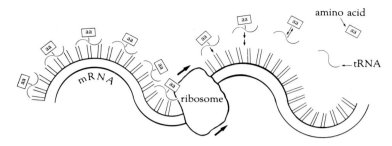

Fig. 5-6   Ribosomes, the cell's "protein factories," travel along the mRNA "rails" linking tRNAs and their corresponding amino acids in the proper sequences to produce the proteins appropriate to providing for the needs of the cell.

and their corresponding amino acids in the correct orders so that the proteins appropriate to providing for the needs of the cell will be produced (Fig. 5-6).

Many of the proteins produced in the ribosomes are enzymes, which cause vital chemical reactions to take place within the cell at the appropriate times. Some of the enzymes produced are called *repair enzymes*. These enzymes can mend damaged molecules and are therefore capable of helping the cell to recover from a small amount of radiation-induced damage. Both the catalytic and repair capabilities of enzymes are of vital importance to the survival of the cell.

Chromosomes are tiny rod-shaped bodies, which under a microscope appear to be long-threadlike structures. Chromosomes are composed of DNA. In a normal human being there are 46 different chromosomes. The DNA making up each chromosome is divided into hundreds of segments called *genes*. Each segment contains information responsible for directing cytoplasmic activities, controlling growth and development of the cell, and transmitting hereditary information. Thus genes are the basic units of heredity (Fig. 5-7).

Inorganic compounds

Inorganic compounds may be defined as compounds that do *not* contain carbon. The inorganic compounds found in the body occur in nature independent of living things; they are acids (hydrogen-containing compounds that can attack and dissolve metal, e.g., HNO_3, nitric acid), bases (alkali or alkaline earth* OH compounds that can neutralize acids, e.g., $Mg(OH)_2$, otherwise known as milk of magnesia), and salts (chemical compounds that result

---

*See Glossary.

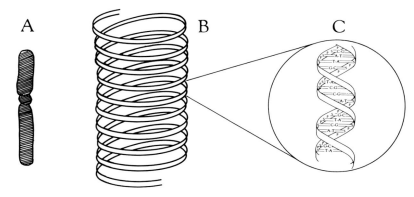

Fig. 5-7   A chromosome viewed under a microscope appears rod-shaped *(A)*; when further magnified, a chromosome appears as a tightly wound spiral structure *(B)* that is composed of hundreds of genes each of which is a segment of the DNA macromolecule *(C)*.

from the action of an acid and a base on each other). Salts are sometimes referred to as *electrolytes*. Water is the major inorganic substance contained in the human body; it comprises approximately 80% of the body's weight. Within the cell, water is indispensable for metabolic activities because it is the medium in which the chemical reactions that are the basis of these activities occur; it also functions as a solvent by dissolving chemical substances within the cell. Outside of the cell water functions as a transport vehicle for materials the cell uses or eliminates. In addition, water acts as the medium in which acids, bases, and salts are dissolved. Once in solution, the concentration of these substances may be regulated. Water is also responsible for maintaining a constant body temperature of 98.6°F (37°C).

Mineral salts exist in smaller quantities to maintain the correct proportion of water in the cell. These salts are also necessary for proper cell function, creation of energy, and conduction of impulses along nerves. Basically, the constituents of salts exist as ions (particles carrying a positive or negative electric charge) in the cell. They cause materials to be altered, broken down, and recombined to form new substances. Potassium (K) constitutes most of the positive ions (cations) present in cells, whereas phosphate (P) constitutes the majority of negative ions (anions). Potassium is of primary importance in maintaining adequate amounts of intracellular fluid. Water tends to move across cell surfaces or "membranes" into areas in which there is a high concentration of ions. This motion is referred to as "osmosis." Thus, by balancing the concentration of the potassium (K) ion (as well as the sodium [Na]

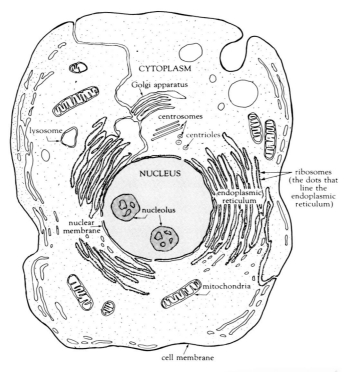

Fig. 5-8   Diagram of a typical cell demonstrating its basic components.
(From Brachet, J., *The living cell,* Sept. 1961, Scientific American, with permission.)

and chloride [Cl] ions), the cell can balance the amount of fluid it contains. Potassium also aids in maintaining acid-base balance (a state of equilibrium or stability between acids and bases).

CELL STRUCTURE
The normal cell (Fig. 5-8) has several components:
  1. cell membrane
  2. cytoplasm
  3. cytoplasmic organelles
      a. endoplasmic reticulum
      b. Golgi apparatus
      c. mitochondria
      d. lysosomes
      e. ribosomes
      f. centrosomes
  4. nucleus

Cell membrane

The cell membrane is a frail structure encasing and surrounding the cell. It functions as a barricade to protect cellular contents from their environment and controls the passage of water and other materials into and out of the cell. Because the cell membrane selects the substances that will penetrate it and regulates the speed at which these substances travel within the cell, it plays an important role in the cell's transport system. When a substance moves through a cell membrane by the process of osmosis, the transport system is classified as passive, because the movement depends more on the concentrations of particles in fluid than it does on the cell membrane. When the movement of a substance across a cell membrane is controlled more by the properties and powers of the cell membrane than it is by the relative concentrations of particles in fluid, the transport system is classified as active. In active transport, the cell must expend energy to pump substances into and out of itself.

Cytoplasm

Cytoplasm is the protoplasm that exists outside of the cell's nucleus. It makes up the majority of the cell and contains large amounts of all the molecular components with the exception of DNA. All metabolic functions in the cell occur in the cytoplasm.

Cytoplasmic organelles

With the exception of DNA, the cytoplasm contains all the miniature components of the cell. These tiny tubules,* vesicles,* granules,* and fibrils* are referred to as *cytoplasmic organelles,* the little organs of the cell. Together, these intercellular structures perform various functions for the cell. DNA determines the function of each cytoplasmic organelle, and RNA carries the instructions into the cytoplasm.

Endoplasmic reticulum

The endoplasmic reticulum (ER) is a vast, irregular network of tubules and vesicles spreading in all directions throughout the cytoplasm. It enables the cell to communicate with the extracellular environment and to transfer food from one part of the cell to another. Thus, the ER functions as the highway system of the cell. For example, messenger RNA travels from the nucleus to the cytoplasm through the endoplasmic reticulum.

Cells have two types of endoplasmic reticulum: rough-surfaced (gran-

---

*See Glossary.

ular) and smooth (agranular). If ribosomes are present on the surface of the endoplasmic reticulum, the surface is rough or granular. If they are not present, the surface is smooth or agranular. This observation can be made when various types of cells are seen through an electron microscope. The cell type appears to determine the type of endoplasmic reticulum. For example, cells that actively manufacture proteins for export, such as the pancreatic cells, which produce insulin, have a lot of rough or granular endoplasmic reticulum. A lesser amount of rough or granular endoplasmic reticulum is found in cells that synthesize proteins mainly for their own use.*

Golgi apparatus

The Golgi apparatus extends from the nucleus to the cell membrane and consists of tubes and tiny sacs located near the nucleus. It unites large carbohydrate molecules and then combines them with proteins to form glycoproteins. Also, when the cell manufactures enzymes and hormones, the Golgi apparatus transports them through the cell membrane so that they can exit the cell and enter the bloodstream and be carried to areas of the body where they are required.

Mitochondria

Large, bean-shaped structures called *mitochondria* function as "powerhouses" of the cell. They contain highly organized enzymes in their inner membrane that produce energy for cellular activity by breaking down nutrients through a process of oxidation. Some of the enzymes combined in the mitochondria are essential in the production of adenosine triphosphate (ATP), a high-energy phosphate compound essential for sustaining life. This compound plays a role in active transport within the cell. In active transport, molecules are moved through cell membranes regardless of the relative concentrations of particles. This requires energy, which is supplied by ATP.

Lysosomes

Lysosomes are small pealike sacs containing digestive enzymes, which break down organic compounds by adding water. Lysosomes are the digestive organs of the cell. They function as "cellular garbage disposals" by disposing of large particles such as bacteria and food stuffs. Lysosomes are sometimes referred to as "suicide bags," because the enzymes they contain can break

---

*For more detail refer to Travis EL: *Primer of medical radiobiology,* ed 2, Chicago, 1989, Yearbook Medical Publishers, p 6.

down and digest not only proteins and certain carbohydrates but also, under certain conditions, the cell itself. Exposure to radiation can cause lysosomes to rupture, in which case the cell dies.

Ribosomes

Ribosomes are small, spherical organelles that attach to the endoplasmic reticulum. They consist of two thirds RNA and one third protein and are essential for cellular function. Ribosomes are commonly referred to as the cell's "protein factories" because their job is to manufacture (synthesize) the various proteins that cells require using the "blueprints" provided by messenger RNA.

Centrosomes

Centrosomes are located in the center of the cell near the nucleus. They contain the centrioles, which are pairs of small, hollow, cylindrical structures believed to play some part in the formation of the mitotic spindle during cell division. Cell division is discussed later in this chapter.

Nucleus

The nucleus forms the heart of the cell. It is a spherical mass of protoplasm containing the genetic material (DNA), which is stored in its molecular structure. The nucleus also contains a rounded body called the nucleolus, which holds a large amount of RNA. The nucleus controls cell division and multiplication and also biochemical reactions that occur within the cell. By directing protein synthesis, the nucleus plays an essential role in active transport, metabolism, growth, and heredity. A summary of cell components may be found in Table 5-1.

CELL DIVISION

Cell division is the multiplication process whereby one cell divides to form two or more cells. Mitosis and meiosis are the two types of cell division that occur in the body. When somatic cells (all cells in the human body except the germ cells) divide, they undergo mitosis. Genetic cells (the oogonium, the female germ cell, and the spermatogonium, the male germ cell) undergo meiosis.

Mitosis

Through the process of mitosis (Fig. 5-9), a parent cell divides to form two daughter cells identical to the parent cell. This process results in an approximately equal distribution of all cellular material between the two daughter

Table 5-1 **Summary of Cell Components**

Title	Site	Activity
Cell membrane	Cytoplasm	Functions as a barricade to protect cellular contents from their environment and controls the passage of water and other materials into and out of the cell
Endoplasmic reticulum	Cytoplasm	Enables the cell to communicate with the extracellular environment and transfers food from one part of the cell to another
Golgi apparatus	Cytoplasm	Unites large carbohydrate molecules and then combines them with proteins to form glycoproteins and also transports enzymes and hormones through the cell membrane so that they can exit the cell and enter the bloodstream and be carried to areas of the body where they are required
Mitochondria	Cytoplasm	Produce energy for cellular activity by breaking down nutrients through a process of oxidation
Lysosomes	Cytoplasm	Dispose of large particles such as bacteria and food and contain enzymes that can break down and digest proteins and certain carbohydrates but also, under certain conditions, the cell itself
Ribosomes	Cytoplasm	Manufacture the various proteins that cells require
Centrosomes	Cytoplasm	Believed to play some part in the formation of the mitotic spindle during cell division
DNA	Nucleus	Contains the genetic material, controls cell division and multiplication and also biochemical reactions that occur within the cell
Nucleolus	Nucleus	Holds a large amount of RNA

cells. The cellular life cycle may be pictured as in Fig. 5-10. Different phases of cell growth, maturation, and division occur in each cell cycle. Four distinct phases of the cellular life cycle are identifiable. They are: M, G_1, S, and G_2. M (mitosis) can be divided into four subphases: prophase, metaphase, anaphase, and telophase.

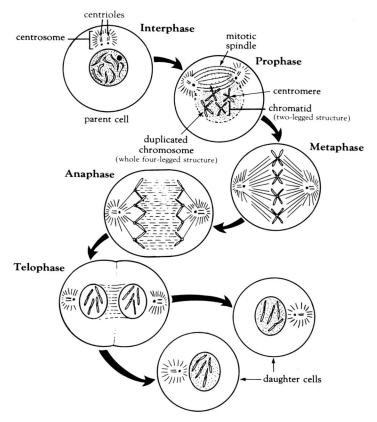

Fig. 5-9   Diagram of mitosis. An animal cell with four chromosomes first multiplies (duplicates its DNA) and then divides forming two new daughter cells each of which contains exactly the same genetic material as the parent cell.

M is the division phase of the cellular life cycle. It is actually the last phase of the cycle. Once it has commenced, it takes only about 1 hour to complete in all cells. Interphase, the period of cell growth that occurs before actual mitosis, consists of three phases: G_1, S, and G_2. G_1, the earliest phase, is the phase between reproductive events. It is the "gap" or interval in the growth of the cell that occurs between mitosis (M) and DNA synthesis (S). Depending on the type of cells involved, this phase may take just a few minutes or it may take several hours. G_1 is designated as the pre-DNA synthesis phase. During G_1, a form of RNA is synthesized in cells that are to reproduce. This RNA is needed before actual DNA synthesis can efficiently begin. S is the actual DNA synthesis phase. While this phase is taking place, each DNA molecule is copied and then divides (replicates) into corresponding

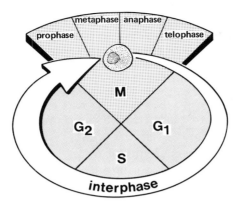

Fig. 5-10   The cellular life cycle may be pictured as four distinct, identifiable phases: M, G_1, S, and G_2. M can be divided into four subphases: prophase, metaphase, anaphase, and telophase.
(From Bushong, S.C., *Radiologic science for technologists: physics, biology and protection, ed 5,* St. Louis: Mosby–Year Book, 1992, p 530; with permission.)

daughter DNA molecules. The chromosome changes in shape from a figure with two chromatids (highly coiled duplicate strands of DNA) connected to a centromere (region on a chromosome serving as a junction point) to a figure with four chromatids connected to a centromere (Fig. 5-11). Two pairs of chromatids having exactly the same DNA substance and form result. When compared to phases G_1 and G_2, the S phase is relatively long. It takes a maximum of 15 hours. G_2 is the post-DNA manufacturing interval in the cellular life cycle. It is a relatively short period occupying approximately 1 to

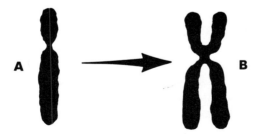

Fig. 5-11   While the S phase is taking place, chromosomes change in shape from a figure with two chromatids connected to a centromere to a figure with four chromatids connected to a centromere. *A,* Two-chromatid figure. *B,* Four-chromatid figure.
(From Bushong, S.C., *Radiologic science for technologists: physics, biology and protection, ed 5,* St. Louis: Mosby–Year Book, 1992, p. 530; with permission.)

5 hours of the whole cycle. During this phase, cells manufacture certain proteins and RNA molecules needed to enter and complete the next mitosis. When G_2 is complete, cells enter the first phase of mitosis, the prophase, and the process of division commences.

Interphase

Interphase is the period of cell growth that occurs before actual mitosis. As previously stated, G_1, S, and G_2 are the phases of the cell cycle that compose interphase. Cells are not yet undergoing division during this phase. If a cell is viewed through a microscope during interphase, the nucleus looks somewhat odd. DNA can be demonstrated by using a specific stain designed to make it visible; it appears as clumps of material shaped in different patterns. These patterns are seen throughout the nucleus. Individual chromosomes are not visible during interphase. During the synthesis portion of interphase (S), each chromosome reproduces itself and splits longitudinally forming two chromatids attached to each other at the centromere. Hence, the cell's DNA molecules have duplicated in preparation for cell division. Genetic information is also transcribed into different kinds of RNA molecules, such as messenger and transfer, which, after passing into the cytoplasm, will translate the genetic information by promoting the synthesis of specific proteins.

Prophase

During prophase, the nucleus enlarges and the DNA complex (the chromatid network of threads) coils up more tightly and the chromatids become more visible on stained microscopic slides. Chromosomes enlarge, and the DNA begins to take structural form. The nuclear membrane disappears, and the centrioles (small hollow cylindrical structures) migrate to opposite sides of the cell and begin to regulate the formation of the mitotic spindle, the delicate fibers of which are attached to the centrioles and extend from one side of the cell to the other.

Metaphase

As this phase begins, the fibers collectively referred to as the mitotic spindle form between the organelles called centrioles. Each chromosome (which now consists of two chromatids) lines up in the center of the cell attached by its centromere to the mitotic spindle. This forms the equatorial plate. The centromeres then duplicate, and each chromatid attaches itself individually to the spindle. At the end of metaphase, the chromatids are strung out along the mitotic spindle much like laundry hung out on a clothesline. It is during metaphase that cell division can be stopped and chromosomes can be examined under a microscope. Chromosome damage caused by radiation can then be evaluated.

Anaphase

During anaphase, the duplicate centromeres migrate in opposite directions along the mitotic spindle carrying the chromatids to opposite sides of the cell.

Telophase

During telophase, the chromatids undergo changes in appearance by uncoiling and becoming long, loosely-spiraled threads. They are now referred to as new, complete chromosomes. Simultaneously, the nuclear membrane reforms and two nuclei (one for each new daughter cell) appear. The cytoplasm also divides near the equator of the cell to surround each new nucleus. With the completion of this cell division, each daughter cell contains exactly the same genetic material (46 chromosomes) as the parent cell.

Meiosis

Meiosis (Fig. 5-12) is a special type of cell division that reduces the number of chromosomes in each daughter cell to half the number of chromosomes in the parent cell. Male and female germ cells, sperm and ova, each begin meiosis with 46 chromosomes. However, before the male and female germ cells unite to produce a new organism, the number of chromosomes in each must be reduced by one half to ensure that the daughter cells ("zygotes") formed when they unite will contain only the normal number of 46 chromosomes. Hence, meiosis is really a process of reduction division (Fig. 5-13).

Paradoxically, meiosis begins with a doubling of the amount of genetic material; as in mitosis, DNA replication occurs during interphase. As a result of DNA replication, each one-chromatid chromosome duplicates, forming a two-chromatid chromosome. This means that sperm and egg cells begin meiosis with twice the amount of genetic material as the original parent germ cell. Thus, at the beginning of meiosis, the number of chromosomes increases from $2n$ to $4n$ [$n = 23$].

The various phases of meiosis are similar to those occurring in mitosis. The major difference between the two types of cell division begins at the end of the telophase. In meiosis, after the parent germ cell has formed two daughter cells, each of which (in humans) contains 46 chromosomes, the daughter cells divide but without DNA replication; chromosome duplication

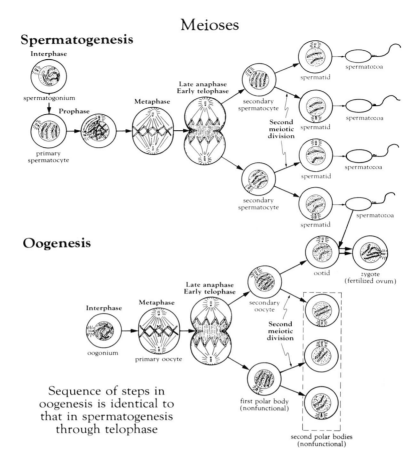

Fig. 5-12 Diagram of meiosis. Four cells result from one germ cell. In spermatogenesis, four spermatids become mature spermatozoa. In oogenesis, one ootid can be fertilized, while three second polar bodies remain nonfunctional.

does not occur at this phase of the division. These two successive divisions result in the formation of four granddaughter cells each of which contains only 23 chromosomes. This means that the proper number of 46 chromosomes will be produced when a female ovum containing 23 chromosomes is fertilized by a male sperm containing 23 chromosomes.

During meiosis, the sister chromatids exchange some chromosomal material (genes). This process, called crossing-over, results in changes in genetic composition and traits that can be passed on to future generations.

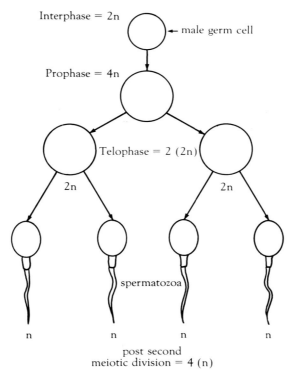

Interphase = 2n

male germ cell

Prophase = 4n

Telophase = 2 (2n)

2n

2n

spermatozoa

n   n   n   n

post second
meiotic division = 4 (n)

Fig. 5-13 Meiosis as a process of reduction division. If we use the letter n to represent the number of chromosomes in a germ cell that is capable of uniting with another germ cell to produce a new organism, then $n = 23$ for a human. Before meiosis the germ cell contains $2n$, or 46, chromosomes.

SUMMARY

In this chapter the fundamentals of cell biology were reviewed. The reader should be able to discuss cell structure, composition, and function and also be prepared to learn how these can be affected adversely by the organism's being exposed to ionizing radiation.

REVIEW QUESTIONS

1. In a DNA macromolecule, the sequence of _____ determines the characteristics of every living thing.
   a. sugars
   b. phosphates
   c. nitrogenous bases
   d. hydrogen bonds

2. Where does protein synthesis occur in the human cell?
   a. in the nucleus
   b. in the mitochondria
   c. in the ribosomes
   d. in the endoplasmic reticulum

3. DNA regulates cellular activity indirectly by reproducing itself in the form of _____ to carry genetic information from the cell nucleus to ribosomes located in the cytoplasm.
   a. messenger DNA
   b. messenger RNA
   c. messenger REM
   d. transfer RNA

4. Which of the following is a process of reduction cell division?
   a. mitosis
   b. meiosis
   c. molecular synthesis
   d. amniocentesis

5. Human cells contain four major organic compounds:
   a. nucleic acids, water, protein, and mineral salts
   b. mineral salts, carbohydrates, lipids, and proteins
   c. carbohydrates, lipids, nucleic acids, and water
   d. proteins, carbohydrates, lipids, and nucleic acids

6. Interphase consists of:
   a. M, G_1, and S
   b. G_1, S, and G_2
   c. S, G_2, and M
   d. G_2, M, and G

7. Radiation-induced chromosome damage can be evaluated during:
   a. prophase
   b. metaphase
   c. anaphase
   d. telophase

8. Which human cell component controls cell division and multiplication and also biochemical reactions that occur within the cell?
   a. endoplasmic reticulum
   b. mitochondria
   c. lysosomes
   d. nucleus

9. Antibodies are produced by the:
    a. erythrocytes
    b. lymphocytes
    c. thrombocytes
    d. platelets

10. Carbohydrates may also be referred to as:
    a. lipids
    b. nucleic acids
    c. hormones
    d. saccharides

Bibliography

Anthony CP: *The textbook of anatomy and physiology,* ed 6, St Louis, 1963, Mosby—Year Book.

Anthony CP, Thibodeau GA: *Textbook of anatomy and physiology,* ed 13, St Louis, 1989, Mosby—Year Book.

Boyd W: *A textbook of pathology structure and function in disease,* ed 8, Philadelphia, 1970, Lea & Febiger.

Burke SR: *Human anatomy and physiology for the health sciences,* New York, 1980, John Wiley & Sons.

Bushong S: *Radiologic science for technologists: physics, biology, and protection,* ed 2, St Louis, 1980, Mosby—Year Book.

Bushong SC: *Radiologic science for technologists: physics, biology and protection,* ed 5, St Louis, 1993, Mosby—Year Book.

Casarett AP: *Radiation biology,* Englewood Clifts, NJ, 1968, Prentice-Hall.

Chabner DE: *The language of medicine,* Philadelphia, 1976, WB Saunders.

Crouch JE: *Functional human anatomy,* ed 4, Philadelphia, 1985, Lea & Febiger.

Crouch JE, McClintic JR: *Human anatomy and physiology,* ed 2, New York, 1976, John Wiley & Sons.

DeRobertis EDP, DeRobertis EMF: *Cell and molecular biology,* ed 8, Philadelphia, 1987, Lea & Febiger.

Frankel R: *Radiation protection for radiologic technologists,* New York, 1976, McGraw-Hill.

Hegner B: *Pathophysiology,* Long Beach, CA, 1980, Elot.

Jacob SW, Francone CA, Lossow WJ: *Structure and function in man,* ed 4, Philadelphia, 1978, WB Saunders.

Mallett M: *A handbook of anatomy and physiology for students of medical radiation technology,* ed 3, Mankato, MN, 1979, Burnell.

Memmler RL, Wood DL: *The human body in health and disease,* ed 4, Philadelphia, 1977, JB Lippincott.

Memmler RL, Wood DL: *Structure and function of the human body,* ed 2, Philadelphia, 1977, JB Lippincott.

Nourse AE and the Editors of Time-Life Books: *The body,* Life Science Library, New York, 1968, Time-Life Books.

Pfeiffer J and the Editors of Time-Life Books: *The cell,* Life Science Library, New York, 1964, Time-Life Books.

Ritenour ER: *Radiation protection and biology: a self-instructional multi-media learning series,* Denver, 1985, Multi-Media Publishing.

Selman J: *Elements of radiobiology,* Springfield, IL, 1983, Charles C Thomas.

Thomas CL, editor: *Taber's cyclopedic medical dictionary,* ed 13, Philadelphia, 1977, FA Davis.

Travis EL: *Primer of medical radiobiology,* ed 2, Chicago, 1989, Mosby—Year Book.

6

Radiation Biology

OBJECTIVES

Upon completion of this chapter, the reader will be able to:

- define *radiation biology* and explain its relevance to radiation protection
- describe how ionizing radiation produces damage in living systems
- explain how linear energy transfer affects the amount of biological damage produced in living matter by ionizing radiation
- explain the concept of relative biological effectiveness
- differentiate between the three levels of biological damage that can occur in living systems as a result of exposure to ionizing radiation
- describe the direct and indirect effects of ionizing radiation upon the molecular structure of living systems
- explain the target theory
- describe the effects of ionizing radiation upon the cell
- state and describe the law of Bergonié and Tribondeau
- describe the effects of ionizing radiation upon various types of cells
- explain the significance of organic damage resulting from exposure of living systems to ionizing radiation
- draw diagrams demonstrating the various radiation dose-response relationships
- identify the factors upon which somatic and genetic damage depend
- list and describe the various early somatic effects of ionizing radiation upon living systems
- recall the LD 50/30 for human adults and explain its significance

- identify and describe the various late somatic effects of ionizing radiation upon living systems
- discuss the concept of radiation-induced genetic effects
- give examples of both stochastic and nonstochastic effects
- describe the concept of risk for radiation-induced malignancies
- give historical examples of late somatic effects of ionizing radiation and discuss each example
- discuss the somatic and genetic effects associated with low-level ionizing radiation

Radiation biology is defined as the branch of biology concerned with the effects of ionizing radiations on living systems. Areas of study included in this science are the sequence of events occurring after the absorption of energy from ionizing radiation, the action of the living system to make up for the consequences of this energy assimilation, and the injury to the living system that may be produced.

The human body is a living system composed of large numbers of various types of cells most of which can be damaged by radiation. Because the potential harmful effects of ionizing radiation on living systems occur primarily on the cellular level, those who administer ionizing radiation to humans for medical purposes should possess a basic understanding of cell structure, composition, and function, and the adverse effects on these by ionizing radiation. This chapter provides the reader with a basic knowledge of aspects of radiation biology relevant to the subject of radiation protection.

IONIZING RADIATION

Ionizing radiation produces damage in living systems by ionizing (removing electrons from) the atoms composing the molecular structures of these systems. X-ray and gamma-ray photons can impart energy to orbital electrons in atoms if the photons happen to pass near to the electrons. High-energy charged particles such as alpha and beta particles and protons can also ionize atoms by interacting electromagnetically with orbital electrons. For example, the alpha particle* with a charge of plus two strongly attracts the negative electron as it passes by.

Biological damage, then, begins with the ionizations produced by vari-

---

*A positively charged particle composed of two protons and two neutrons.

ous types of radiation. An ionized atom will *not* bond properly into the molecules necessary for the normal functioning of an organism.

LINEAR ENERGY TRANSFER (LET) AND ITS RELATIONSHIP TO BIOLOGICAL DAMAGE

When ionizing radiation passes through a medium, it interacts with the medium and, as a result, deposits energy along its path. The average energy deposited per unit path length is called *linear energy transfer* (LET). LET is generally described in units of kiloelectron volts (keV) per micron (1 micron (μm) $= 10^{-6}$ m). Because the amount of ionization produced in an irradiated object is related to how much energy it absorbs and because both chemical and biological effects in tissue coincide with the degree of ionization experienced by the tissue, it can be seen that LET is an important concept in assessing potential tissue and/or organ damage from exposure to ionizing radiation.

Although LET is a function of both mass and charge, the concept of LET is equally applied to both indirectly and directly ionizing radiation. The first category includes electromagnetic radiation (x-rays and gamma rays, which have neither mass nor charge) and neutrons, which also have no electrical charge. X-rays and gamma rays* generate fast electrons, which act as directly ionizing radiation. However, x-rays and gamma rays are considered to be a low-LET radiation.

Unlike electromagnetic radiations, particulate radiations possessing substantial mass and/or charge, such as alpha particles, ions of heavier nuclei, and charged particles released from interactions between neutrons and nuclei, have a far greater chance of interacting with tissue. These kinds of radiation lose energy quickly in the process, rendering countless ionizations across a small space. Such particulate radiations, therefore, are considered to be high-LET radiations.

X-rays and gamma rays produce fewer ionizations in each small space than are produced by charged particles. Even though the electrons set in motion by the x-rays and gamma rays produce more interactions, the x-rays and gamma rays themselves are considered low-LET radiations.

When large amounts of energy from ionizing radiations are transferred to atoms and molecules composing human tissue, the molecular structure of that tissue is disrupted. If the affected molecules are of vital importance for maintaining a normal level of cellular function, the irradiated cells may suffer

---

*Short wavelength, high-energy electromagnetic wave emitted by the nuclei of radioactive substances.

serious injury. If this injury is in excess of that which can be reversed by the cell's repair enzymes, the cell may suffer a loss of function, may function abnormally, or may die.

RELATIVE BIOLOGICAL EFFECTIVENESS

Biological damage produced by radiation escalates as the LET of radiation increases. Consequently, different LET radiations produce different degrees of the same biologic reaction so that identical doses of radiations of various LETs do not render the same biologic effect. The relative biologic effect (RBE) describes the relative capability of radiations with various LETs to produce a particular biologic reaction. It may be defined as the dose of a reference radiation quality,* stated in Gray,† that is necessary to produce the same biologic reaction in a given experiment that is produced by a dose of the test radiation, also stated in Gray. The determination of RBE values for the various types of radiation has been undertaken by many laboratories, and their efforts with this extremely difficult task continue. The RBE for neutrons,‡ in particular, has presented a special challenge.

Because different types of radiation differ in their biological effectiveness per unit quantity of absorbed dose, this concept of RBE is not practical for specifying radiation protection dose levels. To overcome this limitation, the quality factor (QF) or modifying factor has been used in the calculation of the absorbed dose equivalent to determine the ability of a dose of any kind of ionizing radiation to cause biological damage. Quality factors are basically a measure of RBE. Typically, they have been selected in a conscientious fashion on the basis of measured values of the RBE of the radiation in question for a variety of biological effects at low doses. In general, a large QF is associated with a large value of RBE. Quality factors for different types of ionizing radiations are listed in Table 3-1 of this text.

MOLECULAR EFFECTS OF IRRADIATION

In living systems, biological damage resulting from exposure to ionizing radiation can be observed on three levels: molecular, cellular, and organic. Any *visible* radiation-induced injuries to living systems at the cellular or organic level *always* begin with damage at the molecular level. Molecular damage re-

---

*Conventionally, this has been chosen to be 250 kVp x-rays.
†SI unit of absorbed dose equal to one joule of energy absorbed from any type of ionizing radiation in one kilogram of any irradiated object.
‡See Glossary.

sults in the formation of structurally changed molecules that can impair cellular functioning.

Cells of the human body are highly specialized, with each cell having a predetermined task to perform; each cell's function is determined and defined by the structures of its constituent molecules. Since exposure to ionizing radiation can alter the structures of the cell's constituent molecules, such exposure can disturb the cell's chemical balance and hence its functioning. When this occurs, the cell no longer performs its tasks. If a sufficient quantity of somatic cells ("soma" is the Greek word for "body"; hence, "somatic cells" refers to all cells in the body except the female and male germ cells) are affected, body processes may be disrupted. If radiation damages the germ (reproductive) cells, the damage may be passed on to future generations in the form of genetic mutations (changes in the genes). (More information pertaining to somatic and genetic effects are presented later in this chapter.)

When ionizing radiation interacts with a cell, ionizations and excitations (the addition of energy to a molecular system transforming it from a calm to an excited state) are produced in either vital biologic macromolecules (such as DNA) or water (H_2O), the medium in which the cellular organelles are suspended. Based on the site of the interaction, the action of radiation on the cell is classified as either direct or indirect.

The direct effect can result after exposure with any type of radiation. However, it is more likely to happen after exposure to high-LET radiations, such as alpha particles, which, in a very short distance of travel, produce countless ionizations, rather than after exposure to low-LET radiations, such as x-rays, which are sparsely ionizing.

Direct effect

When ionizing particles interact directly with (transfer their energy to) vital biologic macromolecules such as DNA, RNA, proteins, or enzymes, damage occurs as a result of what is called *direct action*. The ionization or excitation of the atoms of these macromolecules results in breakage of the macromolecules' chemical bonds, causing them to become abnormal structures, which may, in turn, lead to inappropriate chemical reactions. When enzyme molecules are damaged as a result of destructive interaction with ionizing particles, essential biochemical reactions may not occur in the cell at the appropriate time. This interferes with normal cell functioning. If an enzyme is inactivated by radiation, it will fail to bring about its proper biochemical reaction. If this reaction is involved in the synthesis of a particular protein, the protein will not be manufactured, and, if this protein was intended to perform a specific function, its nonexistence hinders that function. In the event that other functions depend on the suppressed function, these functions sustain some type of damage as well.

If ionizing particles interact directly with a DNA macromolecule, the subsequent ionization of that critical macromolecule can break one of its chemical bonds, thereby severing one of the sugar-phosphate chain side-rails or strands of the DNA ladder-like molecular structure (Fig. 6-1). Repair enzymes can reverse this damage.

Further exposure of the affected DNA macromolecule to ionizing radiation can result in additional breaks in the sugar-phosphate molecular chain(s). These breaks can also be repaired, but double-strand breaks (one or more breaks in each of the two sugar-phosphate chains) (Fig. 6-2) are not repaired as easily as single-strand breaks. If repair does not take place, further separation can occur in the DNA chains, threatening the life of the cell.

When two direct interactions (hits), one on each of the two sugar-phosphate chains, occur within the same rung of the DNA ladder-like configuration (Fig. 6-3, A), complete chromosome breakage occurs. This results in the formation of a cleaved or broken chromosome (Fig. 6-3, B), with each new portion containing an unequal amount of genetic material. If this damaged chromosome divides, each new daughter cell will receive an incorrect

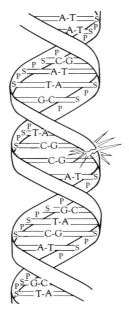

Fig. 6-1   Single-strand break in ladder-like DNA structure.

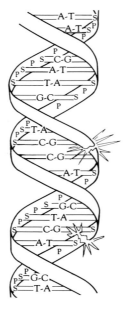

Fig. 6-2   A widely-spaced double-strand break in the ladder-like DNA structure.

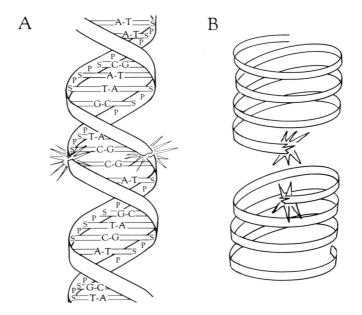

Fig. 6-3   Double-strand break in same rung of DNA ladder-like structure *(A)* causes complete chromosome breakage, resulting in a cleaved or broken chromosome *(B)*.

amount of genetic material. This will result in the death or impaired functioning of the new daughter cells.

When high-energy radiation interacts directly with a DNA molecule, it can damage that molecule by causing a loss or change of a nitrogenous base on the DNA chain. The consequence of this damage is an alteration of the base sequence (Fig. 6-4). The genetic information to be passed on to future generations is contained in the sequence of these bases and, therefore, the loss or change of a base in the DNA chain is called a *mutation*. It may not be reversible and can have acute consequences to the cell. More important, though, if the cell remains viable, incorrect genetic information will be transferred to one of the two daughter cells when the cell divides.

Covalent (chemical union created between atoms sharing one or more pairs of electrons) crosslinks involving DNA can also be produced by high-energy radiation.* A crosslink can be constructed between two places on the same DNA strand. This joining is termed an *intrastrand* crosslink. Crosslinking can also occur between complementary DNA strands (Fig. 6-5) or between entirely different DNA molecules. These joinings are termed *interstrand* crosslinks. DNA molecules can also become covalently linked to a protein molecule.† These linkages may be of considerable concern if they are not properly repaired by the cell.

Radiolysis of water (interaction of radiation with H₂O)

X-ray photons can interact with and ionize (remove electrons from) water molecules contained within the human body. Such an interaction between an x-ray photon and a water molecule creates an ion pair consisting of a wa-

---

*At low energies, covalent crosslinks are most probably caused by indirect action. Indirect action will be discussed subsequently.
†From Travis EL: *Primer of medical radiobiology,* ed 2, St. Louis, 1989, Mosby–Year Book, p 35.

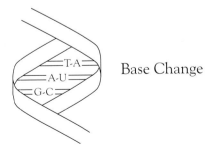

Base Change

Fig. 6-4 Alternation of the nitrogen base sequence on the DNA chain caused by the interaction of high energy radiation impacting directly upon a DNA molecule.

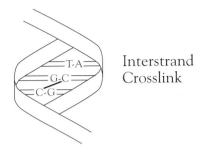

Fig. 6-5   Interstrand covalent crosslink produced by high energy radiating interacting directly upon a DNA molecule.

ter molecule with a positive charge (HOH^+) and an electron (e^-). Both of these components are unstable.

After the original ionization of the water molecule, several reactions can occur. First, the positively charged water molecule (HOH^+) can recombine with the electron (e^-) to reform a stable water molecule ($HOH^+ + e^- = H_2O$). If this happens, no damage occurs. Second, if the two components of the ion pair do not rejoin, the electron (the negative ion) can join with another water molecule and create an unstable water molecule with a negative charge ($H_2O + e^- = HOH^-$).

The positive water molecule (HOH^+) and the negative water molecule (HOH^-) are basically unstable. Hence, they can break apart into smaller molecules. HOH^+ becomes a hydrogen ion (H^+) and a hydroxyl radical ($OH*$), while HOH^- becomes a hydroxyl ion (OH^-) and a hydrogen radical ($H*$). The "*" implies a "free radical." A free radical has no electrical charge but quickly reacts with other molecules because it has an unpaired electron in the valence or outermost electron shell symbolized by the "*". Hence, the final result of the interaction of radiation with water is the formation of an ion pair, H^+ and OH^- (hydrogen ion and hydroxyl ion), and two free radicals, $H*$ and $OH*$ (a hydrogen radical and a hydroxyl radical; Fig. 6-6).

Since the hydrogen and hydroxyl ions can recombine to form a normal water molecule, they may not cause any biological damage; hence, the existence of these ions as free agents within the human body is insignificant in terms of biological damage. The presence of the hydrogen and hydroxyl free radicals, however, is *most significant*. As free radicals (molecules containing an unpaired electron), they are very reactive. They can produce undesirable chemical reactions within the human body and cause biological damage by transferring their excess energy to other molecules, thereby destroying these

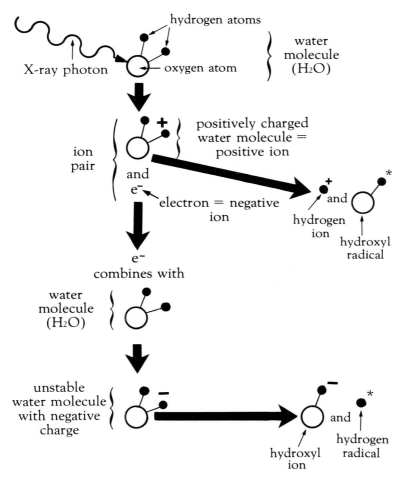

Fig. 6-6 Radiolysis of water. The final result of the interaction of radiation with water is the formation of an ion pair (H^+ and OH^-) and two free radicals (H^* and OH^*).

other molecules' chemical bonds and creating point or molecular lesions (injured areas in molecules caused by the breaking of a single chemical bond) in the molecules.

In addition, since free radicals have excess energy and can travel through the cell, they are capable of interacting with and creating point lesions in other molecules located at some distance from their place of origin.

Hydrogen and hydroxyl radicals are not the only destructive substances that can be produced during the radiolysis of water. A hydroxyl radical

(OH*) can bond with another hydroxyl radical (OH*) and form hydrogen peroxide (OH* + OH* = H_2O_2), a substance that is poisonous to the cell. In addition, a hydroperoxyl radical (HO_2*) is formed when a hydrogen free radical (H*) combines with molecular oxygen (O_2). This radical and hydrogen peroxide are believed to be the main substances that produce biological damage after the interaction of radiation with water.

Absorption of radiation can also cause an organic molecule (RH) to form the free radicals, R*† and H*. Without oxygen or a force to attract an electron, these radicals can react with one another to reform the organic molecule (RH). When oxygen is present, R* and H* may react with the oxygen to form the radicals RO_2* and HO_2*. Hence, the organic molecule (RH) is destroyed. Moreover, the radicals, RO_2* and HO_2* can react with other organic molecules to cause biological damage.

Indirect effect

Destructive chemical changes in body molecules can result from what is called *indirect action of ionizing radiation*. When a vital molecule such as DNA is acted upon by free radicals previously produced by the interaction of radiation with water molecules, the destructive action of the ionizing radiation on the vital biologic macromolecule is "indirect" in the sense that the radiation is *not* the immediate cause of the damage to the critical biologic macromolecule. The free radicals are the immediate cause of this damage. The human body contains an abundance of water molecules (water constitutes approximately 80% of the body's total weight), so more destructive chemical change results from indirect than from direct action of ionizing radiation. Approximately 95% of the effects of x- and gamma radiation in macromolecules of living systems (in vivo) occur as a result of indirect action.

During the process of indirect action (Fig. 6-7), after the water molecule has been excited and ionized by absorbing radiation energy, the molecule breaks down into smaller molecules and produces ions and free radicals. As explained previously, the ions formed are insignificant because they can recombine to reform water and will produce no biological damage. The free radicals produced, however, can recombine to form hydrogen peroxide, a cellular poison, and a hydroperoxyl radical, another toxic substance. Since these toxic agents are highly reactive and can oxidize (remove one or more electrons from) other molecules, they are capable of producing biological damage. Free radicals can also transfer their excess

---

†Organic neutral free radical.

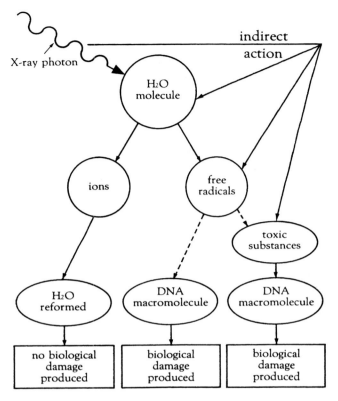

Fig. 6-7 Diagram of indirect action resulting in indirect effect of ionizing radiation on biologic molecules. X-ray photon interacts directly with a water (H_2O) molecule and ionizes it. The H_2O molecule breaks down into ions and free radicals. The ions can recombine to form a water molecule, thereby creating no biological damage. The free radicals can migrate to another molecule, such as a DNA molecule, located at some distance from the site of the initial ionization and interact with, ionize, destroy the chemical bonds of and thereby create molecular or point lesions in the DNA macromolecule. Free radicals can create further biological damage by combining with other molecules to form toxic substances which can also migrate to distant DNA molecules and destructively interact.

energy to other molecules thereby destroying their chemical bonds. This results in molecular or point lesions, which can cause the molecules to malfunction in the cell. When free radicals migrate to and interact with DNA, they transfer their energy to these critical macromolecules, which results in a partial destruction of the macromolecule and also in the destruction of the genes it contains.

Target theory

In addition to a variety of different types of molecules that exist in large numbers in the cell, each cell is believed to contain a sensitive master or key molecule, which maintains normal cell function. This master molecule is necessary for survival of the cell. Since there is only one master molecule in any one cell and no other similar molecules available to replace it and perform its functions, if the master molecule is inactivated by exposure to radiation, the cell will die (Fig. 6-8). Experimental data strongly support this concept and indicate that DNA is the irreplaceable master or key molecule that serves as the vital target.

Destruction of some of the molecules that are plentiful in the cell does not result in cell death after irradiation. The reason is simply that

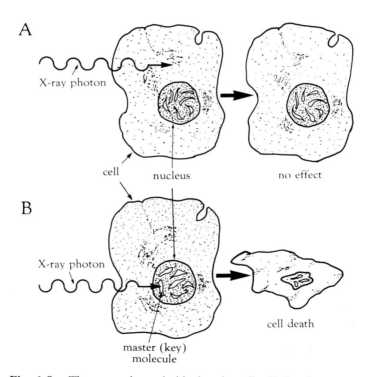

Fig. 6-8   The target theory holds that the cell will die after exposure to ionizing radiation only if the master or key molecule (DNA) is inactivated in the process. In *(A)*, the x-ray photon passes through the cell without interacting with the master molecule (DNA), which is located in the cell nucleus; no measurable effect results. In *(B)*, the x-ray photon enters the nucleus and interacts with and inactivates the master molecule; as a result, the cell dies.

many of the plentiful molecules have other similar molecules to take over and perform necessary functions for them in the event of their demise. Hence, if only a few non-DNA cell molecules are destroyed by radiation exposure, the cell will most likely not show any evidence of injury after irradiation.

In its passage through the molecular structures of living systems, radiation does *not* seek out master molecules in cells to destroy them; it interacts with these key molecules *by chance* in a *random* fashion. The reason why the cell is so sensitive to inactivation of its master molecule by radiation is that this molecule plays an essential part in directing the life support mechanisms of the cell.

The target theory can be used to explain cell death as well as nonfatal cell abnormalities caused by radiation exposure.

Interactions between ionizing radiation and molecular targets (master molecules) such as DNA occur through both the direct and the indirect effect. It is virtually impossible, however, to determine which of the two types of effects or actions has been at work in any given case of cell death.

CELLULAR EFFECTS OF IRRADIATION

Ionizing radiation can affect the cell adversely. Damage to the cell's nucleus reveals itself in one of the following ways:
1. Instant death
2. Reproductive death
3. Interphase death
4. Mitotic or genetic death
5. Mitotic delay
6. Interference of function
7. Chromosome breakage

Instant death

Instant death of large numbers of cells occur when a volume is irradiated with an x-ray or gamma ray dose of about 1000 Gy (100,000 rad) in a period of seconds or a few minutes. This large influx of energy causes gross disruption of cellular form and structure and severe changes in chemical machinery. As a result of receiving such a massive dose of ionizing radiation, a cell's DNA macromolecule breaks up and cellular proteins rapidly coagulate. Radiation doses high enough to cause this type of damage are vastly greater than those used for diagnostic examinations.

Reproductive death

Reproductive death on average results from exposure of cells to moderate doses of ionizing radiation (1 to 10 Gy or 100 to 1000 rad). Although the cell does not die when reproductive death occurs, it *permanently* loses its ability to procreate. Even though the cell has lost its reproductive capacity, it continues to live and metabolize and synthesize nucleic acids and proteins.

Interphase death

Interphase death occurs when a cell that has been irradiated dies without attempting division; hence the term *interphase death*. Two synonymous terms are *nonmitotic* or *nondivision death*. Radiosensitivity of the individual cell governs the dose required to cause interphase death; the more radiosensitive the cell, the smaller the dose required to cause death during interphase. A few hundred centigray (rad) can kill very sensitive cells such as lymphocytes or spermatogonia. Interphase death of less radiosensitive cells, such as those in bone, may on average require radiation doses of several thousand centigray (rad).

Mitotic or genetic death

Ionizing radiation can affect cell division adversely. It can retard the mitotic process or permanently inhibit it; cell death can occur after permanent inhibition. Mitotic or genetic death occurs when a cell dies after one or more divisions. Even small doses of radiation can cause this type of cell death. The radiation dose required to produce mitotic death is less than the dose needed to produce interphase death in slowly dividing cells or in nondividing cells.

Mitotic delay

Exposing a cell to as little as 0.01 Gy (1 rad) of ionizing radiation just before it begins dividing can cause mitotic delay, the failure of the cell to start dividing on time. After this delay, all else being equal, the cell resumes its normal mitotic function.

Interference of function

Permanent or temporary interference of cellular function independent of the cell's ability to divide can occur as a result of exposure to ionizing radiation. If repair enzymes can fix the damage, the cell can recover and continue to function.

Chromosome breakage

Chromosome breakage occurs when ionizing radiation interacts directly with a DNA macromolecule. These breaks can occur in either one or both strands (sugar-phosphate chains) of the DNA ladder-like structure and have been discussed previously (see "Direct effect").

If cells are irradiated during mitosis and chromosome breakage occurs, permanent chromosome abnormalities will be evident in future mitotic cycles. Since chromosome breakage results in a loss of genetic material, this can lead to genetic mutations in succeeding generations.

CELL RADIOSENSITIVITY

The human body is composed of different types of cells and tissues, which vary in their degree of radiosensitivity. Immature cells are nonspecialized (undifferentiated) and undergo rapid cell division, whereas more mature cells are specialized in their function (highly differentiated) and divide at a slower rate or else they do not divide. These factors affect the cell's degree of radiosensitivity. Since both immature and mature cells in various ratios form the various body tissues and organs, radiosensitivity varies from one tissue and organ to another.

When ionizing radiation interacts with cell atoms and molecules, the amount of radiation energy transferred (absorbed in the tissue) determines the biological response. As LET increases (as the radiation transfers more energy per unit length of travel), the ability of the radiation to cause biological effects also increases until it reaches a maximum value. Hence, LET affects cell radiosensitivity.

Oxygen enhances the effects of ionizing radiation on biologic tissue by increasing tissue radiosensitivity. If oxygen is present when a tissue is irradiated, more free radicals (which possess the ability to attack and damage organic molecules) are formed in the tissue; this increases the indirect damage potential of the radiation.

During diagnostic radiologic procedures, fully oxygenated human tissues are exposed to x-radiation. However, diagnostic radiologic and nuclear medicine procedures employ low doses of radiations (x-rays and/or gamma rays), which are also low in LET. Hence, very few cells are killed by the radiations used in these procedures.

The presence of oxygen becomes significant (in terms of radiosensitivity) in radiotherapy. When radiation is used to treat certain types of cancerous tumors, high-pressure (hyperbaric) oxygen has sometimes been used in conjunction with it to increase tumor radiosensitivity. Cancerous tumors can contain hypoxic cells (cells that lack an adequate amount of oxygen) in addition to normally aerated cells. These hypoxic cells severely inhibit the "indirect" mechanism of radiation interaction with cells and therefore are radioresistant (particularly to low LET radiations); hence, they are more difficult to destroy than normally oxygenated cells. When oxygen tensions in capillaries are increased by hyperbaric oxygenation, hypoxic cells may reoxygenate and become sensitive to radiation and consequently their chances of being destroyed by therapeutic radiation increase. Radiosensitization can also be accomplished with chemical enhancing agents such as misonidazole.*

Law of Bergonié and Tribondeau

In 1906, two scientists, J. Bergonié and L. Tribondeau, established a law that states: "the radiosensitivity of cells is directly proportional to their reproductive activity and inversely proportional to their degree of differentiation." This means that the *greatest* radiation effects occur in cells having the *least* maturity and specialization or differentiation, the *most* reproductive activity, and the *longest* mitotic phases. This law applies for *all* types of cells in the human body. Within the realm of diagnostic radiology, this law indicates that the embryo and the fetus, which contain a large number of immature, nonspecialized cells, are *more* susceptible to radiation damage than is the child or the adult. The law also indicates which cells in the adult are most and which cells are least radiosensitive.

Effects of ionizing radiation on various types of cells

Equal doses of ionizing radiation produce different degrees of damage in different kinds of human cells because of differences in radiosensitivity between different kinds of cells. The more mature and specialized in performing specific functions a cell is, the less sensitive it is to radiation.

Blood cells

Ionizing radiation adversely affects blood cells by depressing the number of cells in the peripheral circulation. A whole-body dose of 0.25 Gy (25 rad) produces a measurable hematologic depression. Most blood cells are manufactured in bone marrow. Radiation causes a decrease in the number of immature blood cells (stem or precursor blood cells) produced there and hence a reduction, ultimately, of the number of mature blood cells in the bloodstream. The *higher* the radiation dose received by the bone marrow, the *greater* the severity of the resulting cell depletion.

   If the bone marrow cells have not been destroyed by exposure to ionizing radiation, they can repopulate after a period of recovery. The amount of time necessary for recovery depends on the severity of the radiation dose received. If a low dose (below 1 Gy or 100 rad) of radiation was received, bone marrow repopulation occurs within a few weeks after irradiation. Moderate (1 to 10 Gy or 100 to 1000 rad) to high (10 or more gray or 1000 or

*Hall EJ: *Radiobiology for the radiologist,* ed 3, Philadelphia, 1988, JB Lippincott, p 182.

more rad) doses, which severely deplete the number of bone marrow cells, require a longer recovery period. Very high doses of radiation can cause a permanent decrease in the number of stem cells.

All stem cells existing in bone marrow vary in their degree of radiosensitivity. Erythroblasts (red blood stem cells) are more radiosensitive than myeloblasts (white blood stem cells), and myeloblasts are more radiosensitive than megakaryoblasts (platelet stem cells).

Red blood cells (erythrocytes) live about 120 days and are the most numerous of the formed elements in blood. Erythrocytes have no nucleus. Their function is to transport oxygen and carbon dioxide through the bloodstream. In the human male, the normal red blood count (RBC) is about 5,500,000/mm^3, whereas the female has a normal RBC of about 4,800,000/mm^3. Because these cells have a longer life span (divide less rapidly) than other blood cells, their depression resulting from radiation exposure is less severe and, hence, they are less sensitive to radiation than other blood cells. As erythrocytes mature, their radiosensitivity decreases. A dose of ionizing radiation above 0.5 Gy (50 rad) can cause a decrease in the number of red blood cells in the circulating blood. Depending on the actual dose received, these blood cells can begin to repopulate about a month after their irradiation. Depletion of erythrocytes as a result of radiation exposure leads to anemia (blood deficiency accompanied by a lack of vitality), which worsens by hemorrhages throughout the body.

White blood cells are collectively called leukocytes. A subgroup of this group of blood cells are lymphocytes, which perform a special function for the human body by playing an active role in producing immunity. These cells defend the body against foreign antigens by producing antibodies to combat disease. Because lymphocytes only live for about 24 hours, they have the shortest life span of all of the blood cells. Lymphocytes are the *most radiosensitive* blood cells in the human body. A radiation dose as low as 0.1 Gy (10 rad) is sufficient to depress the number of these cells present in the circulating blood. When lymphocytes are damaged by radiation exposure, the body loses its natural ability to combat infection and becomes more susceptible to bacterial or viral antigens.

The normal white blood cell count for an adult ranges from 5000 to 10,000/mm^3 of blood. The number of lymphocytes present in circulating blood decreases when low doses of radiation (0.25 Gy or less or 25 rad or less) are received. At this dose level, complete blood cell recovery occurs shortly after irradiation. However, when a moderate dose of radiation (0.5 to 1 Gy or 50 to 100 rad) is received, the lymphocyte count decreases to zero within a few days. Recovery generally occurs within a few months after the exposure.

Neutrophils, another kind of white blood cell, also play an important role in fighting infection. If radiation exposure causes a decrease in the number of these cells, a person's susceptibility to infection increases. A dose of 0.5 Gy (50 rad) of ionizing radiation can cause a decrease in the number of neutrophils present in the circulating blood. When they receive moderate doses of radiation, however, these cells decrease in number to the lowest level possible within a period of a few weeks after irradiation. A few months after the exposure, the number of neutrophils present in the blood returns to its original value.

Granulocytes are a type of white blood cell that fights bacteria. They remain alive in the circulating blood for only a few days. These cells respond to irradiation by suddenly increasing in number. After this sudden increase, the granulocytes decrease in number, rapidly at first and then more slowly. Depending upon the dose of radiation received, these cells may recover within about 2 months after their irradiation.

Thrombocytes or platelets initiate blood clotting and prevent hemorrhage. They have a life span of about 30 days. The normal platelet count in the human adult ranges from 150,000 to 350,000/mm^3 of blood. A dose of radiation above 0.5 Gy (50 rad) can decrease the number of platelets in the circulating blood. When exposed to moderate radiation doses, these cells begin to recover about two months after being irradiated.

Neither the blood nor the blood-forming organs of patients should suffer appreciable damage from radiation exposure received during a diagnostic radiologic procedure. However, there have been studies in which chromosome aberrations (changes) were noticed in circulating lymphocytes after the lymphocytes had received radiation doses within the diagnostic radiology range.

A therapeutic dose of ionizing radiation causes a decrease in the blood count. Patients who are undergoing radiation therapy treatment are monitored frequently (in the form of weekly or biweekly blood counts) to determine whether the platelet count is adequate.

A periodic blood count is *not* recommended as a method for monitoring occupational radiation exposure because biological damage has already been sustained when an irregularity is seen in the blood count. Since one of the objectives of radiation monitoring is to discover elevated exposure levels before they present a biological hazard, blood count results are not as useful as other methods. Also, blood count is a relatively insensitive test, being unable to indicate exposures of less than 10 cGy (10 rad). Film badges (p. 246) can detect exposures of a milliroentgen and can therefore be used to discover potentially hazardous working conditions before actual hazards appear.

Epithelial tissue

Epithelial tissue lines and covers body tissue. The cells of these tissues lie close together, with little or no intercellular substances coming between them. Epithelial tissue contains no blood vessels, and it regenerates through the process of mitosis. These cells are found in the lining of the intestines, in the mucous lining of the respiratory tract, in the pulmonary alveoli, and in the lining of blood and lymphatic vessels. Because epithelial tissue is constantly being regenerated by the body, the cells comprising this tissue are highly radiosensitive.

Muscle tissue

Muscle tissue contains fibers that effect movement of an organ or part of the body. Because muscle tissue cells are highly specialized and do not divide, they are relatively *insensitive* to radiation.

Nervous tissue

Nervous tissue is found in the brain and spinal cord. A nerve cell (neuron) (Fig. 6-9) consists of a cell body and two kinds of processes: dendrites (processes extending out from the cell body that carry impulses toward it) and an axon (a long single process extending out from the cell body that carries impulses away from it). Nerve cells relay messages to and from the brain. A message enters the nerve cell through the dendrites. It passes through the cell body and exits the cell through the axon, which transmits the message across a synapse, the communication area leading to the next nerve cell in the chain.

In the adult, nerve cells are highly specialized. They perform specific functions for the body, and, like muscle cells, do not divide. Nerve cells contain a nucleus. If the nucleus of one of these cells is destroyed, the cell will die and never be restored. If the cell nucleus has been damaged but not destroyed by exposure to radiation, the damaged nerve cell may still be able to function; however, its function may be somewhat impaired. Radiation can also cause temporary or permanent damage to a nerve's processes (dendrites and axon). When this occurs, communication with and control of some areas of the body may be disrupted. Whole-body exposure to very high doses of radiation can cause severe damage to the central nervous system. A single exposure in excess of 50 Gy (5000 rad) of ionizing radiation in humans can lead to death within a few hours or days after irradiation.

Compared to nerve cells in the adult, the nerve cells contained within the embryo or the fetus are extremely radiosensitive. The most critical period in terms of exposure of these cells to ionizing radiation is during

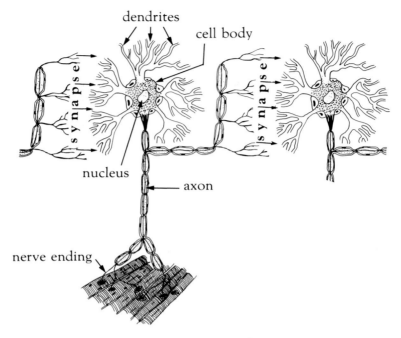

Fig. 6-9   A nerve cell (neuron). Nerve cells relay messages to and from the brain. A message enters a nerve cell through its dendrites, passes through the cell body, and exits the cell through the axon, which transmits the message across a synapse, the communication area leading to the next nerve cell in the chain.

organogenesis (the second through the eighth week after conception), because this is the time when the nerve cells in the brain and spinal cord are developing. Exposure of these developing structures to large amounts of radiation during this time can result in severe damage (congenital abnormalities*).

Reproductive cells

Human reproductive cells (germ cells) are relatively radiosensitive, although the exact responses of male and female germ cells to ionizing radiation differ because their processes of development from an immature to a mature state differ. The male testes contain both mature and immature spermatogonia. Because the mature spermatogonia are specialized and do not divide, they are relatively insensitive to ionizing radiation. The immature sper-

*Defects existing at birth that are not inherited but acquired during development in utero.

matogonia, however, are unspecialized and divide rapidly; hence, these germ cells are very radiosensitive. A radiation dose of 2 Gy (200 rad) can cause temporary sterility for up to 12 months, while a dose of 5 or 6 Gy (500 to 600 rad) can cause permanent sterility. Even small doses of ionizing radiation, doses as low as 0.1 Gy (10 rad), can depress the male sperm population. Male reproductive cells that have been exposed to a radiation dose of 0.1 Gy (10 rad) or more may be able to cause genetic mutations in future generations. To prevent mutations from being passed on to an offspring, males receiving this level of testicular radiation dose should refrain from procreation for a few months after such an exposure. By that time, cells that were irradiated during their most sensitive stages will have matured and disappeared. It should be noted that germ cells of patients undergoing diagnostic radiologic procedures *almost never* receive doses of as much as 0.1 Gy (10 rad). Medical radiographers, working under normal occupational conditions, would *never* receive a gonadal dose of this level.

The ova, the mature female germ cells, do not divide constantly. After puberty, one of the two ovaries expels a mature ovum about every 28 to 36 days (the exact number of days varies from one female to another). During the reproductive life of a woman from approximately age 12 to 50, about 400 to 500 mature ova are produced. Radiosensitivity of ova varies considerably throughout the lifetime of the germ cell. Immature ova are very radiosensitive, while more mature ova have little radiosensitivity. After irradiation, a mature ovum can still unite with a male germ cell during conception. However, these irradiated cells may contain damaged chromosomes. If fertilization of an ovum with damaged chromosomes occurs, genetic damage may be passed on to an offspring. If the offspring receives damaged chromosomes, the child may be born with congenital abnormalities. In general, whenever chromosomes in male or female germ cells are damaged by exposure to ionizing radiation, mutations can be passed on to succeeding generations. Even low doses received from diagnostic procedures *can* potentially cause chromosome damage.

Exposure to ionizing radiation can also cause female sterility. Age somewhat governs the dose necessary to produce this consequence. Sterility occurs when radiation exposure destroys new ova and/or mature ova. The ovaries of the female fetus and a young child are very radiosensitive because they contain a large number of stem cells (oogonia) and immature cells (oocytes). As the female child matures from birth to puberty, the number of immature cells (oocytes) decreases. Hence, the ovaries become less sensitive. This decrease in sensitivity continues up to the age of 30 years. Actually, women between the ages of 20 and 30 are at the lowest level in sensitivity.

After a woman reaches age 30, the sensitivity of the ovaries increases constantly until menopause because there is no replenishment of the new ova being destroyed. Because the ovaries of a younger woman are less sensitive than the ovaries of an older woman, a higher dose of radiation is required to cause sterility in the younger woman.

Temporary sterility can result from a radiation dose of 2 Gy (200 rad) to the ovaries. A dose of 5 Gy (500 rad) can cause permanent sterility in the mature female. Even small doses of ionizing radiation, doses as low as 0.1 Gy (10 rad), received by the ovaries can cause menstrual irregularities such as delay or suppression of menstruation. Although some evidence suggests that immature ova are capable of repair of radiation damage, it is sometimes recommended that women who have received 0.1 Gy (10 rad) or more postpone conception for 30 days or more after such an exposure to allow the damaged immature ova to be expelled. Yet since all the ova a woman will ever possess are present from birth until the time they are fertilized or expelled, it would be wise to avoid large exposures in the first place.

ORGANIC DAMAGE FROM IONIZING RADIATION

Radiation-induced damage at the cellular level can lead to measurable somatic and genetic damage in the organism as a whole. Some examples of measurable biological damage are cataracts, leukemia, and genetic mutations.

Radiation dose-response relationship

Radiation dose-response relationship may be demonstrated graphically through a curve with distinct characteristics. The curve is either linear (straight line) or nonlinear (curved to some degree) and depicts either a threshold dose or nonthreshold dose. Although, in its 1980 Report, the Committee on the Biological Effects of Ionizing Radiation (BEIR) under the auspices of the National Academy of Sciences revealed that the majority of somatic effects* and genetic effects at low dose levels from low-LET radiations† appear to follow a linear-quadratic, nonthreshold curve, a more conservative approach for establishing radiation protection standards is still maintained. This conservative approach is reflected in the continued use of the linear, nonthreshold curve of radiation dose-response. The linear, nonthreshold curve implies that the biological response to ionizing radiation is directly proportional to the dose (Fig. 6-10).

---

*Examples of somatic effects that exhibit a linear-quadratic, nonthreshold behavior include leukemia and cancer.

†Such as those employed in diagnostic radiology.

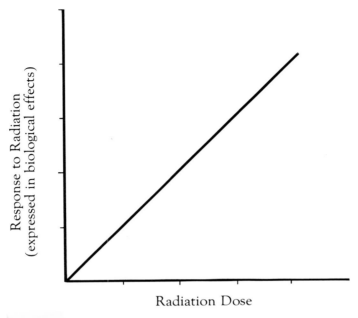

Fig. 6-10   Linear (straight-line), nonthreshold curve of radiation dose-response relationship. The straight-line curve passing through the origin in this graph indicates both that the response to radiation (in terms of biological effects) is directly proportional to the dose of radiation and that there is no known level of radiation dose below which one has absolutely no chance of sustaining biological damage. In contrast to the case of a cell survival curve both the vertical and horizontal axes of a dose-response curve are ordinary linear scales.

The term *threshold* may be defined as the point at which a response or reaction to an increasing stimulation first occurs. If ionizing radiation functions as the stimulus and the biological effects it produces are the response, and if there is a linear, *nonthreshold* relationship between radiation dose and biological response (Fig. 6-10), some biological effects will be caused in living organisms by even the smallest doses of ionizing radiation. From this it follows that *no* radiation exposure level is *absolutely* safe. Because currently it is theorized that all radiation exposure levels possess the potential to cause biological damage, medical radiographers must employ thoughtful radiation safety measures whenever humans are subjected to radiation exposure during diagnostic radiologic procedures. The linear-quadratic, nonthreshold curve (Fig. 6-11) estimates the risk associated with low-level radiation. As previously stated, it is perceived by the BEIR Committee to reflect more accurately the somatic and genetic effects at low dose levels from low-LET radi-

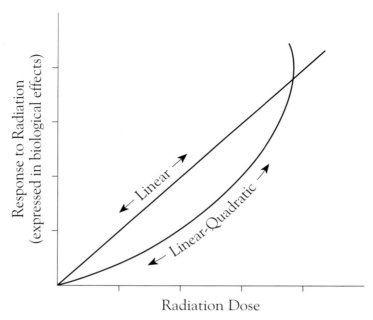

Fig. 6-11   Linear-quadratic, nonthreshold dose-response relationship. The curve estimates the risk associated with low dose levels from low-LET radiations.

ations. The linear-quadratic, nonthreshold curve is supported by an analysis of the leukemia occurrences in Nagasaki and Hiroshima using a recent reevaluation of the radiation dose distribution in these two cities.*†

The continued use of the linear dose-response model for radiation protection standards potentially exaggerates the reality of radiation effects at lower dose levels from low-LET radiations. However, it accurately reflects the effects of high-LET radiations (neutrons and alpha rays) at higher doses. In establishing radiation protection standards, the regulatory agencies have chosen to remain traditional and implement changes in a most cautious manner.

Effects of significant radiation exposure such as skin erythema and hematological depression can be graphically demonstrated through the use of a linear, threshold curve of radiation dose-response (Fig. 6-12). Here, a biological response does *not* occur below a specific dose level. Labora-

*Webster EW: In *Proceedings No. 3, Critical issues in setting radiation dose limits,* Washington, DC, 1982, National Council on Radiation Protection, p. 239, Fig. 13.
†Straume T, Dobson RL: *Health Phys* 41:666, 1981.

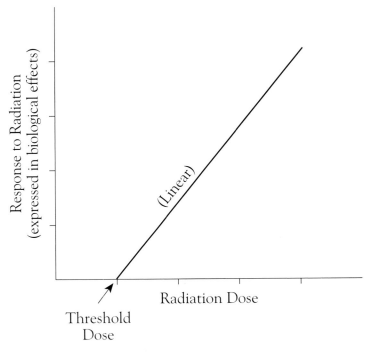

Fig. 6-12   Linear, threshold curve of radiation dose-response. This depicts those cases for which a biological response does not occur below a specific radiation dose.

tory experiments on animals and data of human populations observed after acute high doses of radiation have provided the foundation for this curve.

Factors upon which the amount of somatic and genetic damage depend

The amount of somatic and genetic biological damage a human suffers as a result of radiation exposure depends upon several factors. The most important are:

1. The quantity of ionizing radiation to which the subject is exposed.
2. The ability of the ionizing radiation to cause ionization of human tissue.
3. The amount of body area that is exposed.
4. The specific parts of the body that are exposed.

Ionizing radiation produces the *greatest* amount of biological damage in the human body when a *large* dose of *highly ionizing* (high LET) radiation is delivered to a *large or radiosensitive* area of the body.

Somatic effects

When living organisms (such as humans) that have been exposed to radiation suffer biological damage as a result of this exposure, the effects of this exposure are classified as *somatic effects*. Depending upon the length of time from the moment of irradiation to the first appearance of symptoms of radiation damage involved, the effects are classified as either *early or late somatic effects*.

Early somatic effects

Early or acute somatic effects are defined as effects that appear within minutes, hours, days, or weeks of the time of radiation exposure. A substantial dose of ionizing radiation is required to produce biological effects so soon after irradiation. Diagnostic radiologic procedures *do not* impose radiation doses sufficient to cause early effects. The high-dose effects include: nausea, fatigue, erythema (abnormal redness of the skin), epilation (loss of hair), blood disorders, intestinal disorders, fever, dry and moist desquamation (shedding of the outer layer of skin), depression of the sperm count in the male, temporary or permanent sterility of the male and female, and injury to the central nervous system (at extremely high radiation doses). These various types of organic damage can be related to the cellular effects discussed previously in this chapter. For example, intestinal disorders are brought about by damage to the sensitive epithelial tissues that line the intestines. When the whole body is exposed to a super lethal dose of 6 Gy (600 rad) of ionizing radiation, many of these manifestations of organic damage occur in succession. This early somatic effect is called *acute radiation syndrome*.

Acute radiation syndrome. Acute radiation syndrome or radiation sickness occurs in humans after whole-body reception of *large* doses of ionizing radiation delivered over a *short* period of time. *Syndrome* is a medical term that means a collection of symptoms. Hence, this disorder is actually a collection of symptoms associated with high-level radiation exposure. Three separate dose-related syndromes occur as part of the total-body syndrome: *hematopoietic syndrome, gastrointestinal syndrome,* and *central nervous system syndrome*. Each of these syndromes will be described in greater detail subsequently.

The acute radiation syndrome manifests itself in four major stages: prodromal, latent period, manifest illness, and recovery or death. The prodromal stage, also called the *prodromal syndrome,* occurs within hours after a whole-body absorbed dose of 1 Gy (100 rad) or more. Nausea, vomiting, diarrhea, fatigue, and leukopenia (an abnormal decrease of white blood corpuscles usually below 5000/mm^3) characterize this initial stage. The severity of these symptoms is dose-related. The higher the dose, the more severe are the symptoms. The length of time involved for this stage to run its course may be just hours to a few days. After the prodromal stage, there is a period of about one week during which there are no visible symptoms. Hence, it is considered a relatively asymptomatic period. Towards the end of the first week, the next stage begins. This phase is called *manifest illness* because it is the period during which symptoms become visible. Some of these symptoms are apathy, confusion, decrease in the number of red and white blood cells and platelets in the circulating blood, dehydration, epilation, exhaustion, vomiting, severe diarrhea, fever, headaches, infection, hemorrhage, and cardiovascular collapse. After this stage, emaciated humans eventually die. Hence, a primary effect of the acute radiation syndrome is shortening of the life span.

If, after a whole-body sublethal dose such as 2 or 3 Gy (200 to 300 rad), exposed persons pass through the first three stages but show less severe symptoms than those seen after super lethal dosages of 6 to 10 Gy (600 to 1000 rad), recovery may occur within about three months. However, those who recover may show some signs of radiation damage and may experience late effects. Late effects will be discussed subsequently in this chapter.

The massive explosion that blew apart a reactor at the nuclear power station in Chernobyl, Russia, on April 26, 1986, provides a recent example of humans suffering from acute radiation syndrome. During the explosion, several tons of burning graphite, uranium dioxide fuel, and other contaminants such as cesium-137, iodine-131, and plutonium-239, were ejected vertically into the atmosphere in a three-mile-high, radioactive plume of intense heat.

Out of 444 people working at the power plant at the time of the explosion, 2 died instantly and 29 died within 3 months of the accident as a consequence of thermal trauma (burns) and severe injuries from doses of whole-body ionizing radiation of approximately 6 Gy (600 rad) or more.*†‡

Without effective physical monitoring devices, biological criteria, such as the occurrence of nausea and vomiting, played an important role in the identification of radiation casualties during the first 2 days after the nuclear disaster. The acute radiation syndrome caused the hospitalization of at least

---

*Gale RP: Immediate medical consequences of nuclear accidents: lessons from Chernobyl, JAMA 258(5):625, 1987.
†Perry AR, Iglar AF: The accident at Chernobyl: radiation doses and effects, *Radiol Technol* 61(4):290, 1990.
‡Finch SC: Acute radiation syndrome, JAMA 258(5):666, 1987.

203 people.§‖ A determination of the lapse of time from the incidental exposure of the victims to the onset of nausea and/or regurgitation completes the biological criteria. Dose assessment was determined from biological dosimetry. This included serial measurements of levels of lymphocytes and granulocytes in the blood, and a quantitative analysis of dicentric chromosomes (chromosomes having two centromeres) in blood and hematopoietic cells coming from bone marrow. The data were compared to doses and effects from earlier radiation mishaps.#**

Historically, the Japanese atomic bomb survivors of Hiroshima and Nagasaki provide examples of a human population afflicted with the acute radiation syndrome as a consequence of war. Follow-up studies of the survivors who did not die of the acute radiation syndrome, however, have demonstrated late effects of ionizing radiation. These late effects will be addressed further on in this chapter.

The atomic bombing of Japan and the nuclear accident at Chernobyl have made the medical community recognize the need for a thorough understanding of the acute radiation syndrome and for appropriate medical support of persons afflicted.

Hematopoietic syndrome. The hematopoietic form of acute radiation syndrome, or "bone marrow syndrome," occurs when humans receive whole-body doses of ionizing radiation ranging from 1 to 10 Gy (100 to 1000 rad).

The hematopoietic system manufactures the corpuscular elements of the blood and is the *most radiosensitive* vital organ system in humans. Radiation exposure causes the number of red cells, white cells, and platelets in the circulating blood to decrease. Dose levels that cause this syndrome can also damage other cells in other organ systems causing the affected organ or organ system to fail to function. For example, radiation doses ranging from 1 to 10 Gy (100 to 1000 rad) can cause a decrease in the number of bone marrow stem cells. When the cells of the lymphatic system are damaged, the body loses some of its ability to combat infection. Since the number of platelets also decreases with a loss of bone marrow function, the body loses a corresponding amount of its ability to clot blood when exposed to radiation doses within this range. This makes the body more susceptible to hemorrhage.

---

§Linnemann RE: Soviet medical response to Chernobyl nuclear accident, JAMA 258(5):639, 1987.
‖Perry AR, Iglar AF: The accident at Chernobyl: radiation doses and effects, *Radiol Technol* 61(4):293, 1990.
#Gale RP: Immediate medical consequences of nuclear accidents: lessons from Chernobyl, JAMA 258(5):626, 1987.
**Perry AR, Iglar AF: The accident at Chernobyl: radiation doses and effects, *Radiol Technol* 61(4):292, 1990.

For persons affected with this syndrome, survival time decreases as the radiation dose increases. Since more bone marrow cells are destroyed as radiation dose increases, the body becomes more susceptible to infection, mostly from its own intestinal flora, and more prone to hemorrhage. When death occurs, it results as a consequence of bone marrow destruction.

Death may occur 6 to 8 weeks after irradiation in some sensitive people who receive a whole-body dose of 2 Gy (200 rad). As the whole-body dose increases from 2 to 10 Gy (200 to 1000 rad), irradiated individuals will die sooner. If the radiation exposure is not lethal, perhaps in the 1 to 2 Gy (100 to 200 rad) range, bone marrow cells repopulate to a level necessary to support life in most individuals. Many of these people recover between 3 weeks to 6 months after irradiation. The actual dose of radiation received and the irradiated person's general state of health at the time of irradiation determine the possibility of recovery.

Survival of hematopoietic patients can be enhanced by intense supportive care and special hematologic procedures. As an illustration, victims like those of the nuclear power station accident in Chernobyl, who received doses in excess of 5 Gy (500 rad), benefitted from bone marrow transplants from appropriate histocompatible donors. During the operation, hematopoietic stem cells were transplanted to facilitate bone marrow recovery. This operation, however, is not an absolute cure for victims suffering from the hematopoietic syndrome, because many of these individuals undergoing bone marrow transplant die of burns or other damages of radiation they sustained before the transplanted stem cells have had a chance to "take" and support the individual.

Gastrointestinal syndrome. In humans, the gastrointestinal form of the acute radiation syndrome appears at a threshold dose of 6 Gy (600 rad) and peaks after a dose of 10 Gy (1000 rad). Without medical support to sustain life, exposed persons receiving doses between 6 and 10 Gy (600 to 1000 rad) die within 3 to 10 days after being exposed. Even if medical support is provided, the exposed person will only live a few days longer. Survival time does not change with dose in this syndrome.

After the dose required to cause the gastrointestinal syndrome has been received, the prodromal stage occurs within a few hours. Severe nausea, vomiting, and diarrhea persist up to 24 hours. This is followed by a latent period, which lasts up to 5 days. During this time, the symptoms disappear. The manifest illness stage, however, follows this period of false calm. Again, there is severe nausea, vomiting and diarrhea. Other symptoms that can occur are fever (as in the hematopoietic syndrome), fatigue, loss of appetite, lethargy, anemia, leukopenia (a decrease in the number of white blood cells), hemorrhage (gastrointestinal tract bleeding occurs because the body loses its ability to clot blood), infection, electrolyte imbalance, and emaciation. Death occurs primarily because of catastrophic damage to the epithelial cells that line the gastrointestinal tract. Such severe damage to these cells results in the exposed person dying from infection, fluid loss, or electrolyte imbalance within three to five days of irradiation. Death from the gastrointestinal syndrome results not only from damage to the bowel but can also result from damage to the bone marrow. The latter, incidentally, is usually sufficient to cause death from the hematopoietic syndrome.

In the gastrointestinal tract, the small intestine is the most severely affected part. Because epithelial cells function as an essential biological barrier, their breakdown leaves the body vulnerable to infection (mostly from its own intestinal flora), dehydration, and severe diarrhea. Some epithelial cells do regenerate before death occurs. However, due to the large number of epithelial cells damaged by the radiation, death may occur before cell regeneration can be accomplished.

Central nervous system syndrome. The central nervous system form of acute radiation syndrome results from receiving doses of 50 Gy (5000 rad) or more of ionizing radiation. From a dose of this magnitude, death may occur anywhere within a few hours to several days (2 or 3) after exposure. After irradiation, the prodromal stage begins. Symptoms include excessive nervousness, confusion, severe nausea and vomiting, diarrhea, loss of vision, burning sensation of the skin, and loss of consciousness. A latent period lasting up to 12 hours follows. During this time, symptoms lessen or disappear. After the latent period, the manifest illness stage occurs. During this period, the prodromal syndrome reoccurs with increased severity and other symptoms present. These symptoms are disorientation and shock, periods of agitation alternating with stupor, ataxia (confusion and lack of coordination), edema, loss of equilibrium, fatigue, lethargy, convulsive seizures, electrolyte imbalance, meningitis, prostration, respiratory distress, vasculitis, and coma. Damaged blood vessels and permeable capillaries permit fluid to leak into the brain, causing an increase in fluid content. This causes an increase in intracranial pressure, which, in turn, causes more tissue damage. The final result of this damage is failure of the central nervous system, which causes death in a matter of minutes. Because the gastrointestinal and hematopoietic systems are more radiosensitive than the central nervous system, they also will be severely damaged and fail to function after a dose of this magnitude. However, because death occurs quickly after irradiation of this magnitude, the consequences of the failure of these two systems will not be demonstrated.

LD 50/30. The term *LD 50/30* signifies the whole-body dose of radiation that can be lethal to 50% of the exposed population within 30 days. For adult humans, LD 50/30 is about 3.0 Gy (300 rad) midline absorbed dose. For x-rays and gamma rays, this is equal to a dose equivalent of 3.0 Sv (300 rem). Whole-body doses above 6 Gy (600 rad) could be sufficient to cause death of the entire population within 30 days without medical support.

If an exposed human population is observed after a whole-body lethal exposure for 60 days rather than 30 days, lethality may be expressed as LD 50/60. In this instance, 50% of the exposed subjects would be expected to die within 60 days after irradiation. Usually, there is not much quantitative difference between the LD 50/60 and LD 50/30 doses.*

Repair and recovery

Because cells contain a repair mechanism inherent in their biochemistry (repair enzymes), repair and recovery can occur when cells are exposed to sublethal doses of ionizing radiation. After irradiation, surviving cells begin to repopulate. This permits an organ that has sustained functional damage as a result of radiation exposure to regain some or most of its functional ability. However, the amount of functional damage sustained determines the organ's potential for recovery. In the repair of sublethal damage, oxygenated cells have a better prospect for recovery than do hypoxic (i.e., poorly oxygenated) cells. Consequently, if both oxygenated and hypoxic cells receive a comparable dose of low-LET radiation, the oxygenated cells will be more severely damaged. Those that survive will repair themselves and recover from the injury. The hypoxic cells, which are less severely damaged, do not repair and recover.

It has been proven that repeated radiation injuries have a *cumulative* effect. Hence, a percentage (about 10%) of the radiation-induced damage becomes nonrepairable, whereas the remaining 90% may be repaired over time. When the processes of repair and repopulation work together, they aid in healing the body from radiation injury and promote recovery.

Late somatic effects

Late effects are defined as effects that appear after a period of months or years after exposure to ionizing radiation. These effects may result from previous whole- or partial-body acute, high radiation doses, or they may be the product of individual low doses and chronic low level doses sustained over a period of several years.

These low level doses are a consideration for both patients and personnel receiving exposure from ionizing radiation as a result of diagnostic radio-

---

*Bushong SC: *Radiologic science for technologists: physics, biology, and protection*, ed 5, St Louis, 1992, Mosby–Year Book, p. 563.

logic procedures. The risk estimate of humans contracting cancer from low-level radiation exposure is still controversial. There is as yet *no conclusive proof* that low-level ionizing radiation causes a significant increase in the *risk* of malignancy. The *risk*, in fact, *may be negligible.*

To encompass the various sources of ionizing radiation such as x-ray and radioactive materials used for diagnostic purposes in the healing arts, employment-related exposures in both medicine and industry, and natural background exposure, low-level radiation must be defined in broad terms. Such low-level radiation has been defined as "an absorbed dose of 10 rem or less delivered over a short period of time," or "a larger dose delivered over a long period of time, for instance, 50 rem in 10 years."* Numerous laboratory experiments on animals and studies on human populations exposed to high doses of ionizing radiation have been conducted to determine health effects. From all data available on high radiation exposure, members of the scientific and medical communities have determined that there are three health effects categories that require study at low-level exposures: cancer induction, damage to the unborn from irradiation in utero, and genetic effects. Each of these effects is discussed later in the chapter.

Cells that survive the initial irradiation and then retain a "memory" of that event are responsible for producing late effects. Such effects are *nonthreshold* and are referred to as *stochastic events*. For these, it is the probability of their occurrence rather than the severity that is proportional to the dose. This means that the *greater* the dose received by a individual, the *greater* is the chance that a specific late effect will be seen. However, the severity of the effect does *not* increase as a consequence of increased dose. Cancer and genetic defects are examples of stochastic effects. When the biological effects demonstrate the existence of a *threshold* (a dose below which an individual has a negligible chance of sustaining specific biological damage) and the severity of that biological damage *increases* as a consequence of *increased* absorbed dose, the *threshold effects* are considered to be *nonstochastic* effects. Cataract formation and reproductive cell damage leading to impaired fertility are examples of nonstochastic effects. These effects usually occur at much higher doses than those causing stochastic effects.

The four major types of late somatic effects are carcinogenesis, cataractogenesis, life span shortening, and embryological or birth effects.

Risk estimates for causing cancer in humans. Exposure to ionizing radiation involves some risk of causing cancer as a late effect. Both high and low doses possess this potential. Risk estimates may be specified in terms of

*Ritenour ER: In Hendee WR, editor: *Health effects of low-level radiation*, Norwalk, CT, 1984, Appleton-Century-Crofts, p 13.

the "absolute risk" or the "relative risk." Absolute risk establishes a number of cancers in a specific group of people within a period of 1 year for a given level of absorbed dose (i.e., the above average number of cancer cases in 1 million [10^6] humans exposed to 1 rem). Relative risk assumes exposure to radiation will end in a steady percentage increase of cancers over the normal risk of malignancy occurrence in people of all ages. Epidemiologists now favor this model.

The knowledge gained from epidemiological studies such as those done on the Japanese atomic bomb survivors and radiation workers exposed occupationally to radiation indicates that radiation-induced malignancies in humans are probably the *most important* effect produced by exposure to low doses of radiation. Hence, there is concern over low doses of radiation such as those encountered in diagnostic radiology. Still with this consideration in mind, the benefits to be obtained in terms of information gained from a radiologic examination should far outweigh the minimal risk of developing cancer as a late effect. The risk associated with radiation-induced malignancies from low doses of ionizing radiation can only be estimated by extrapolating from high-dose data, using either a linear or linear-quadratic model. If the linear model (Fig. 6-13, *A*) is used, both high and low doses have the same risk per rad. This means that the occurrence of cancer follows a straight-line or proportional progression throughout the entire dose range. Although this model suits current high-dose information satisfactorily, it exaggerates the actual risk or danger at low doses and dose rates. The linear-quadratic model (Fig. 6-13, *B*) also suits high-dose information; however, if this model is used, the risk per rad at low doses is less but may be underestimated. The BEIR III report uses the linear-quadratic model as its model of choice.* The 1989 BEIR V Report supports the linear-quadratic model as its model of choice for leukemia *only*. For all other cancers, the BEIR V Report supports the linear model.†

Carcinogenesis. Cancer is the *most important* late somatic effect caused by exposure to ionizing radiation. Laboratory experiments with animals and statistical studies of human populations exposed to ionizing radiation prove that radiation induces cancer. In humans, these radiation-induced cancers may take 5 or more years to develop. It is difficult to distinguish radiation-induced cancer by its physical appearance, because it *does not* appear different

---

*National Research Council, Advisory Committee on Biological Effects on Ionizing Radiation (BEIR III): *The effect on populations of exposure to low levels of ionizing radiation,* Washington, DC, 1980, National Academy of Science.

†National Research Council, Commission of Life Sciences, Committee on Biological Effects on Ionizing Radiations (BEIR V), Board on Radiation Effects Research: *Health effects of exposure to low levels of ionizing radiation,* Washington, DC, 1989, National Academy Press.

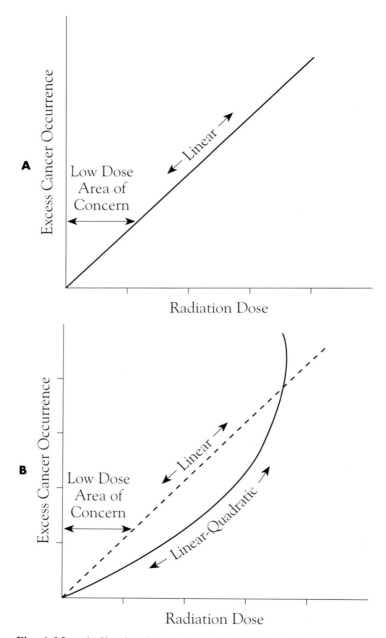

Fig. 6-13   *A,* Simple schematic of the linear model used to extrapolate the occurrence of cancer from high dose information to low doses. This model suits current high dose information satisfactorily but exaggerates the actual risk or danger at low doses and dose rates. *B,* Simple schematic of the linear-quadratic model used to extrapolate the occurrence of cancer from high dose information to low doses. This model suits current high dose information satisfactorily, but risks at low doses may be underestimated.

from cancers that arise from other causes. Because cancer from natural causes frequently occurs and the number of cancers induced by radiation is small when compared to the natural incidence of malignancies, cancer caused by low-level radiation is hard to discover. Human evidence for radiation carcinogenesis comes from observation of irradiated humans and from epidemiologic studies done over a period of many years after exposure to high doses of ionizing radiation. Examples of these data follow.

Radium-dial painters. During the early years of this century, a prosperous radium-dial painting industry existed in some factories in New Jersey. Young girls employed in these factories hand-painted the luminous numerals on watches and clocks with a radium-containing paint. The girls used sable brushes to apply the paint. To do the fine work required, some would place the paint-saturated brush tip to their lips to draw the bristles to a fine point. The girls who followed this procedure ingested large quantities of radium. Since it is chemically similar to calcium, the ingested radium localized in the bone. The accumulation of this toxic substance eventually caused osteoporosis (decalcification of the bone), osteogenic sarcoma (bone cancer), and other malignancies to develop in several of the girls. The bones most frequently affected include the pelvis, femur, and mandible. The number of head carcinomas attributed to the radium-dial painting industry is significant. Out of 1474 women in the industry, there were 61 diagnosed cancers of the paranasal sinuses and 21 cancers of the mastoid air cells. Studies attribute the death of at least 18 of the female radium-dial painters to "radium poisoning."

Uranium miners. During the early years of this century, people worked in European mines to extract pitchblend, a uranium ore. Uranium is a radioactive element with a very long half-life (for U-238, the half-life is 4.5×10^9 yr); it decays through a series of radioactive nuclides by emitting alpha, beta, and gamma radiation.

One of the most important members of its decay family is radium (atomic number = 88). Radium, itself radioactive, decays with a half-life of 1622 years to the radioactive element radon (atomic number = 86). Radon, unfortunately, is a gas that decays with a half-life of 3.8 days by way of alpha particle emission. This gas emanated through tiny gaps in the rocks being worked on by the miners, creating an insidious airborne hazard. Many miners throughout the course of many years of employment inhaled significant amounts of radon. Possessing high LET, alpha particles passing through a person's lungs have high probability of producing a great deal of cellular damage. About 50% of the miners eventually succumbed to lung cancer.

During the 1950s and 1960s, at the height of the Cold War between the United States and Russia, the US government needed fuel for nuclear weapons and plants. The Navajo Indians in Arizona and New Mexico mined uranium to meet this need. Because no action was taken by the government to regulate working conditions in the mines to ensure safety from exposure, even though there was an awareness of risk, some 15,000 Navajos and Caucasians who worked in the uranium mines suffered a lethal dose of ionizing radiation from radioactive dust and from water they drank. Experts estimate individual miners unknowingly received an approximate dose equivalent of 10 Sv (1000 rem) or more per miner.* This resulted in an alarmingly high rate of miners dying predominantly from cancer and other respiratory diseases. To add to this tragedy, the families of the miners were also affected. Because the miners had no knowledge of the adverse effects of ionizing radiation, they did not change their work clothing, which was contaminated with radioactive material, before going home. Hence, their spouses and children were also contaminated by radioactive material, making them vulnerable to radiation-induced cancers from substantial exposures.

Early medical radiation workers. A number of the early radiation workers (radiologists, dentists, and technologists) were exposed to large amounts of ionizing radiation. This resulted in some severe radiation injuries. Many radiologists and dentists developed cancerous skin lesions on the hands as a result of their occupational exposure. When compared to their nonradiologist counterparts, many early radiologists showed a higher incidence of blood disorders such as aplastic anemia and leukemia. Because early radiologists functioned without the benefit of protective devices, that they sustained these radiation-induced injuries is understandable. As a result of the advancement in radiation safety education and the development and use of acceptable, effective protective devices, radiation workers employed in the radiology industry today need not suffer any adverse health effects as a consequence of their work. Studies of radiographers and physicians who began their careers in radiology after the 1940s reveal that these radiation workers have shown no increase in adverse health effects as a result of their occupational exposure. This can be attributed to increased knowledge and use of proper protective measures and devices.

Thyroid nodules and carcinoma. During the 1940s and early 1950s, physicians diagnosed thymus gland enlargement in many infants suffering from respiratory distress. The thymus is located adjacent to the thyroid in the mediastinal cavity, which extends up into the neck as far as the lower edge of the thyroid gland. Functioning as a vital part of the immune mechanism, this

---

*Tilke B: Navajo miners battle long-term effects of radiation, *Advances for Radiologic Technologists* 3(31):3, 1990.

gland plays a critical role in the body's defense against infection. Shortly after birth, the thymus glands in these infants responded to infection by enlarging. To reduce the size of the gland, the infants were treated with therapeutic doses (1.2 to 60 Gy, or 120 to 6000 rad) of x-radiation. Because the thyroid gland is adjacent to the thymus, it also received a substantial radiation dose. This resulted in the development, some 20 years later, of thyroid nodules and carcinomas in many of the children whose thymuses had been irradiated.

Thyroid cancer also occurred in the children of the Marshall Islanders who were inadvertently subjected to high levels of fallout during an atomic bomb test (code-named BRAVO) on March 1, 1954. During the detonation of a 15-megaton thermonuclear device on Bikini Atoll, the wind shifted and carried the fallout over the neighboring islands. As a consequence of this exposure, the children received substantial absorbed doses to the thyroid from both external exposure and internal ingestion of radioiodine. Estimates indicate that inhabitants of Rongelap Atoll received a mean dose of radiation to the thyroid gland of 21 Gy (2100 rad), while the inhabitants of Utrik Atoll received 2.80 Gy (280 rad).*†

Japanese atomic bomb survivors. Epidemiological studies of approximately 100,000 Japanese survivors of the atomic bombings at Hiroshima and Nagasaki indicate that ionizing radiation causes leukemia (proliferation of the white blood cells). It is estimated that atomic bomb survivors *(hibakusha)* exposed to radiation doses of about 1 Gy (100 rad) or more showed a significant increase in the incidence of leukemia. When compared with the *spontaneous* incidence of leukemia in the Japanese population at the time of the bomb, the incidence of leukemia in the irradiated population increased about 100 times after the high dose of radiation was received. "Studies of the atomic bomb survivors in both Hiroshima and Nagasaki show a statistically significant increase in leukemia incidence in the exposed population as compared to the nonexposed population. In the period 1950-1956, 117 new cases of leukemia were reported in the Japanese survivors; approximately 64 of these can be attributed to radiation exposure."‡

The incidence of leukemia has slowly declined since the late 1940s and early 1950s. However, there are other radiation-induced malignancies whose occurrence rates have continued to escalate since the late 1950s and early

---

*Hamilton TE, vanBelle G, LoGerfo J: Thyroid neoplasia in Marshall Islanders exposed to nuclear fallout, *JAMA* 258(5):629, 1987.

†Lessard E et al: Thyroid absorbed dose for people at Rongelap, Utrik, and Sifo on March 1, 1954. US Department of Energy publication (BNL) 51-882, Upton, NY, 1985, Brookhaven National Laboratory.

‡Travis EL: *Primer of medical radiobiology,* ed 2, Chicago, 1989, Mosby–Year Book, p 170.

1960s. Among these are a variety of solid tumors such as thyroid, breast, lung, and bone cancers.

Although studies from Hiroshima and Nagasaki confirm that high doses of ionizing radiation cause cancer, radiation is really not a highly effective cancer-causing agent. For example, follow-up of approximately 82,000 atomic bomb survivors studied from 1950 to 1978 reveal an excess of only 250 cancer deaths attributed to radiation exposure. Instead of the expected 4500 cancer deaths, there actually were 4750. This means that out of about every 300 atomic bomb survivors, one died of a malignancy blamed on an average whole-body radiation dose of approximately 0.14 Sv (14 rem).

Epidemiological data on the Hiroshima atomic bomb survivors also indicate that there is a linear relationship between radiation dose and radiation-induced leukemia. That is, the chance of suffering leukemia as a result of being exposed to radiation is directly proportional to the magnitude of the radiation exposure. Available information of the kind necessary to establish the existence of a threshold dose/response (whether or not there is a harmless dose) is inconclusive. Hence radiation-induced leukemia follows a *linear-nonthreshold* dose-response relationship when compared with a population who have *not* been exposed to ionizing radiation.†

Recent re-evaluation of the quantity and type of radiation that was released in the cities of Hiroshima and Nagasaki provides a better foundation for radiation dose and damage assessment. Originally, neutrons were credited with the damage in Hiroshima. However, when recent studies revealed that the uranium-fueled bomb dropped on Hiroshima provided more gamma radiation exposure and less neutron exposure than previously believed, data on the survivors were updated to reflect more accurate information. It has been established that gamma radiation and neutrons each provided about 50% of the radiation dose inflicted on the population of Hiroshima. On the other hand, the population of Nagasaki, who were exposed to a plutonium bomb, received only 10% of their exposure from neutrons and 90% from gamma radiation. Based on revised atomic bomb data, radiation-induced leukemias and solid tumors occurring in the survivors may be attributed predominantly to gamma radiation exposure.

Evacuees from the Chernobyl nuclear power station disaster. The 1986 nuclear power station accident at Chernobyl requires long-term follow-up studies to assess the magnitude and severity of late effects on the exposed population. Detailed observations investigating potential increases in

---

†Bushong SC: *Radiologic science for technologists: physics, biology and protection,* ed 5, St Louis, 1992, Mosby–Year Book, pp. 584-588.

the incidence of leukemia, thyroid problems, and other possible radiation-induced malignancies must be made.

Within 36 hours of the nuclear catastrophe, 45,000 people residing in Pripyat, a city 2 miles from the plant, were evacuated. An additional 90,000 people, most of whom were living in a 10-mile (30-km) radial zone of Chernobyl, were also evacuated over a period of 14 days after the disaster.

In general, the 135,000 evacuees received an average absorbed dose equivalent of 0.12 Sv (12 rem) per person. Out of the 135,000, approximately 24,000 people received an absorbed dose equivalent of about 0.45 Sv (45 rem). The remaining 111,000 people received from 0.03 to 0.06 Sv (3 to 6 rem).*† If the evacuees are monitored for at least the next 30 years, important estimates of radiation-induced leukemias and other malignancies may be obtained.

There is worldwide concern about the possibility of late effects occurring from the Chernobyl power station disaster. Because winds carried the radioactive plume in several different directions during the 10 days after the accident, more than 20 countries received fallout as a consequence of the catastrophe. Approximately 400,000 people received some exposure from fallout. In February 1989, Dr. Richard Wilson, Professor of Physics at Harvard University in Cambridge, Massachusetts, estimated "that about 20,000 people throughout the world"‡ will develop a radiation-induced malignancy from the Chernobyl accident.

Iodine-131 is one of the radioactive materials that became airborne in the radioactive plume. Iodine-131 concentrates in the thyroid gland. It possesses the ability to cause cancer many years after the initial exposure. In an attempt to prevent thyroid cancer as a consequence of accidental overdose to iodine-131, potassium iodide was administered to children in Poland and some other countries after the Chernobyl accident. The potassium iodide, by offering a substitute for take-up by the thyroid gland, is intended to block effectively the gland's uptake of iodine-131. The degree of effectiveness of this preventive treatment needs to be determined. In other accidentally exposed populations, thyroid cancer has been caused in some individuals at doses of 1 Gy (100 rad) or less. The approximate time for the appearance of

*Gale RP: Immediate medical consequences of nuclear accidents: lessons from Chernobyl, *JAMA* 258(5):625, 1987.

†Perry AR, Iglar, HF: The accident at Chernobyl: radiation doses and effects, *Radiol Technol* 61(4):293, 1990.

‡WGBH Transcripts: Back to Chernobyl, *Nova* #1604, Boston, MA, 1989 (television program originally broadcast on PBS on February 14, 1989).

such radiation-induced thyroid malignancies is usually between 10 and 20 years after exposure.

Through appropriate studies, a great deal of knowledge can be acquired about the link between ionizing radiation and cancer. A more thorough understanding of the effects of low-level ionizing radiation can also be gained. However, because the actual levels of risk from the accident are still unknown due to the limited data provided by the Russians, it is difficult to determine the chances for development of radiation-induced malignancies.

Cataractogenesis. The lens of the eye contains transparent fibers that transmit light. The retina receives the light focused by the lens and permits the image formed by the lens to be received. A single threshold dose of ionizing radiation of about 2 Gy (200 rad) or higher doses induce the formation of cataracts (opacity of the eye lens). This causes a loss of vision. Laboratory experiments with mice prove that cataracts can be induced with doses as low as 0.1 Gy (10 rad). Highly ionizing neutron radiation is extremely efficient for inducing cataracts. A dose as low as 0.01 Gy (1 rad) has been known to cause the formation of cataracts in mice. Radiation-induced cataracts in humans follow a threshold, nonlinear dose-response relationship. Evidence for human radiation cataractogenesis comes from observation of small groups of people who accidentally received substantial doses to the eyes. These groups include Japanese atomic bomb survivors, nuclear physicists working with cyclotrons (units that produce high-energy particles such as protons) between 1932 and 1960, and radiotherapy patients who received exposures to the eyes from application of radium plaques during therapeutic treatment.

Life span shortening. Laboratory experiments with small animals indicate that animals exposed to both acute and chronic doses of ionizing radiation die younger than animals that have never been irradiated. Both exposed and unexposed animals die of the same diseases; however, the exposed animals develop disease at an earlier age and also die at an earlier age. Since there are no specific, distinguishable diseases associated with radiation-induced life span shortening, this reduction in the life cycle is termed "nonspecific life span shortening."

It appears that radiation, in addition to causing tissue degeneration, also accelerates the aging process. Premature aging seems to make animals more susceptible to a number of diseases. Early demise of the experimental animals results from the induction of cancer.

Evidence of radiation-induced life span shortening in humans comes from studies of physicians practicing radiology during the early years (before 1940) of the profession. Studies indicate that, when compared with the general population and nonradiologist physicians, early radiologists experienced an average life span shortening of about 5 years. At the present time, the life spans for radiologists and nonradiologists appear to be the same. This may be attributed to the implementation of appropriate radiation protection procedures and the use of modern equipment designed with safety considerations in mind. The average life expectancy of those employed as radiation workers today remains unshortened. It appears that life span shortening is not a consequence of occupational exposure in this day and age.

Embryological effects. All life forms seem to be most vulnerable to radiation during their embryonic stage of development. The period of gestation during which the embryo or fetus is exposed to radiation governs the effects (death or congenital abnormality) of the radiation upon it.

Since embryonic cells begin dividing and differentiating after conception, they are extremely radiosensitive and hence can easily be damaged by exposure to ionizing radiation during this period. The *first trimester* seems to be the *most critical* period as far as irradiation of the embryo or the fetus is concerned, since both the embryo and the fetus contain a large number of stem cells during this period of gestation. Since the central nervous system and related sense organs consist of many of these stem cells, they are extremely radiosensitive and can suffer radiation-induced damage. Irradiation of the embryo during the first 8 weeks of development to dose equivalents in excess of 200 mSv (20 rem), frequently results in death or causes congenital abnormalities. During the preimplantation stage (about 9 days), embryonic death is the major consequence. Malformations resulting from radiation exposure do not occur at this stage. Because organogenesis occurs between the second and the eighth week after conception, the developing fetus is *most susceptible* to radiation-induced congenital abnormalities during this time. These abnormalities can include growth inhibition, mental retardation, microcephaly, genital deformities, and sense organ damage. Skeletal damage from radiation exposure occurs most frequently during the period from the third to the twentieth week of development. Cancer development during childhood is another possible effect of first trimester fetal irradiation.

Fetal radiosensitivity decreases as gestation progresses. Hence, during the second and third trimesters, the developing fetus is *less sensitive* to ionizing radiation exposure than it is during the first trimester. However, even in these later trimesters, congenital abnormalities and functional disorders such as sterility can be caused by radiation exposure. A great deal of the human evidence for radiation-induced congenital abnormalities comes from follow-up studies of children exposed in utero during the atomic bomb detonations in Hiroshima and Nagasaki.

Although the *risk* of radiation-induced leukemia is *greater* when the embryo or fetus is irradiated during the *first trimester*, leukemia may also be induced by exposure to radiation during the second and third trimesters. Although some studies of children irradiated in utero* indicate an excess of cancer and leukemia deaths, studies of children exposed in utero during the atomic bomb detonations in Hiroshima and Nagasaki have *not* demonstrated any excess cancer and leukemia deaths.

Of the 135,000 evacuees from the 18-mile (30-km) radial zone of the Chernobyl nuclear power plant, approximately 2000 were pregnant women. Each received an average total-body dose equivalent of 0.43 Sv (43 rem). No obvious abnormalities were observed in the 300 live babies born by August of 1987. On the television program *Nova,* Dr. Yelena Lukinova stated, "1950 babies were born after the accident from pregnant women in the zone. All are as healthy as 600 born before the accident."†

Fetal effects such as mortality, induction of malformations, mental retardation, and childhood cancer were reviewed and considered by the United Nations Scientific Committee on the Effects of Atomic Radiation (UNSCEAR).‡ This group has proposed an upper limit combined radiation risk for the aforementioned fetal effects "of 3 chances per 1000 children for each rem of fetal dose."§ If each effect was estimated individually, the estimate would be a little lower. Without radiation, these fetal effects have an estimated normal total risk of "60 chances per 1000 children (6%)."§

The effect of low-level ionizing radiation on the embryo/fetus can only be estimated. Documentation on the effects of low-level radiation on the unborn irradiated in utero is still insufficient, because there is always some type of abnormality occurring in a small percentage of all live births in the United States. In addition, no birth abnormalities unique to high levels of radiation have been produced. The abnormalities that occur are the same as those that happen naturally. However, if the exposure occurs during a period of major organogenesis, the abnormality may be more pronounced. Assessment of radiation-induced birth abnormalities from low-level exposure(s) may also be

---

*The Oxford Survey by Dr Alice Stewart and associates is a study of childhood cancers in England, Scotland, and Wales resulting from fetal irradiation. See Stewart A et al: A survey of childhood malignancies, *Br Med J* 1(5086):1495, 1958.

†WGBH Transcripts: Back to Chernobyl, *Nova* #1604, Boston, MA, 1989 (television program originally broadcast on February 14, 1989).

‡United Nations Scientific Committee on the Effects of Atomic Radiation (UNSCEAR): Biological effects of pre-natal irradiation, 35th Session of UNSCEAR, Vienna, April 1986, New York, United Nations.

§Webster EW et al: AAPM Report No. 18, *A primer on low-level ionizing radiation and its biological effects,* New York, 1986, American Institute of Physics (published for the American Association of Physicists in Medicine).

more difficult because human genes may vary naturally or as a consequence of the environment.

Because the embryo/fetus is relatively sensitive to radiation, it is prudent to exercise caution and employ appropriate safety measures when performing diagnostic radiographic procedures that result in any dose to the unborn. Most diagnostic procedures would result in dose equivalents less than 0.01 Sv (1 rem). Such doses are not usually considered to be dangerous to the unborn.

Genetic effects

Biological effects of ionizing radiation on generations yet unborn are termed *genetic effects*. These effects occur as a result of radiation-induced damage to the DNA molecule in the sperm or ova of an adult. When these germinal mutations occur, faulty genetic information is transmitted to the offspring. This faulty genetic information may manifest itself in offspring as various diseases or malformations.

Normally, mutations in genetic material occur spontaneously without a known cause. Such mutations in genes and DNA that occur at random as a natural phenomenon are called spontaneous mutations. Because these genetic alterations are permanent and heritable, they can be transmitted from one generation to another. Spontaneous mutations in human genetic material cause a large variety of disorders or diseases, some of which include hemophilia, Huntington's chorea, Down's syndrome (mongolism), Duchenne muscular dystrophy, sickle cell anemia, cystic fibrosis, and hydrocephalus. Some genetic disorder is present in about 10% of all live births in the United States.

In each generation, some genetic mutations occur as part of the natural order of events. However, certain agents, such as elevated temperatures, ionizing radiations, viruses, and chemicals, can increase the frequency of occurrence of mutation. These agents are called *mutagens,* with ionizing radiation being one of the more effective mutagens known. Any nonlethal radiation dose received by the germ cells can cause chromosome mutations, which can be transmitted to successive generations.

When radiation interacts with DNA macromolecules, it can modify the structure of these molecules by causing breaks in the chromosomes, or it may change the amount of DNA that a cell contains by causing a deletion or an alteration in the sequence of nitrogen bases. Such modifications change the cell's genetic information. A mutation of this type can eventually lead to genetic disease in subsequent generations.

Enzymes attempt to repair cellular damage by mending structural breaks in chromosomes that have been hit by ionizing radiation. If repair is successful, the cell continues to function normally. If repair does not occur, the cell may suffer some functional impairment or die.

Mutant genes cannot properly govern the cell's normal chemical reactions nor can they properly control the sequence of amino acids in the formation of specific proteins. These incapacities of mutant genes result in various genetic diseases. For example, sickle cell anemia results from the defective synthesis of hemoglobin (a protein). About 300 amino acids combine to form the hemoglobin molecule; sickle cell anemia is caused by the substitution of only one vital amino acid.

Point mutations (genetic mutations at the molecular level) can be either dominant (probably expressed in the offspring) or recessive (probably not expressed for a number of generations). Radiation is thought to cause primarily recessive mutations, if any. For a recessive mutation to appear in the offspring, both parents must have the same genetic defect. This means that the defect must be located on the same part of a specific DNA base sequence in each parent. Since this rarely occurs, the effects of recessive mutations are not very likely to appear in a population. However, by irradiating more individuals it becomes more likely that two individuals having the same type of mutation will have offspring. Therefore, it is prudent not only to limit the amount of radiation that an individual might receive but also to limit the radiation exposure of the entire population. Damage from recessive mutations sometimes manifests itself more subtly and may take the form of allergies, a slight alteration in metabolism, decreased intelligence, nonspecific life span shortening, or predisposition to certain diseases.

The only concrete evidence available that indicates that ionizing radiation causes genetic effects comes from extensive experimentation with flies and mice. The data obtained from these experiments indicate that genetic effects do not have a threshold dose, that is, a dose of ionizing radiation at which genetic effects begin to occur and below which they cannot occur as a result of exposure to ionizing radiation. Because this means that even the smallest radiation dose can cause some genetic damage, there is no such thing as a "100% safe" gonadal radiation dose.

Existing data on radiation-induced genetic effects in humans are inconclusive. Some of the data accumulated come from observation of test groups of children conceived after one or both parents had been exposed to radiation resulting from the atomic bomb detonation in Hiroshima or Nagasaki. As of the third generation, there are no known radiation-induced genetic effects. However, this does not mean that effects will not be seen in subsequent generations. J.F. Crow, a geneticist who spent many years experimenting with fruit flies, stated that it is possible that "the most frequent mutations in man are not those leading to freaks or obvious hereditary diseases, but those causing minor impairments leading to higher embryonic death rates, lower life expectancy, increase in disease, or decreased fertility."*

Animal studies of radiation-induced genetic effects have led to the development of the *doubling dose* concept. This dose measures the effectiveness of ionizing radiation for causing mutations. Doubling dose may be defined as the radiation dose that causes the number of spontaneous mutations occurring in a given generation to increase to two times the original number (i.e., to double). Thus, in a particular generation, the frequency of genetic mutations would double after receiving a doubling dose. For example, if 7% of the offspring in each generation are born with mutations, the doubling dose would eventually increase the number of mutations to 14%. The radiation doubling dose for humans is estimated to be in the range of 0.5 Gy (50 rad) to 2.5 Gy (250 rad). For this reason, the administering of even low doses of radiation to the gonads must be minimized to reduce the risk of genetic damage in future generations. This will help to preserve the biological fitness of the human race.

SUMMARY

This chapter presented the principles of radiation biology relevant to radiation protection. The reader should be able to discuss the concept of destructive ionizing radiation interaction with the cell and identify the molecular, cellular, and organic effects of such destructive interactions. Early and late somatic and genetic effects of radiation have been identified and described. The reader should be able to discuss those effects.

REVIEW QUESTIONS

1. Radiation damage is observed on three levels:
   a. molecular, cellular, and osmotic
   b. molecular, cellular, and organic
   c. microscopic, molecular, and organic
   d. organic, inorganic, and cellular

2. The term "LD 50/30" denotes the radiation dose required to kill:
   a. 50% of the exposed population in 30 days
   b. 30% of the exposed population in 50 days
   c. 50% of the exposed population in 50 days
   d. 30% of the exposed population in 30 days

---

*Crow JF: Genetic effects of radiation. *Bulletin of the Atomic Scientists* 14:19, 1958.

3. The effect of ionizing radiation that is *most* harmful to the human body is the:
   a. direct effect
   b. indirect effect
   c. epidemiological effect
   d. mitotic effect

4. With respect to the law of Bergonié and Tribondeau, which of the following would *best* complete this statement? "The *greatest* radiation effects occur in cells having the:
   a. least reproductive activity, shortest mitotic phases, and most maturity."
   b. most reproductive activity, shortest mitotic phases, and most maturity."
   c. most reproductive activity, longest mitotic phases, and least maturity."
   d. least reproductive activity, shortest mitotic phases, and least maturity."

5. Which of the following groups of cells are *most* radiosensitive?
   a. lymphocytes
   b. adult nerve cells
   c. erythrocytes
   d. muscle cells

6. Which molecules in the human body are *most commonly* directly acted on by ionizing radiation to produce molecular damage through an indirect effect?
   a. protein
   b. carbohydrate
   c. fat
   d. water

7. Which of the following is considered to be a low-LET radiation?
   1. x-rays
   2. alpha particles
   3. gamma rays
   a. 1 only
   b. 2 only
   c. 1 and 3 only
   d. 2 and 3 only

8. Ionizing radiation causes complete chromosome breakage when:
   a. a single strand of the sugar-phosphate chain sustains a direct hit
   b. two direct hits occur in the same rung of the DNA macromolecule
   c. two direct hits occur in different rungs of the DNA macromolecule
   d. two direct hits are sustained at opposite ends of the DNA macromolecule

9. Which of the following is *most* radiosensitive?
   a. a mature person
   b. the embryo or fetus during the first trimester of gestation
   c. the fetus during the third trimester of gestation
   d. a 5-year-old child

10. Which of the following are classified as *early* somatic effects of ionizing radiation?
    a. erythema, cataractogenesis, life span shortening
    b. nausea, epilation, intestinal disorders
    c. male and female sterility, embryological effects, carcinogenesis
    d. blood disorders, fever, nonspecific life span shortening

11. Which of the following is *not* a form of the acute radiation syndrome?
    a. carcinogenic syndrome
    b. hematopoietic syndrome
    c. gastrointestinal syndrome
    d. central nervous system syndrome

12. Uranium miners in the Colorado plateau who developed lung cancer after a period of years provide an example of:
    a. early somatic effects
    b. late somatic effects
    c. early genetic effects
    d. late genetic effects

13. Cancer and genetic defects are examples of _____ effects.
    a. stochastic
    b. nonstochastic
    c. birth
    d. early

14. Radiation can induce genetic damage by:
    a. interacting with somatic cells of only one parent
    b. interacting with somatic cells of both parents
    c. altering the essential base coding sequence of DNA
    d. none of the above

15. Most radiation-induced genetic mutations are:
    a. dominant mutations
    b. expressed in first-generation offspring
    c. spontaneous mutations that are unique to radiation only
    d. recessive mutations

16. Based on current data, which of the following would be considered a *safe* radiation dose for the gonads?
    a. 5 Gy
    b. 3 Gy
    c. 1 Gy
    d. 0 Gy

17. Which of the following groups of cells are *least* radiosensitive?
    a. adult nerve cells
    b. nerve cells in the embryo or fetus
    c. lymphocytes
    d. immature spermatogonia

18. Which of the following gonadal radiation doses will cause *permanent* sterility in a human male?
    a. 0.01 Gy
    b. 1 Gy
    c. 2.0 Gy
    d. 6 Gy

19. Upon which of the following factors does somatic or genetic radiation-induced damage depend?
    1. the amount of body area exposed
    2. quantity of ionizing radiation to which the subject is exposed
    3. the specific parts of the body that are exposed
    a. 1 only
    b. 2 only
    c. 3 only
    d. 1, 2, and 3

20. Revised atomic bomb data for Hiroshima and Nagasaki have led to the conclusion that radiation-induced leukemias and solid tumors occurring in the survivors may be attributed to exposure from:
    a. x-rays
    b. gamma radiation
    c. neutrons
    d. various nonionizing radiations

21. To estimate the number of radiation-induced leukemias and other malignancies that may occur in some of the 135,000 evacuees from the 1986 nuclear power station accident in Chernobyl, Russia, the exposed population must:
    a. not be permitted to receive any additional medical radiation exposure for the next 20 years
    b. not be permitted to intermingle with the unexposed population
    c. be monitored for only the next 10 years
    d. be monitored for at least the next 30 years

22. The acute radiation syndrome manifests itself in four major stages. The order of occurrence of these stages is:
    a. latent period, prodromal, manifest illness, recovery or death
    b. manifest illness, prodromal, latent period, recovery or death
    c. prodromal, latent period, manifest illness, recovery or death
    d. manifest illness, latent period, prodromal, recovery or death

23. Which of the following systems is the *most* radiosensitive vital organ system in humans?
    a. central nervous
    b. gastrointestinal
    c. hematopoietic
    d. skeletal

24. If an exposed human population is observed for 60 days after a whole-body lethal dose of ionizing radiation rather than for 30 days, and 50% of the people receiving the dose die within the 60 days, lethality may be expressed as:
    a. LD 50/30/30
    b. LD 50/60
    c. LD 100/60
    d. LD 30/60

25. Of the following late somatic effects caused by exposure to ionizing radiation, which is considered to be *most* important?
    a. cataract formation
    b. embryological or birth effects
    c. cancer
    d. life span shortening

26. Which of the following groups of people exposed to ionizing radiation provide proof that low-level radiation exposure produces late effects?
    a. 135,000 evacuees from the 1986 nuclear power station accident in Chernobyl, Russia
    b. Japanese atomic bomb survivors
    c. children of the Marshall Islanders who were inadvertently subjected to fallout during the atomic bomb test in 1954
    d. none of the above

27. When an assumption is made that exposure to radiation will end in a steady percentage increase of cancers over the normal risk of malignancy occurrence in people of all ages, the risk is termed:
    a. absolute
    b. excess
    c. quadratic
    d. relative

28. Studies of the Japanese atomic bomb survivors demonstrate that the incidence of leukemia has _____ since the late 1940s and early 1950s while the incidence of solid tumors has continued to _____ since the late 1950s and early 1960s.
    a. slowly declined, escalate
    b. increased rapidly, decrease
    c. increased slowly, decrease
    d. rapidly declined, decrease

29. Radiation-induced cataracts in humans follow a _____ dose-response relationship.
    a. nonlinear, nonthreshold
    b. linear, nonthreshold
    c. linear, threshold
    d. nonlinear, threshold

30. After the 1986 nuclear power station accident in Chernobyl, Russia, an attempt was made to prevent thyroid cancer in children in Poland and some other countries as a consequence of accidental overdose to iodine-131. _____ was administered as a substitute for take-up by the thyroid gland to effectively block its uptake of iodine-131.
    a. potassium bromide
    b. sodium chloride
    c. sodium bicarbonate
    d. potassium iodide

31. Genetic effects from exposure to ionizing radiation occur as a result of radiation-induced damage to the DNA molecule in the:
    1. sperm of an adult male
    2. ova of an adult female
    3. somatic cells of male and female adults
    a. 1 only
    b. 2 only
    c. 3 only
    d. 1 and 2 only

32. Large doses of ionizing radiation sustained by the Japanese children in utero at the time of the atomic bomb detonation at Hiroshima and Nagasaki have resulted in some congenital abnormalities. These abnormalities include:
    a. mental retardation
    b. microcephaly
    c. growth inhibition
    d. a, b, and c

33. Existing data on radiation-induced genetic effects in humans:
    a. prove conclusively that radiation causes major genetic effects
    b. prove conclusively that radiation causes only minor genetic effects
    c. are still inconclusive
    d. prove conclusively that radiation does not cause any genetic effects

34. $OH^* + OH^* =$
    a. H_2O
    b. HOH^+
    c. HOH^-
    d. H_2O_2

35. The radiation doubling dose for humans is estimated to be:
    a. 0.05 Gy (5 rad) to 0.25 Gy (25 rad)
    b. 0.5 Gy (50 rad) to 2.5 Gy (250 rad)
    c. 3 Gy (300 rad) to 4.5 Gy (450 rad)
    d. 5 Gy (500 rad) to 6 Gy (600 rad)

36. Early effects of ionizing radiation are *not* caused by doses:
    a. above 3 Gy (300 rad)
    b. above 6 Gy (600 rad)
    c. resulting from atomic bomb detonation
    d. encountered in diagnostic radiology

37. The dose of a reference radiation quality, stated in grays, necessary to produce the *same* biological reaction in a given experiment that is produced by a dose of the test radiation, also stated in grays, simply defines:
    a. linear energy transfer
    b. relative biological effectiveness
    c. quality factor
    d. low-level radiation effectiveness

38. While passing through a human cell, an x-ray photon interacts with and inactivates the cell's master molecule. The consequence to the cell is:
    a. a loss of intracellular fluid
    b. increased pressure upon the cell membrane
    c. disruption of its chemistry
    d. death

39. Radiation dose-response may be demonstrated graphically through the use of curves. Which of the following curves would express a linear-quadratic, non-threshold dose response?
    a.
    b.
    c.
    d.

40. 1 micron (μm) =
    a. 10^{-6} m
    b. 10^{+6} m
    c. 10^{-3} m
    d. 10^{+3} m

Bibliography

American Broadcasting Companies: 20/20 Transcript, Chernobyl: through a doctor's eyes, ABC News, Show 634, August 28, 1986. J Diamond, Producer; B Walters, correspondent. Transcript produced by Journal Graphics, New York.

Anthony CP, Thibodeau GA: *Textbook of anatomy and physiology*, ed 13, St Louis: 1989, Mosby–Year Book.

Ballinger PW: *Merrill's atlas of radiographic positions and radiologic procedures*, ed 6, vol 1, St Louis, 1986, Mosby–Year Book, p 15.

Ballinger PW: *Merrill's atlas of radiographic positions and radiologic procedures*, ed 7, vol 1, St Louis, 1991, Mosby–Year Book, p 18.

Barannov A et al: Bone marrow transplantation after the Chernobyl nuclear accident, *N Engl J Med* 321(4):205, 1989.

Baron J et al: *Radiation biology: a survey of the measurement of ionizing radiation and the latent effects of low levels of radiation*, Chicago, American Society of Radiologic Technologists.

Bushong S: *Radiologic science for technologists: physics, biology, and protection*, ed 2, St Louis, 1980, Mosby–Year Book.

Bushong SC: *Radiologic science for technologists: physics, biology and protection*, ed 5, St Louis, 1993, Mosby–Year Book.

Casarett AP: Radiation biology, Englewood Clifts, NJ, 1968, Prentice-Hall.

Cobb Jr CE: Living with radiation, *National Geographic* 175(4):403, 1989.

Commission of Life Sciences, Advisory Committee on Biological Effects of Ionizing Radiation: *Biological effects of radiation, 1989 (BEIR V Report)*, Washington, DC, 1989, National Academy Press.

Committee on Biological Effects of Ionizing Radiation, National Research Council, Commission of Life Sciences, Board on Radiation Research: *Health effects of exposure to low levels of ionizing radiation (BEIR V Report)*, 1989, National Academy Press.

Committee on the Biological Effects of Ionizing Radiation, National Academy of Sciences, National Research Council: *The effects on populations of exposure to low levels of ionizing radiations, 1980 (BEIR III Report)*, Washington, DC, 1980, National Academy Press.

Crouch JE: *Functional human anatomy*, ed 4, Philadelphia, 1985, Lea & Febiger.

Crow JF: Genetic effects of radiation, *Bulletin of the Atomic Scientists* 14:19, 1958.

DeRobertis EDP, DeRobertis EMF: *Cell and molecular biology*, ed 8, Philadelphia, 1987, Lea & Febiger.

Edwards M: Chernobyl—one year after, *National Geographic* 171(5):632, 1987.

Fabrikant JI: *Radiobiology*, Chicago, 1972, Yearbook Medical.

Frankel R: *Radiation protection for radiologic technologists*, New York, 1976, McGraw-Hill.

Finch SC: Acute radiation syndrome, JAMA 258(5):664, 1987.

Fullerton GD et al, editors: *Medical Physics Monograph No. 5*, New York, 1980, American Institute of Physics (published for the American Association of Physicists in Medicine).

Gale RP: Immediate medical consequences of nuclear accidents: lessons from Chernobyl, JAMA 258(5):625, 1987.

Gurley LT, Callaway WJ, editors: *Introduction to radiologic technology*, ed 3, St Louis, 1992, Mosby–Year Book.

Hall EJ: *Radiobiology for the radiologist*, ed 3, Philadelphia, 1988, JB Lippincott.

Hamilton TE, vanBelle G, LoGerfo JP: Thyroid neoplasia in Marshall Islanders exposed to nuclear fallout, JAMA 258(5):629, 1987.

Hendee WR, editor: *Health effects of low-level radiation,* Norwalk, CT, 1984, Appleton-Century-Crofts.

Howl B: *Simplified radiotherapy for technicians,* Springfield, IL, 1972, Charles C Thomas.

Lessard E et al: *Thyroid absorbed dose for people at Rongelap, Utrik, and Sifo on March 1, 1954,* US Department of Energy publication (BNL) 51-882, Upton, NY, 1985, Brookhaven National Laboratory.

Linnemann RE: Soviet medical response to the Chernobyl nuclear accident, JAMA 258(5): 637, 1987.

Mallett M: *A handbook of anatomy and physiology for students of medical radiation technology,* ed 3, Mankato, MN, 1979, Burnell.

March HC: Leukemia in radiologists, *Radiology* 43:275, 1944.

Meck BJ: The effects of radiation on the eye, *RT Image* 1(11):1, 1988.

Miller PE: Biological effects of diagnostic irradiation, *Radiologic Technology* 48:11, 1976.

Miller RW: Delayed radiation effects in atomic-bomb survivors, *Science* 166:569, 1969.

Miller RW: Effects of ionizing radiation from the atomic bomb on Japanese children, *Pediatrics* 41:257, 1968.

National Council on Radiation Protection and Measurements (NCRP): Report #39, Basic radiation protection criteria, Washington, DC, 1971, NCRP Publications.

National Council on Radiation Protection and Measurements (NCRP): Report #43, *Review of the current state of radiation protection philosophy,* Washington, DC, 1975, NCRP Publications.

National Council on Radiation Protection and Measurements (NCRP): Report #54, *Medical radiation exposure of pregnant and potentially pregnant women,* Washington, DC, 1977, NCRP Publications.

National Council on Radiation Protection and Measurements (NCRP): Report #91, *Recommendations on limits for exposure to ionizing radiation,* Bethesda, MD, 1987, NCRP Publications.

Noz ME, Maguire Jr GQ: *Radiation protection in radiologic and health sciences,* ed 2, Philadelphia, 1985, Lea & Febiger.

Perry AR, Iglar HF: The accident at Chernobyl: radiation doses and effects, *Radiol Technol* 61(4):290, 1990.

Pizzarello DJ, Witcofski, RL: *Medical radiation biology,* ed 2, Philadelphia, 1982, Lea & Febiger.

Pizzarello DJ, Witcofski RL: *Basic radiation biology,* ed 2, Philadelphia, 1975, Lea & Febiger.

Polednak AP, Stehney AF, Rowland RE: Mortality among women first employed before 1930 in the US radium dial-painting industry, *Am J Epidemiol* 107:179, 1978.

Rafla S, Rotman M: *Introduction to radiotherapy,* St Louis, 1974, Mosby–Year Book.

Reimenschneider J: Rethinking radiation protection standards, *RT Image* 3(6):1990.

Ritenour ER: Radiation protection and biology: a self-instructional multi-media learning series, Denver, 1985, Multi-Media Publishing.

Rowland RE, Stehney AF, Lucas Jr HF: Dose-response relationships for female radium dial workers, *Radiat Res* 76:368, 1978.

Russell LB, Russell WL: Radiation hazards to the embryo and fetus, *Radiology* 58:369, 1962.

Saccomanno G et al: Lung cancer of uranium miners on the Colorado plateau, *Health Physics* 10:1195, 1964.

Selman J: *Elements of radiobiology,* Springfield, IL, 1983, Charles C Thomas.

Seltser R, Sartwell PE: The influence of occupational exposure to radiation on the mortality of American radiologists and other medical specialists, *Am J Epidemiol* 81:2, 1965.

Stewart AM: *An epidemiologist takes a look at radiation risk,* DHEW Publication No. (FDA-BRH) 73-8024, 1973, Department of Health, Education and Welfare, p 37.

Stewart A et al: A survey of childhood malignancies, *Br Med J* 1(5086):1495, 1958.

Stewart A, Kneale GW: Radiation dose effects in relation to obstetric x-ray and childhood cancers, *Lancet* 1:1185, 1970.

Straume T, Dobson RL: *Health Physics* 41:666, 1981.

Sullivan CA: Chromosome aberrations as a means to determine occupational exposure: an alternative, *Radiol Technol* 52:185, 1980.

Thomas CL, editor: *Taber's cyclopedic medical dictionary,* ed 13, Philadelphia, 1977, FA Davis.

Tilke B: Navajo miners battle long-term effects of radiation, *ADVANCE for Radiologic Technologists,* 3(31):3, 1990.

Travis EL: *Primer of medical radiobiology,* ed 2, Chicago, 1989, Year Book Medical Publishers.

Tsuya A et al: Capillary microscopic observation of the superficial minute vessels of atomic bomb survivors, Hiroshima, 1972-73, *Radiat Res* 72:353, 1977.

US Department of Health, Education, and Welfare, Public Health Service, Food and Drug

Administration, Bureau of Radiological Health and Barnett MH: *The biological effects of ionizing radiation: an overview,* HEW Publication FDA 77-8004. Rockville, MD, 1976, HEW.

Vinocur B: New data rekindle radiation debate, *Diagnostic Imaging,* November:94, 1983.

Watkins GL: Public health risks from low dose medical radiation, *Radiol Technol* 59(2):160, 1987.

Webster EW et al: AAPM Report No. 18, *A primer on low-level ionizing radiation and its biological effects,* New York, 1986, American Institute of Physics (published for the American Association of Physicists in Medicine).

Webster EW: In *Proceedings No. 3, Critical issues in setting radiation dose limits,* Washington, DC, 1982, National Council in Radiation Protection, p 239, Fig. 13.

WGBH Transcripts: Back to Chernobyl. NOVA #1604. Boston, MA, 1989 (television program was originally broadcast on February 14, 1989).

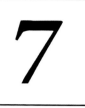

Protection of the Patient During Diagnostic Radiologic Procedures

OBJECTIVES

Upon completion of this chapter, the reader will be able to:

- explain the need for effective communication between Radiology Department personnel and the patient
- explain the significance of adequate immobilization of the patient during a radiographic exposure
- describe the various beam-limiting devices and identify the device that best confines the radiographic beam
- state the requirement for good coincidence between the radiographic beam and the localizing light beam when using a variable rectangular collimator
- explain the function of x-ray beam filtration in diagnostic radiology
- describe half-value layer (HVL) and give examples of HVLs required for selective peak kilovoltages
- state the reason for using gonadal shielding during radiologic examinations and identify the types of shields used
- discuss the need for using appropriate radiographic exposure factors for all radiologic procedures
- explain how radiographic exposure factors can be adjusted to reduce patient dose

- explain how the use of high speed film-screen combinations reduces radiographic exposure for the patient
- discuss the value of good radiographic processing techniques in reducing radiographic exposure for the patient
- explain how radiographic grids increase patient dose
- state the reason for reducing the number of repeat radiographs
- identify the benefits of repeat analysis programs
- explain how to limit the effects of the inverse square falloff of radiation intensity with distance when performing mobile radiography
- explain how patient exposure can be reduced during fluoroscopic procedures
- list three ways to indicate patient dose from diagnostic radiologic procedures
- discuss radiographic techniques employed for mammography and explain the patient dose consequences of each technique
- compare the patient dose received from a succession of adjacent CT scans with the patient dose received from an ordinary series of diagnostic radiographs of the adult cranium
- explain why children require special radiation protection when undergoing diagnostic radiologic procedures
- describe special precautions employed in medical radiography to protect the pregnant or potentially pregnant patient

A holistic approach to patient care (treating the whole person rather than just the area of concern) during a diagnostic radiologic procedure is essential. This begins with "real communication" between the patient and the radiographer, which alleviates patient uneasiness and increases the chances for successful completion of the procedure. Hence, the reader must develop effective communication skills, which he or she can use when dealing with adult or pediatric patients.

Radiographers must know how to limit exposure of the patient to ionizing radiation by correctly employing the techniques and devices suited to this purpose. Patient exposure can be limited by proper immobilization, use of appropriate beam limitation devices, correct filtration, use of gonadal shielding, selection of appropriate exposure factors used in conjunction with high speed film-screen combinations, good radiographic processing techniques, and a minimum number of repeat radiographs. This chapter provides an overview of how to protect the patient from radiation exposure during diagnostic radiologic procedures.

EFFECTIVE COMMUNICATION

Total patient care during a radiologic procedure begins with effective communication between the radiographer and the patient. When verbal (words) and nonverbal (unconscious actions or body language) messages are understood as intended, communication is effective. Communication encourages closeness, reduces anxiety or emotional stress, enhances the professional image of the radiographer as a person who "cares," and increases the chance for successful completion of the radiologic examination.

Patient protection during a diagnostic radiologic procedure should begin with clear, concise instructions (Fig. 7-1). When responsibilities are adequately defined through effective communication, the patient understands what must be done and can more fully cooperate. When procedures are not explained or are poorly explained to the patient, he or she faces "the fear of the unknown" and experiences anxiety and nervousness. This stress increases the patient's state of mental confusion and leads to patient depression. To alleviate the problem, the radiographer must take adequate time to explain

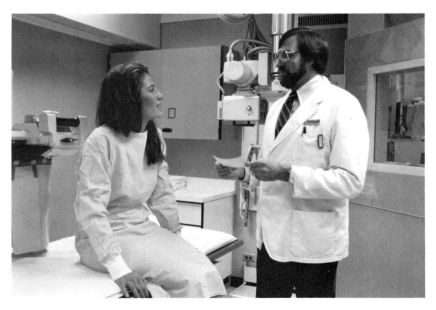

Fig. 7-1   Clear, concise instructions promote effective communication between the patient and the radiographer.

the procedure in simple terms that the patient will understand. Then the patient must be given the opportunity to ask questions. These questions should be answered truthfully by the radiographer within limits that ethics permit. This creates a sense of trust between the patient and the radiographer and encourages further communication.

If the radiographic procedure (for example, angio-catheterization or contrast media injection) will cause pain, discomfort or any strange sensations, the patient should be informed (Fig. 7-2). This prepares the patient for the examination. To prevent the patient from imagining more pain or

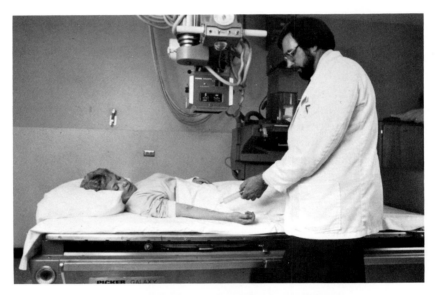

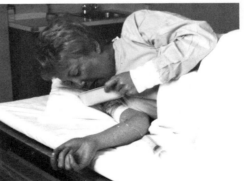

Fig. 7-2   Inform the patient of any pain, discomfort, or strange sensations that will be experienced during the radiologic procedure.

discomfort than the procedure will actually cause, the radiographer should make every attempt not to overemphasize this aspect of the examination.

Everyone within the Radiology Department should always function as a humanistic professional. Words and actions must demonstrate caring, concern, understanding, and respect for human dignity and for the uniqueness of the individual. A feeling of patient compassion must always be provided.

Repeat radiographs can sometimes be attributed to poor communication between the radiographer and the patient. Inadequate or misinterpreted communication can cause a communication gap, which may result in the patient's being unable to cooperate. For example, during an interventional radiographic examination in which the patient will feel some sensations, he or she may not understand this and may move due to surprise or simply to inform the technologist or physician that something is wrong. This would result in an unnecessary repeat exposure. Effective communication between radiographer and patient can prevent this problem from occurring and hence prevent additional, unnecessary radiation exposure.

IMMOBILIZATION

If a patient moves during a radiographic exposure, the radiographic image will be blurred. Such radiographs have little or no diagnostic value. This would necessitate a repeat examination, resulting in additional radiation exposure for the patient and the radiographer.

To eliminate the problem of voluntary motion (motion controlled by will, i.e., skeletal muscle) the radiographer must adequately immobilize the patient during the radiographic exposure (Fig. 7-3). A variety of suitable de-

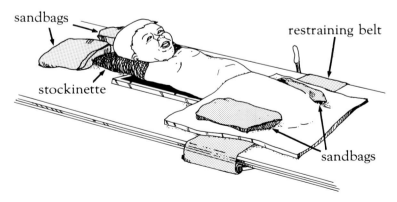

Fig. 7-3 Proper immobilization during radiographic examinations eliminates voluntary motion.

vices are available to immobilize either the whole body or the individual body part to be radiographed. Involuntary motion, caused by muscle not under voluntary control as in the case of the digestive organs, can be reduced by reducing exposure time, not by immobilization.

BEAM LIMITATION DEVICES

X-ray beam limitation devices include aperture diaphragms, cones, and collimators. These devices limit the useful beam (primary beam or umbra) *before* it enters the area of clinical interest, thereby decreasing the quantity of body tissue irradiated. This reduces the amount of scattered and absorbed radiation in the tissue, thereby sparing the surrounding tissue from unnecessary exposure.

Aperture diaphragm

An aperture diaphragm is the simplest of all beam limitation devices. It consists of a flat piece of lead with a hole of a designated size and shape cut in its center. The dimensions of the hole determine the size and shape of the radiographic beam.

Placed directly below the window of the x-ray tube, the aperture dia-

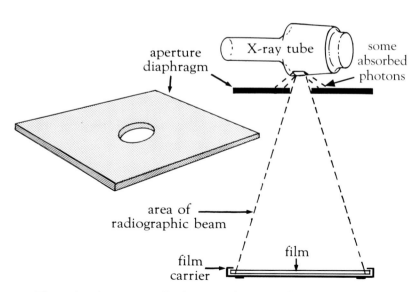

Fig. 7-4 An aperture diaphragm, a flat piece of lead with a hole of a designated size and shape cut in its center, is placed directly below the window of the x-ray tube to limit the radiographic beam to a fixed size so that the beam covers a given size film at a given distance.

phragm limits the radiographic beam to a fixed size suitable to cover a given size film at a given distance (Fig. 7-4). Use of an aperture diaphragm reduces scattered radiation, because the diaphragm limits field size (the area of the body irradiated) and the amount of scattered radiation produced is a function of the volume of tissue irradiated.

Cones

Cones are circular metal tubes that attach to the x-ray tube housing or variable rectangular collimator to limit the beam to a predetermined size and shape. The design of this collimating device is simple, consisting of either a flared metal tube or a straight cylinder (Fig. 7-5, *A* and *B*). Although the

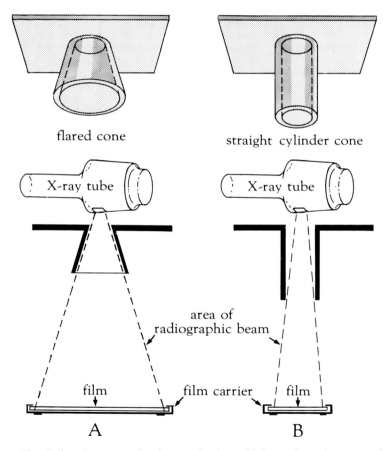

Fig. 7-5 Cones are circular metal tubes which attach to the x-ray tube housing or variable rectangular collimator to limit the radiographic beam to a certain size and shape. *A,* Cone fashioned in the form of a flared metal tube. *B,* Cone fashioned in the form of a straight cylinder.

length and diameter of cones vary, it is primarily the lower rim of the cone that governs beam limitation. Greater beam limitation is achieved when the cone or cylinder is longer and the diameter of the opening is smaller. Field size at selected source-to-image (SID) distances should be indicated on the cone.

Spot, or very small field, radiography is *best* accomplished through the use of extension cylinders, which are cylindrical metal tubes that possess a 10 to 20 inch metal extension at the far end of the barrel (Fig. 7-6). The use of this extension piece further limits the size of the useful beam.

Variable rectangular collimators have replaced cones for most radiographic examinations. However, cones are still frequently used for radiographic examinations of the head and vertebral column and chest.

Beam-defining cones are widely used in dental radiography. Owing to the fact that dental x-ray equipment is usually less bulky than general purpose equipment, a one-piece beam limitation device such as a cone is convenient.

Collimators

The collimator is the *most versatile* device for defining the size and shape of the radiographic beam. The variable rectangular collimator (Fig. 7-7, *A*) is the type of collimator *most often* used with multipurpose x-ray units. It is

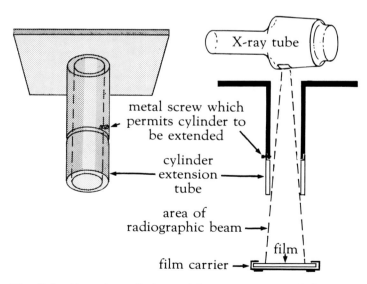

Fig. 7-6   Extension cylinder used for spot or very small field radiography.

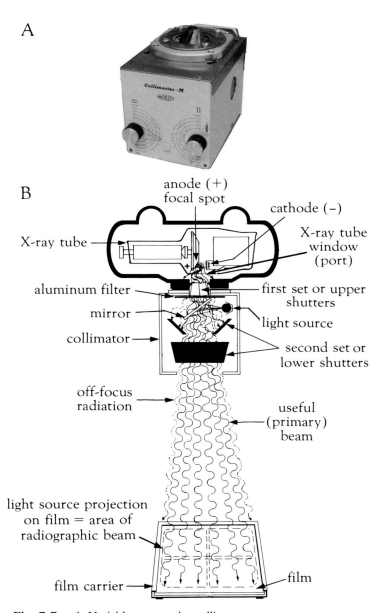

A

B

anode (+)
focal spot

cathode (−)

X-ray tube

X-ray tube
window
(port)

aluminum filter

first set or upper
shutters

mirror

light source

collimator

second set or
lower shutters

off-focus
radiation

useful
(primary)
beam

light source projection
on film = area of
radiographic beam

film carrier

film

Fig. 7-7 *A,* Variable rectangular collimator.
(Courtesy Machlett Labs, Inc., Stamford, Conn.)
B, Diagram of a typical collimator demonstrating radiographic beam-defining
system: (1) anode focal spot; (2) X-ray tube window; (3) mirror; (4) light
source; (5) first set or upper shutters; (6) second set or lower shutters; (7) aluminum filter. The metal shutters collimate the radiographic beam so that it is
no larger than the image receptor (the film). *Continued.*

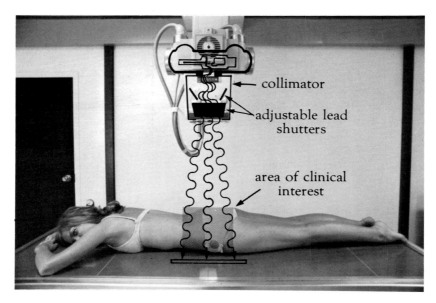

Fig. 7-7, cont'd.   *C,* Collimator containing the radiographic beam-defining system, which establishes the parameters (margins) of the beam. Adjustable lead shutters limit the cross-sectional area of the beam and confine it to the area of clinical interest.

box-shaped and contains the radiographic beam-defining system (Fig. 7-7, *B*), which consists of two sets of adjustable lead shutters mounted within the device at different levels, a light source to illuminate the x-ray field and permit it to be centered over the area of clinical interest, and a mirror to deflect the light beam toward the object to be radiographed.

The first set of shutters, the upper shutters, are mounted as close as possible to the tube window to reduce the amount of off-focus or stem radiation (x-rays emitted from parts of the tube other than the focal spot) coming from the primary beam and exiting at various angles from the x-ray tube window. This radiation can *never* be completely eliminated because the metal shutters *cannot* be placed immediately beneath the actual focal spot of the x-ray tube, but placing the first set or upper shutters as close as possible to the tube window can reduce it significantly. This practice reduces patient exposure resulting from off-focus radiation.

The second set of shutters, the lower shutters, are mounted below the level of the light source and mirror and function to confine further the radiographic beam to the area of clinical interest (Fig. 7-7, *B* and *C*). This set of shutters consists of two pairs of lead plates oriented at right angles to each other. Each set can be adjusted independently so that a variety of rectangular shapes can be selected. In this way, the field is not limited to the circular or square shapes that, in some cases, irradiate areas of the patient that do not need to be viewed.

To protect the patient's skin from exposure to electrons produced by photon interaction with the collimator, the patient's skin surface should be at least 15 cm below the collimator. Some collimator housings contain "spacer bars," which project down from the housing to prevent the collimators from being closer than 15 cm to the patient.

When using a variable rectangular collimator, good coincidence (i.e., both physical size and alignment) between the radiographic beam and the localizing light beam is essential for quality control. Both alignment and length and width dimensions of the radiographic and light beams must correspond to within 2% of the SID. As an example, 40 inches, which is approximately equal to 100 cm, is an SID commonly used in radiography. At this SID, the maximum allowable difference in either length or width dimensions of the projected light field in relation to the radiographic beam at the level of the image receptor must be no more than 2% of 100 cm (40 inches) or 2 cm (2% of 100 cm = 0.02 × 100 = 2 cm).

In the collimation system described so far, it would be possible for the radiographer to use inadvertently a film size much *smaller* than the size of the radiation field. Thus, areas of the patient would be irradiated that would not be recorded on film. Either the radiation field size should be smaller (if the anatomy is not of diagnostic interest) or the film should be larger (if the anatomy is indeed of diagnostic interest). To prevent such a mismatch, radiographic collimators now include a feature called *positive beam limitation* (PBL). The PBL feature consists of electronic sensors in the film cassette holder that send signals to the collimator housing. When the PBL feature is activated, the collimators are automatically adjusted so that the radiation field size matches the film size. The PBL feature may be deactivated by turning a key if some special conditions require that the radiographer have complete control of the system. However, in such a circumstance, a warning light is automatically lit to indicate that the PBL system has been deactivated.

The PBL system illustrates an important principle of patient protection during radiographic procedures. That is, the radiographer must ensure that collimation is adequate by applying the following principle: *Collimate the radiographic beam so that it is no larger than the image receptor (the film)* (Fig. 7-8, *A* to *C*). Accuracy by 2% of the SID is required with PBL.

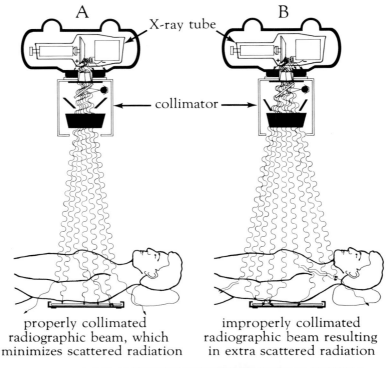

properly collimated
radiographic beam, which
minimizes scattered radiation

improperly collimated
radiographic beam resulting
in extra scattered radiation

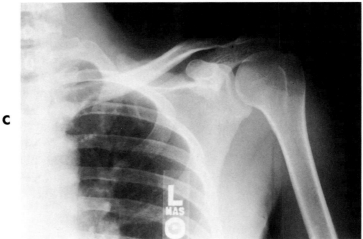

Fig. 7-8   Collimate the radiographic beam so that it is no larger than the image receptor (the film). Limiting the beam to the area of clinical interest decreases the amount of tissue irradiated and thereby minimizes patient exposure by reducing the amount of scattered and absorbed radiation. *A*, Good collimation. *B*, Poor collimation. *C*, AP radiograph of the shoulder demonstrating good collimation.

FILTRATION

Filtration of the radiographic beam reduces exposure to the patient's skin and superficial tissue by absorbing *most* of the lower energy photons (long wavelength or soft x-rays) from the heterogeneous beam (Fig. 7-9). This improves the quality of the beam and increases its mean (average) energy. Such improvement of beam quality is sometimes referred to as "hardening" of the beam.

Because filtration absorbs some of the photons in a radiographic beam, it decreases the intensity (quantity or amount) of radiation. The remaining photons are as a whole more penetrating and therefore have less probability of being absorbed in body tissue. Hence, the absorbed dose to the patient decreases when proper filtration is placed in the path of the radiographic beam. If adequate filtration were not placed in the path of the beam, very low energy photons (20 keV or lower) would always be absorbed in the body regardless of the tissue traversed. They should be removed from the radiographic beam through the process of filtration.

There are two types of filtration:
1. Inherent filtration.
2. Added filtration.

Inherent filtration includes the glass envelope encasing the x-ray tube,

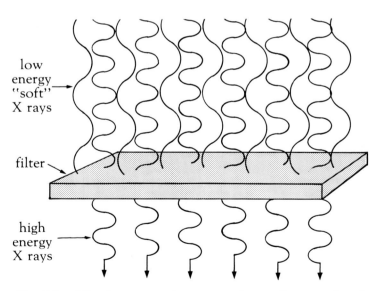

Fig. 7-9   Filtration removes low energy photons (long wavelength or "soft" x-rays) from the beam by absorbing them and permits higher energy photons to pass through. This reduces patient dose.

the insulating oil surrounding the tube, and the glass window in the tube housing.

Added filtration usually consists of sheets of aluminum (or its equivalent) of appropriate thickness. This additional filtration is interposed outside of the glass window of the tube housing. The inherent and added filtration combine to equal the required amount of total filtration necessary to filter adequately the useful beam.

The peak kilovoltage of a given x-ray unit determines the total amount of filtration required. Fixed radiographic equipment requires total filtration of 1.5 mm aluminum-equivalent for x-ray units operating from 50 to 70 kVp and 2.5 mm aluminum-equivalent for x-ray units operating above 70 kVp (Fig. 7-10). Mobile diagnostic units and fluoroscopic equipment each require 2.5 mm aluminum-equivalent total permanent filtration.

In diagnostic radiology, aluminum (atomic number 13) is the metal most widely selected as filter material because, without severely decreasing the x-ray beam intensity, it effectively removes low-energy (soft) x-rays from a polyenergetic (heterogeneous) x-ray beam. Also, aluminum is lightweight, sturdy, relatively inexpensive, and readily available.

In compliance with the Radiation Control for Health and Safety Act of

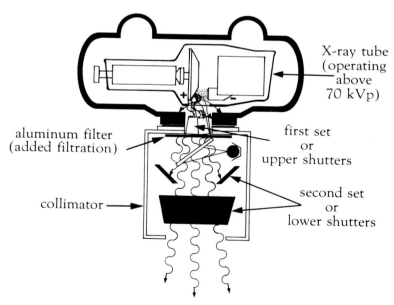

Fig. 7-10   A minimum of 2.5 mm aluminum-equivalent total filtration is required for fixed radiographic units operating above 70 kVp.

1968, a diagnostic x-ray beam must always be adequately filtered.* To verify this, the half-value layer (HVL) of the beam must be measured. HVL may be defined as the thickness of a designated absorber (customarily a metal such as aluminum) required to decrease the intensity (quantity or amount) of the primary beam by 50% of its initial value. This measurement should be obtained by a radiologic physicist at least once a year and also after there have been repairs made on the diagnostic x-ray tube housing or collimation system. For diagnostic x-ray beams, the HVL measurement is obtained and expressed in millimeters of the light metallic element, aluminum (atomic number 13). Because HVL is a measure of beam quality, a certain minimal HVL is required at a given peak kilovoltage. Examples of required HVLs for selective peak kilovoltages are listed in Table 7-1.

GONADAL SHIELDING DEVICES

Gonadal shielding devices are used during radiologic procedures to protect the reproductive organs from exposure to the useful beam when they are in or within close proximity (about 5 cm) of a properly collimated beam. Go-

---

*That is, a sufficient quantity of low-energy photons has been removed from a beam produced at a given peak kilovoltage.

Table 7-1 **HVL Required by the Radiation Control for Health and Safety Act of 1968 and Detailed by the Bureau of Radiological Health* in 1980**

Peak kilovoltage	Required HVL in millimeters of aluminum
30	0.3
40	0.4
50	1.2
60	1.3
70	1.5
80	2.3
90	2.5
100	2.7
110	3.0
120	3.2

*The Bureau of Radiological Health changed in title to the Center for Devices and Radiological Health in 1982.

nadal shielding should be a *secondary* protective measure, *not* a substitute for a *properly* collimated beam. Proper collimation of the radiographic beam (Fig. 7-11) *must always be* the *first step* in gonadal protection.

As a consequence of the anatomical location of the female reproductive organs, these organs receive about three times more exposure during a given radiographic procedure involving the pelvic region than do the male reproductive organs. However, gonadal exposure for both male and female can be greatly reduced through the application of appropriate gonadal shielding. For female patients, the use of a flat contact shield (containing 1 mm of lead) placed over the reproductive organs reduces exposure by about 50%. Primary beam exposure for male patients can be reduced by 90 to 95% through the use of a shaped contact shield (also containing 1 mm of lead). Gonadal shielding should always be used whenever it will not obscure necessary clinical information. Each radiology department should establish a written shielding protocol for each of its radiologic procedures. This contributes to a reduction in the cumulative population gonad dose.

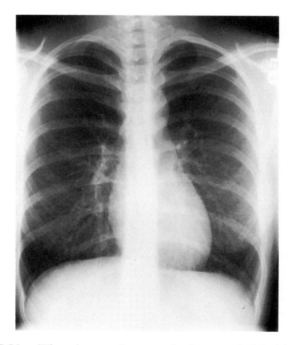

Fig. 7-11   When the gonads are not in the area of clinical interest, proper collimation of the radiographic beam reduces gonadal exposure.

Types of gonadal shielding devices

Four basic types of gonadal shielding devices are used:
1. Flat contact shields.
2. Shadow shields.
3. Shaped contact shields.
4. Clear lead.

Flat contact shields

Flat contact shields are made of lead strips or lead-impregnated materials. These shields can be placed directly over the patient's reproductive organs (Fig. 7-12) or they may be secured to the patient by being taped in place. These shields are most effective when used as protective devices for patients having anteroposterior (AP) or posteroanterior (PA) radiographs while in a recumbent position. Flat contact shields are not well suited for use during fluoroscopy, for nonrecumbent positions, or for projections other than AP or PA.

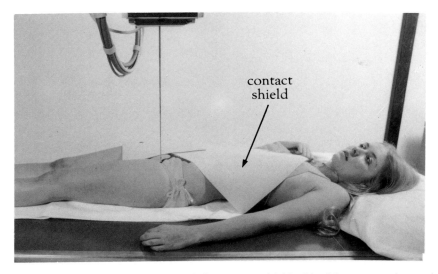

Fig. 7-12 An uncontoured, flat contact shield of lead-impregnated material can be placed over the patient's gonads to provide protection from x-radiation.

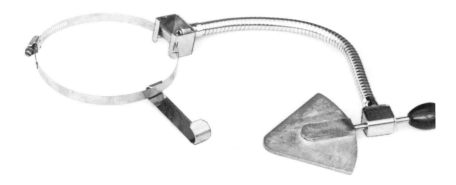

Fig. 7-13 *A,* Shadow shield components.
(Courtesy Nuclear Associates, Carle Place, N.Y.)

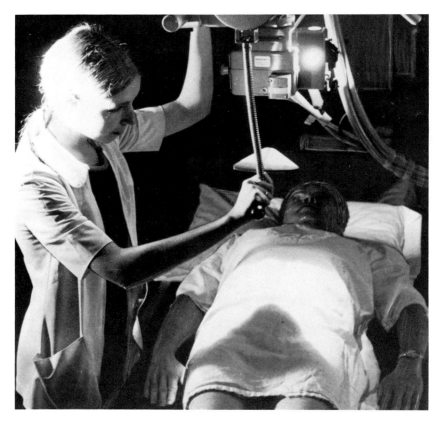

Fig. 7-13 *B,* A shadow shield suspends from above the radiographic beam-defining system and casts a "shadow" over the protected body area, the gonads. (Courtesy Nuclear Associates, Carle Place, N.Y.)

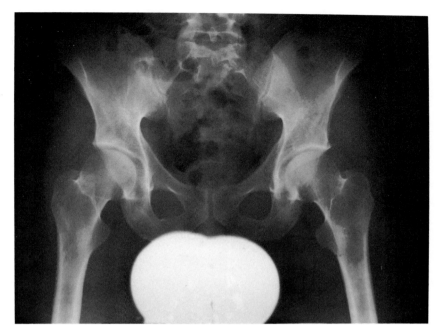

Fig. 7-13, cont'd.   *C*, The radiograph demonstrates effective gonadal shielding resulting from the use of a shadow shield.

Shadow shields

Shadow shields (Fig. 7-13, *A*) are made of a radiopaque material. Suspended from above the radiographic beam-defining system, this shield hangs over the area of clinical interest to cast a shadow in the primary beam over the patient's reproductive organs (Fig. 7-13, *B* and *C*). The beam-defining light casts the shadow of the shield over the anatomy. To ensure proper placement of the shadow shield, the beam-defining light must be accurately positioned. The shadow shield is not suitable for use during fluoroscopy, because there is no localizing light field and the field of view is usually moved about during a study. However, the shadow shield may be used effectively to provide gonad protection in a sterile field or when examining incapacitated patients.

Shaped contact shields

Shaped contact shields are made of radiopaque material contoured to enclose the male reproductive organs. Disposable or washable athletic supporters or jockey style briefs function as carriers for these shields. The carriers each con-

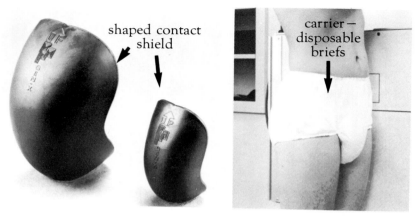

Fig. 7-14 Shaped contact shields (cuplike in shape) can be held in place with the use of a suitable carrier.
(Courtesy Nuclear Associates, Carle Place, N.Y.)

tain a pouch into which the shield is placed (Fig. 7-14). The cuplike shape of the shield permits comfortable placement of the shield over the scrotum and penis whether the patient is in a recumbent or a nonrecumbent position. To ensure privacy and avoid embarrassment, the patient can don the garment containing the shield in the confines of the dressing room.

Because the shaped contact shield is securely held in place by the carrier, AP, oblique, or lateral radiographs may be obtained with maximum gonadal protection. Because it remains in position, this shield is also suitable for use during fluoroscopic examinations. Shaped contact shields are not recommended for use in sterile fields or with incapacitated patients, because problems may occur.

Clear lead

Some of the basic gonadal shielding devices, such as the shaped contact shield and the shadow shield, are being replaced by clear lead gonad and breast shielding (Fig. 7-15). These shields are made of transparent lead-plastic material impregnated with approximately 30% lead by weight. Examples of the gonad and breast shield are provided in Fig. 7-16, *A* and *B,* which demonstrates a full-spinal scoliosis examination. Along with the clear lead gonad and breast shields, a lightweight, fully transparent clear lead filter is incorporated to provide uniform density throughout the spinal canal (Fig. 7-16, *A*).

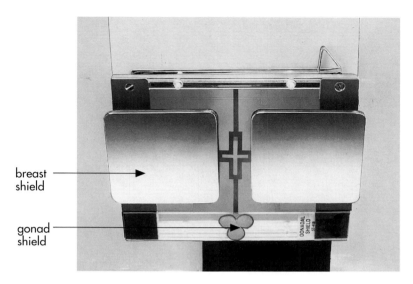

breast
shield

gonad
shield

Fig. 7-15   Clear lead filter with breast and gonad shielding device.
(Courtesy Nuclear Associates, Carle Place, N.Y.)

In summary, effective shielding programs can be established in any facility by providing the appropriate shields. Because substantial gonadal dose
reduction can be achieved through effective shielding, persons possessing reproductive potential should be shielded during radiologic procedures whenever possible. This protective measure minimizes the number of potentially
deleterious x-ray–induced mutations expressed in future generations.

COMPENSATING FILTERS

Dose reduction and uniform radiographic imaging of body parts that vary
considerably in thickness or tissue composition can be accomplished by using compensating filters constructed of aluminum, lead-acrylic, or some
other suitable material. These devices selectively attenuate x-rays that are directed toward the thinner or less dense area while permitting more x-radiation to pass through the thicker or more dense area. For example, the *wedge
filter* (Fig. 7-17) may be used to provide uniform density when radiograph-
ing the foot in the dorsoplantar projection. For this examination the wedge
is positioned with its *thickest* part toward the toes and its *thinnest* part toward the heel. The *trough or bilateral wedge filter*, which is used in some ded-

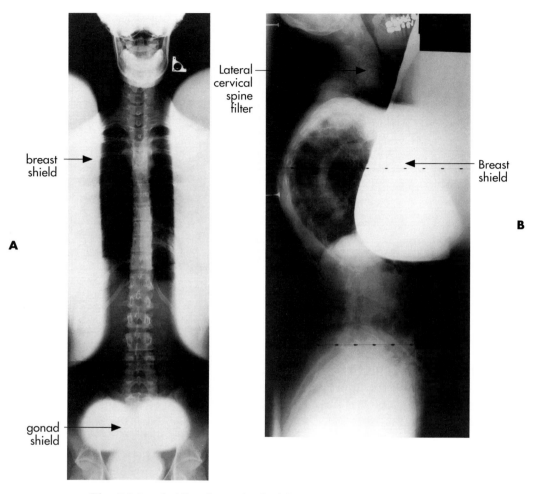

Fig. 7-16 *A,* AP radiograph of a full spine scoliosis examination demonstrating clear lead filter with breast and gonad shields.
(Courtesy Nuclear Associates, Carle Place, N.Y.)
B, Lateral radiograph of full spine scoliosis examination with lateral cervical filter and breast shield.
(Courtesy Nuclear Associates, Carle Place, N.Y.)

icated chest radiographic units, provides another example of a compensating filter. This filter is thin in the center to permit adequate x-ray penetration of the mediastinum and thick laterally to reduce exposure to the aerated lungs. A radiographic image with uniform average density is obtained.

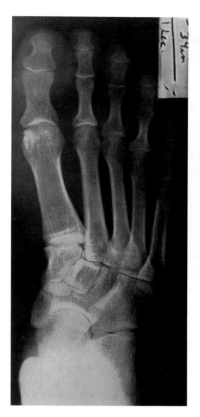
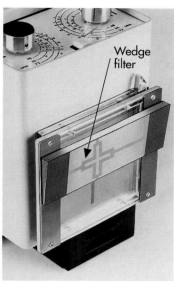

Fig. 7-17 Wedge-shaped clear lead compensating filter used to provide uniform density for a dorsoplantar projection of the foot.
(Courtesy Nuclear Associates, Carle Place, N.Y.)

EXPOSURE FACTORS

Selection of appropriate exposure factors for each radiographic examination is essential to ensure a diagnostic radiograph with minimum patient dose. The technique chosen must ensure sufficient penetration of the area of clinical interest, appropriate film density (exposure), and an adequate amount of radiographic contrast between adjacent tissue densities. The appropriate factors are determined by factors such as (1) the mass per unit volume of tissue of the area of clinical interest, (2) the effective atomic numbers and electron densities of the tissues involved, (3) the film-screen combination, (4) the x-ray SID, (5) the type and quantity of filtration employed, (6) the type of x-ray generator used (single phase or three phase), and (7) the balance of radiographic density and contrast required.

To ensure *uniform* selection of radiographic exposure factors, efficient radiology departments use standardized technique charts for each x-ray unit. It is the responsibility of the radiographer to consult this chart *before* making each radiographic exposure to ensure a diagnostic radiograph with minimum patient dose. Neglecting to use standardized technique charts necessitates exposure factor guesswork, which can result in poor quality radiographs, repeat examinations, and additional, unnecessary exposure for the patient.

Exposure factors that minimize the radiation dose to the patient should be selected whenever possible. The use of higher kilovoltage (kVp) and lower milliamperage and exposure time in seconds (mAs*) reduces patient dose (Fig. 7-18, *A* and *B*). However, this exposure factor combination produces a poorer quality radiograph. As kVp increases and mAs decreases, radiographic contrast is reduced. Consequently, the amount of diagnostically useful information in the image is reduced. To ensure the presence of adequate information in the image and to minimize patient dose, a balance in radiographic exposure factors must be achieved. To achieve this balance, the radiographer must select the *highest* kVp and the *lowest* mAs that will yield sufficient information for each examination (Fig. 7-18, *C*).

RADIOGRAPHIC PROCESSING

Proper radiographic processing enhances image quality by making diagnostic information visible on the finished radiograph. Poorly processed radiographs offer inadequate diagnostic information, necessitating repeat examinations. This results in additional, unnecessary patient exposure.

To ensure standardization in processing techniques, radiology departments should establish a quality assurance program that includes monitoring and maintenance of all processors in the facility. Such a program ensures the production of high-quality radiographs. A number of excellent reviews have been written on this subject. These reviews include step-by-step procedures for performance, monitoring, and quality control.†

---

*mAs (milliampere seconds) is the product of x-ray electron tube current and the amount of time in seconds that the x-ray beam is on.

†Bushong SC: *Radiologic science for technologists: physics, biology and protection*, ed 5, St Louis, 1993, Mosby, pp 203-216.

Gray J et al: *Quality control in diagnostic imaging*, Baltimore, 1983, University Park Press.

Hendee WR, Chaney EL, Rossi RP: *Radiologic physics equipment and quality control*, Chicago, 1977, Year Book Medical Publishers, p 236.

McKinney W: *Radiographic processing and quality control*, Philadelphia, 1988, JB Lippincott.

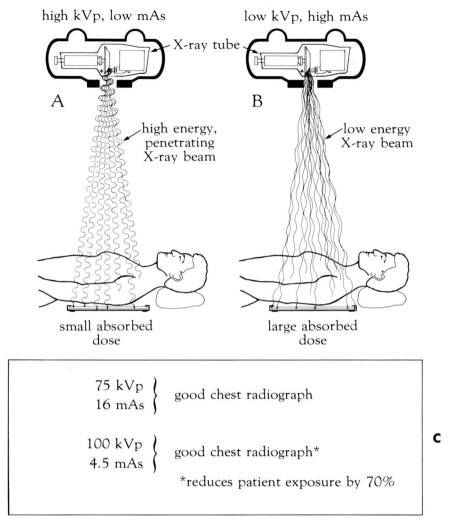

high kVp, low mAs   low kVp, high mAs

X-ray tube

A

high energy,
penetrating
X-ray beam

B

low energy
X-ray beam

small absorbed
dose

large absorbed
dose

75 kVp
16 mAs } good chest radiograph

100 kVp
4.5 mAs } good chest radiograph*

*reduces patient exposure by 70%

C

Fig. 7-18 The use of higher kilovoltage (kVp) and lower milliamperage and exposure time in seconds (mAs) reduces patient dose. *A,* The use of high kVp and low mAs results in a high-energy, penetrating x-ray beam and a small patient absorbed dose. *B,* The use of low kVp and high mAs results in a low-energy x-ray beam, most of which is easily absorbed by the patient. *C,* Example of a higher kVp, lower mAs technique effecting a 70% reduction in patient exposure without significantly compromising radiographic quality.

FILM-SCREEN COMBINATIONS

Choice of film-screen combination affects patient dose. Since high-speed film and screens require *less* x-ray exposure because of their greatly enhanced sensitivity, their use *significantly reduces* patient dose. However, proper radiographic exposure factors must be used to ensure maximum efficiency from the various film-screen combinations. Suggested exposure factors are provided by the manufacturers of film-screen systems and are intended to maximize radiographic quality while minimizing patient dose.

Radiographic film

There are two basic types of radiographic film:
1. nonscreen film (direct exposure film)
2. screen film

Nonscreen film is contained in a cardboard holder or disposable film holder and requires a direct x-ray exposure to produce a latent image. Years ago, this film was used for producing radiographs of relatively thin anatomical areas such as hands and feet. Today, it is seldom used for imaging of such body parts. Imaging can now be accomplished by using single-emulsion film with fine-grain, high-detail screens. When compared with screen film, nonscreen film produces a longer scale of radiographic contrast (more shades of gray in the radiographic image) and, consequently, less radiographic contrast. The use of thicker film emulsion or additional or different chemical dyes increases nonscreen film speed to from two to six times that of screen-type film used without screens.

Screen film is manufactured in different speeds for use with intensifying screens, which enhance the action of x-rays. This film responds mainly to the blue light emitted by calcium tungstate screens or to the green light emitted by rare-earth screens. Film speed influences radiographic exposure time. When the amount of silver bromide crystals contained in the film emulsion is increased, the speed of the film is increased, which means that less radiation exposure is required to obtain an image. As radiographic exposure decreases, patient dose decreases.

Intensifying screens

Intensifying screens accelerate the action of x-rays by converting x-ray energy into visible light. Because a single x-ray photon can produce 80 to 95 light photons, this conversion speeds up the film exposure process. About 95% of the density of the recorded image results from the visible light photons emitted by the intensifying screens. Because more light is emitted from the screens, radiographic exposure can be reduced. This leads to a reduction in patient dose.

Kilovoltage affects screen speed. As kilovoltage increases, screen speed increases. This results in a reduction in patient dose.

When compared to slower speed film-screen combinations, the use of high speed film-screen combinations (with calcium tungstate intensifying screens) drastically reduces patient dose, because less radiation exposure is required to produce a given radiograph. Although the use of high speed film-screen image receptor systems significantly reduces patient dose, it can also result in some loss of radiographic quality, since the recorded image may have poorer resolution. Because of this, the use of high speed film-screen image receptor systems may not be practical for all radiography. To be able to select the appropriate image receptor system for a given radiographic examination, the radiographer must be aware of the capabilities and limitations of the different systems available. Product information of this type can be obtained from manufacturers or distributors.

Rare-earth intensifying screens are more efficient than calcium tungstate intensifying screens in converting x-ray energy into light photons. Made of rare-earth phosphors such as gadolinium, lanthanum, or yttrium, these screens absorb approximately three to five times more x-ray energy than calcium tungstate screens; hence, they emit more light. This results in a significant reduction in the radiographic exposure required to obtain an image of acceptable quality. Because rare-earth screens are from two to ten times as fast as high-speed calcium tungstate screens, their employment may significantly reduce patient dose. An additional benefit of rare-earth screens is that high resolution (the ability of a system to make two adjacent objects visually distinguishable) of the recorded image remains constant. This ensures radiographic quality. Higher speed rare-earth systems do, however, produce quantum mottle (faint blotches) in the recorded image, causing some degradation of the image.

RADIOGRAPHIC GRIDS

When x-rays pass through an object, photons are scattered away from their original path due to coherent and Compton scattering processes. Radiographic quality is *highest* when scattered photons are *not* recorded on the radiograph. If scattered photons *are* recorded, there is a general darkening of the film that detracts from the viewer's ability to distinguish between the different structures of the object being radiographed. Thus, only those photons that have passed through matter with no deviation from their original path should be recorded. To minimize the influence of scattered photons, a "grid" is inserted between the patient and the film. The grid acts as a sieve to block the passage of photons that have been scattered at some angle from their original path (Fig. 7-19).

Grids are made of parallel radiopaque lead strips alternated with radioparent strips of aluminum, plastic, or wood. Because some fraction of the film is covered with lead, mAs must be increased to compensate for the use of the grid. Hence, patient dose *increases* whenever a grid is used. Because more lead is contained in higher ratio grids, patient dose increases as grid ratio increases.

Even though patient dose *increases* with the use of the radiographic

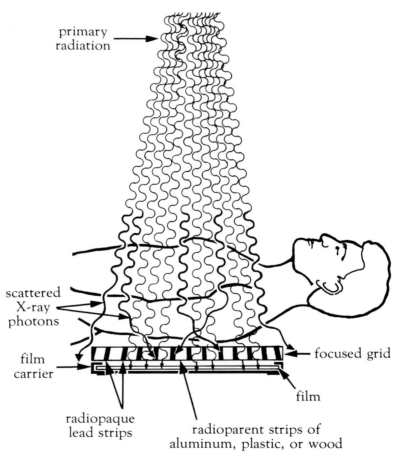

Fig. 7-19   Radiographic grids remove scattered x-ray photons that emerge from the object being radiographed before this scattered radiation reaches the film and decreases radiographic quality.

grid, the benefit obtained (improved radiographic contrast, making available a greater quantity of diagnostic information) makes the use of the grid a fair compromise. However, care must be taken to ensure that the proper type of grid is being used for a particular exam or else a repeat may be necessary, which would negate the benefit of increased image quality.

REPEAT RADIOGRAPHS

The term *repeat radiograph* refers to any radiograph that must be performed more than once because of some human or mechanical error in the process of producing the initial radiograph. This additional exposure increases patient dose. The skin and gonads of the patient receive a double dose whenever a repeat examination occurs. For this reason repeat radiographs must be minimized. An occasional repeat radiograph recommended by the radiologist for the purpose of obtaining additional diagnostic information is permissible. However, repeat examinations resulting from carelessness or poor judgment on the part of the radiographer must be eliminated. The radiographer must select the radiographic techniques and exposure factors that will ensure the production of high-quality radiographs for each examination *the first time.*

Institutions can benefit significantly by implementing and maintaining a repeat analysis program. By determining the number of repeats and the reasons for producing unacceptable radiographs, existing problems and conditions in a Radiology Department can be identified. Repeat analysis studies determine the number of radiographs in a given period of time that must be done more than once because of human or mechanical error. Many categories may be established for discarded radiographs. Among these categories are: radiographs too dark or too light due to inappropriate selection of technique, incorrect patient positioning, improper centering of the radiographic beam, improper collimation, patient motion, and processing artifacts.

The existence of a repeat analysis program in a Radiology Department offers multiple benefits. First, the program increases awareness among staff and student radiographers of the need to produce optimal quality images. Second, radiographers generally become more careful in producing their radiographs because they are aware that the radiographs are being reviewed. Third, when the repeat analysis program identifies problems or concerns, inservice education programs can be designed for radiography personnel to cover the topic of concern.

A repeat analysis program for radiographers can also help to reduce a Radiology Department's repeat volume. A quality control radiographer or other designated person reviews discarded radiographs with coworkers to point out the causes of various repeats. At the very least this should lead to an improvement in technical skills.

UNNECESSARY RADIOLOGIC PROCEDURES

The responsibility for ordering a radiologic examination lies only with the physician. Hence, it becomes his or her responsibility to determine the need for performing any radiologic procedure. To make this decision, the physician must determine whether the benefit to the patient in terms of medical information gained provides sufficient justification to subject that patient to the minimal risk of absorbed radiation dose that will result from the examination.

In the past, some radiographic examinations were performed routinely even though there were no definite medical indications for the examinations. Some of these nonessential radiologic examinations included:

1. A chest x-ray upon scheduled admission to the hospital. This examination should not be performed unless there is some clinical indication of chest disease or other important concern to justify exposing the patient to ionizing radiation. This includes presurgical patients. A panel of physicians appointed by the Food and Drug Administration (FDA)* concluded that a chest x-ray is not necessary for every presurgical patient.

2. A chest x-ray as part of a pre-employment physical. Very little information about previous illness or injury that would be useful to the employer can be gained through this examination.

3. Lumbar spine examinations as part of a pre-employment physical. As with the preemployment chest x-ray, very little information about previous illness or injury that would be useful to the employer can be gained through this examination.

4. Chest x-rays or other unjustified x-rays as part of a routine health check-up. Radiologic procedures should not be performed unless a patient presents symptoms that merit radiologic investigation.

5. Chest x-ray for mass screening for tuberculosis (TB). Such examinations are of little value as a TB testing tool for most people. Testing for TB can be done with more efficient procedures. However, Bushong† indicates that some x-ray screening is still acceptable. This applies to high-risk groups such as members of the medical and para-

---

*FDA Publication No. 86-8265, *Pre-surgical chest x-ray screening examinations,* Superintendent of Documents, U.S. Government Printing Office, Washington, DC.
†Bushong SC: *Radiologic science for technologists: physics, biology and protection,* ed 5, St Louis, 1993, Mosby, pp 647-669.

medical community; people working in occupations, such as educators and food handlers, that could possibly create a health hazard in the community; and in selective groups of workers such as those dealing with materials like asbestos or silica.

MINIMUM SOURCE-SKIN DISTANCE FOR MOBILE RADIOGRAPHY

Mobile radiographic units require special consideration to ensure patient safety. When operating the unit, the radiographer must use a source-skin distance of at least 12 inches (30 cm; Fig. 7-20). The 12 inch distance limits the effects of the inverse square falloff of radiation intensity with distance. This falloff is more pronounced the shorter the source-to-skin distance. When the source-skin distance is *small*, patient entrance exposure is *significantly greater* than exit exposure. Thus, when reasonable techniques are used to obtain an image of midline structures, the entrance surface of the patient receives

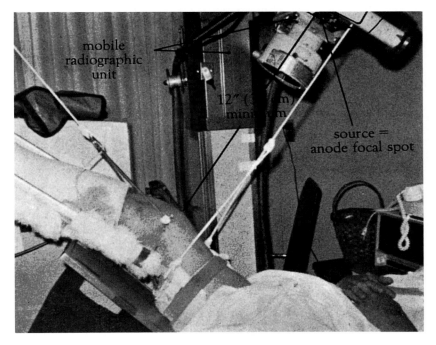

Fig. 7-20 Mobile radiographic examinations require a minimum source-skin distance of 12 inches (30 cm) to limit the effects of the inverse square falloff of radiation intensity with distance.

an unnecessarily high exposure. By increasing source-skin distance, a more uniform distribution of exposure throughout the patient is maintained.

Mobile (portable) units should only be used to perform radiographic procedures on patients who are unable to be transported to a fixed radiographic installation (an x-ray room). They are not designed to take the place of specially designed rooms.

FLUOROSCOPIC PROCEDURES

Fluoroscopic procedures produce the *greatest* patient radiation exposure in diagnostic radiology. In view of this fact, the physician should carefully evaluate the need for a fluoroscopic examination to ascertain whether the potential benefit to the patient in terms of information gained outweighs the potentially adverse somatic or genetic effects of the examination. If the fluoroscopic procedure is necessary, every precaution must be taken to *minimize* patient dose.

Image intensification fluoroscopy

Image intensification fluoroscopy has three significant benefits:
1. Increased image brightness.
2. Saving of time for the radiologist.
3. Patient dose reduction.

The x-ray image intensification system converts the x-ray image pattern into a corresponding amplified visible light pattern. Overall brightness of the fluoroscopic image increases to 7000 times the brightness of the image on a conventional fluoroscopic system operating under the same conditions. This image brightness increase permits the radiologist increased perception of the fluoroscopic image.

Because an image intensification system permits viewing of the fluoroscopic image at ordinary brightness level (regular white light), the radiologist uses photopic or cone vision when viewing the image through this system. Because cone vision can be used, the radiologist does *not* need to go through the process of darkness adaptation; this saves time. Cone vision also considerably improves visual acuity, permitting the radiologist to better discriminate between small fluoroscopic images.

Because an image intensification system significantly increases brightness, image intensification fluoroscopy requires less milliamperage than does conventional fluoroscopy (about 1.5 to 2 mA is required for image intensification systems, whereas 3 to 5 mA is required for conventional fluoroscopy). The consequent decrease in exposure rate results in a reduction in dose for the patient.

Intermittent fluoroscopy

The practice of intermittent fluoroscopy (periodical activation of the fluoroscopic tube by the radiologist rather than lengthy, continuous activation) *significantly* decreases patient dose, especially in long procedures, and helps to extend the life of the tube. Many systems include a "last-image-hold" feature that allows the radiologist to see the most recent image without exposing the patient to another pulse of radiation.

Limitation of the size of the fluoroscopic field

The radiologist must limit the size of the fluoroscopic field to include *only* the area of clinical interest by properly collimating the x-ray beam by adjusting the lead shutters placed between the fluoroscopic tube and the patient. When fluoroscopic field size is limited, patient dose decreases substantially.

Both primary beam length and width need to be confined within the image receptor boundary. Irrespective of the distance from the x-ray source to the image receptor, the useful beam should *not* extend outside the image receptor.

Exposure factors

Proper exposure factors must be selected in fluoroscopic procedures to minimize patient dose. Increases in peak kilovoltage and filtration reduce patient radiation exposure rate. Most fluoroscopic examinations performed with image intensification systems employ a range of from 85 to 120 kVp for adult patients, depending on the area of the body being examined. This optimum peak kilovoltage range produces the proper level of fluoroscopic image brightness. Lower peak kilovoltage results in increased patient dose and reduced brightness of the fluoroscopic image. If lower peak kilovoltage (a less energetic and penetrating x-ray beam) is employed for an adult patient, a higher milliamperage (a larger quantity of x-ray photons in the beam) must be used to provide an adequate exposure. This causes an *increase* in radiation exposure rate leading to an *increase* in patient dose. In addition, to avoid excessive entrance exposure of the patient (see p. 181) and reduce the total exposure of both patient and radiographer, the source-to-tabletop distance must *not* be less than 15 inches (38 cm) for fixed fluoroscopes and *not* less than 12 inches (30 cm) for mobile fluoroscopes. A 12 inch (30 cm) minimum distance is required, but a 15 inch (38 cm) minimum distance is preferred for all image intensification systems.

Exposure factors for fluoroscopic procedures for children necessitate a decrease in peak kilovoltage by as much as 25%. The peak kilovoltage chosen should depend on part thickness just as it does in radiography.

Filtration

The function of a filter in fluoroscopy as in radiographic procedures is to reduce the patient's skin dose. Adequate layers of aluminum-equivalent material placed in the path of the useful beam remove the more harmful lower energy photons from the beam by absorbing them. A minimum of 2.5 mm total aluminum-equivalent filtration must be permanently installed in the path of the useful beam of the fluoroscopic unit. With image intensification systems, a total aluminum-equivalent filtration of 3.0 mm may be preferred. Patient dose decreases by one fourth during fluoroscopic procedures when aluminum filtration increases from 1 mm aluminum to 3 mm aluminum. Although this increase in filtration causes a slight loss of fluoroscopic image brightness, compensation can be made by increasing peak kilovoltage somewhat.

As in radiography, when there is a question of adequate filtration of the x-ray beam, the half-value layer (HVL) of the beam must be measured. In image intensification fluoroscopy, an x-ray beam HVL of 3 mm aluminum is considered acceptable when peak kilovoltage ranges from 90 to 100.

Source-to-tabletop distance

The source-to-tabletop distance must be *not less* than 15 inches (38 cm) for fixed fluoroscopes and *not less* than 12 inches (30 cm) for mobile fluoroscopes. This ensures, as previously discussed (see p. 181), that the entrance surface of the patient does *not* receive excessive exposure. This reduces the exposure of the patient as well as that of the radiographer.

Cumulative timing device

A cumulative timer must be provided and used with each fluoroscopic unit. This device times the x-ray exposure and sounds an audible alarm after the fluoroscope has been activated for 5 minutes. It makes the radiologist aware of the length of time for which the patient receives exposure during each procedure and enables the staff radiographer to determine patient exposure for each fluoroscopic examination. When the fluoroscope is activated for shorter periods of time, the patient and the radiologist and radiographer receive less exposure.

Fluoroscopic unit exposure rate limitation

Current federal standards limit exposure rates of general purpose intensified fluoroscopic units to a maximum of 10 R per minute ($10 \times 2.58 \times 10^{-4}$ C/kg/min), whereas nonintensified units may not exceed 5 R per minute ($5 \times 2.58 \times 10^{-4}$ C/kg/min). Measured at tabletop, these standards have been imposed to give consideration to cumulative small doses of radiation the patient receives throughout a lifetime. Because fluoroscopic procedures result in some of the largest patient doses in diagnostic radiology, fluoroscopic unit exposure rate must be kept within established limits.

C-arm fluoroscopy

C-arm fluoroscopes are frequently used in the operating room for orthopedic procedures (e.g., pinning of a fractured hip). This piece of equipment can be manipulated in almost any position and can be in an energized state for long periods of time to accommodate the surgeon during the procedure. Personnel routinely operating a C-arm fluoroscope or those who are in the immediate area of the unit should wear a protective apron. This garment should be 0.5 mm lead equivalent to ensure adequate protection. Appropriate monitoring of personnel (see Chapter 9) normally involved in C-arm fluoroscopic procedures should be a routine procedure.

Mobile fluoroscopic units are required to have a *minimum* source-to-skin distance of 30 cm. Some type of spacer or frame attachment is usually installed to prevent any part of the patient from violating this minimum distance standard.

Cinefluorography

The techniques that reduce patient dose during fluoroscopy also apply to dose reduction during cinefluorography. In cinefluorography, or cine, a movie camera is used to record the image of the output phosphor of the image intensifier. Dose reduction techniques are especially important in cine, however, because cine procedures tend to result in the *highest* patient doses of all diagnostic procedures. The high dose resulting from cine is due to a relatively high inherent dose rate and the length of the procedure, particularly in cardiology and neuroradiology. Thus, a percentage decrease in cine dose yields greater actual dose reduction than the same percentage decrease in lower dose procedures.

Patient dose may be inferred from tabletop exposure levels. The amount of exposure varies with a number of operator adjustable parameters. Typical cine tabletop exposure is approximately 25 mR/frame for 6 to 7 inch mode. This translates to 45 R/min if a frame rate of 30 frames per second is used. Thus, any limitation of beam-on time is important as long as the efficacy of the procedure is not compromised. Patient exposure increases when a smaller viewing mode (6 inches compared to 9 inches) or a lower speed cine film is used. Exposure increases if the frame rate is increased. For example, switching from a 9 inch to a 6 inch field of view approximately doubles the tabletop exposure rate. If the frame rate is increased from 30 frames per second to 60 frames per second, the exposure rate is doubled. If both adjustments, mode and frame rate, are made at the same time, the exposure rate increases by a factor of four. Other factors, such as image intensifier input phosphor exposure level set by the vendor, grid factor, and source-to-skin distance, play a role in determining typical dose levels for a system.

Collimating to the area of interest has the same effect in cine as in fluoroscopy. Collimation decreases the "integral dose" (product of dose and volume of tissue irradiated) while increasing image quality by reducing scatter.

The radiologist or cardiologist can reduce exposure during cine procedures by limiting the time of the cine run, using fluoroscopy when possible to locate the catheter. When using fluoroscopy, intermittent exposures to verify location and moving the catheter between exposures can limit total fluoroscopy time as well. Some optional equipment features, such as "last-frame-hold," where the most recent fluoroscopic image remains in view as a guide to the radiologist when the x-ray beam is off, also promote lower patient dose.

The typical dose delivered to the patient depends on the procedure. In selective coronary arteriography, most radiation exposure is from the cine. Although the dose rate is lower, the total dose from fluoroscopy may exceed the total dose from cine if the total fluoroscopy time is longer, as is often the case in percutaneous transluminal angioplasty.

PATIENT DOSE

Because more and more people in the United States are undergoing diagnostic radiologic procedures each year, there is great concern about the risk associated with such procedures. It is imperative that risk to patients be reduced whenever possible by employing radiation control practices that ensure safety by minimizing dose.

In general there are three ways that may be used to specify patient dose from diagnostic radiologic procedures: entrance exposure, skin dose, and organ dose. Although each type of specification has significance in estimating the risk to the patient, the entrance exposure is the *most frequently* reported because it is simple to determine.

Skin dose

Thermoluminescent dosimeters (TLD) are the sensing devices *most frequently* used to assess skin dose. The characteristics, components, and function of the TLD are described in Chapter 9.

To assess skin dose a small, relatively thin pack of TLDs is secured to the patient's skin in the middle of the clinical area of interest and is exposed during a radiographic procedure. Because the sensing material in the TLD responds like human tissue when exposed to ionizing radiation, a reasonable determination of dose can be made. Table 1-3 provides a list of permissible skin entrance exposures for various radiographic examinations.

In fluoroscopy, patient dose can be estimated by measuring the radiation exposure rate at tabletop.

Organ dose

Radiation dose absorbed by a specific organ or tissue cannot be measured accurately by a direct method. For examinations in which this dose is of major concern, it can be estimated. For example, breast tissue becomes a critical concern when a mammographic examination is performed. (See Table 1-4 for approximate skin and mean glandular dose per mammographic projection.)

Bone marrow is another organ of major importance because it contains large numbers of stem or precursor blood cells that can be depleted or destroyed by substantial exposure to ionizing radiation. In diagnostic radiology, the mean marrow dose (MMD) can provide a measure of patient absorbed dose even though hematological effects are negligible for doses associated with this discipline. Mean marrow dose may be defined as "the average radiation dose to the entire active bone marrow."† For example, if, in the course of performing a specific radiographic procedure, 25% of the active bone marrow were in the useful beam and received an average absorbed dose of 0.8 mGy (80 mrad), the MMD would be 0.2 mGy (20 mrad).

Bushong states that: "Bone marrow dose is used to estimate the population MMD as an index of the somatic effect of radiation exposure."‡ Table 1-5 provides some typical bone marrow doses for various radiographic exposures. Although each dose listed in the table results from fragmentary exposure of the human body, it is averaged over the whole body.

The possibility of genetic effects occurring as a consequence of exposure to ionizing radiation causes the reproductive organs also to be of concern in diagnostic radiology. Table 1-6 lists some typical gonadal doses from various radiographic examinations. For several examinations identified in the table, there are differences between the dosage received by males and females. Protection of the ovaries by overlying tissue accounts for these differences. In the realm of diagnostic radiology, the relatively low gonadal dose

---

†Bushong SC: *Radiologic science for technologists: physics, biology, and protection,* ed 5, St Louis, 1993, Mosby, p 653.

‡Bushong SC: In Ballinger PW, editor: *Merrill's atlas of radiographic positions and radiologic procedures,* ed 7, vol 1, St Louis, 1991, Mosby, p 27.

for a single human is considered insignificant. However, when the low gonadal dose is applied to the entire population, the dose becomes far more significant. To assess the impact of this dose, the concept of *genetically significant dose (GSD)* is used. GSD is the absorbed dose equivalent to the reproductive organs that, if received by every human, would be expected to bring about an identical gross genetic injury to the total population as does the sum of the actual doses received by exposed individual population members. In other words, if there were a maximum of 500 people inhabiting the earth and each person received an absorbed dose equivalent of 0.005 Sv (0.5 rem) gonadal radiation, the gross genetic effect would be identical to the effect occurring when 50 individual inhabitants each receive 0.05 Sv (5 rem) of gonadal radiation and no absorbed dose equivalent is received by the other 450 inhabitants. In simple terms, the GSD concept suggests that the consequences of substantial absorbed doses of gonadal radiation become significantly less when averaged over an entire population rather than when applied to just a few of its members.

The GSD takes into consideration the fact that some people receive radiation to their reproductive organs during a given year whereas others do not. Also, it takes into account that there is no genetic impact from population members who cannot bear children and from those who are beyond reproductive years. Hence, the GSD is the average annual gonadal absorbed dose equivalent to members of the population who are of childbearing age. It includes the number of children who may be expected to be conceived by members of the exposed population in a given year. The estimated GSD for the population of the United States is about 0.2 mSv (20 mrem).

Fetal dose

It is only possible to estimate fetal dose. This is customarily obtained from phantom measurements or computer-generated calculations. Table 1-7 lists typical fetal doses as a function of the normalized skin exposure. To determine fetal dose according to this table, the reader must first determine the entrance exposure for the radiologic procedure of choice. The fetal dose is given in millirads per roentgen of entrance exposure.§

When the primary x-ray beam passes through the uterus, as it does during radiography of the abdomen or pelvis, fetal dose is highest. However, it is significantly lower when the diagnostic x-ray beam is directed toward a part of the body away from the lower trunk (i.e., head, feet).

---

§Bushong SC: In Ballinger PW, editor: *Merrill's atlas of radiographic positions and radiologic procedures,* ed 7, vol 1, St Louis, 1991, Mosby, p 27.

OTHER IMPORTANT DIAGNOSTIC EXAMINATIONS AND IMAGING MODALITIES
Patient dose in mammography

Mammography can detect breast cancer when it is so small that it is nonpalpable. There is still some concern, however, in certain quarters as to whether the benefit to the patient in terms of detection of early breast cancer from routine screening outweighs the small risk of causing a radiogenic cancer in the future. However, compared with the natural incidence of breast cancer occurring in women, the risk of developing a radiogenic breast cancer years after the diagnostic x-ray examination is miniscule. When breast cancer is detected early with mammography, there is a 90 to 95% chance for survival. Without mammography, if early breast cancer is present and goes unnoticed, the chance for survival decreases considerably. Another benefit to the patient of early detection of breast cancer is when the cancer is still in the pre-lump stage. This gives the patient more treatment options. Frequently, instead of having to undergo a radical mastectomy (complete surgical removal of the breast and axillary lymph nodes), the patient may be able to choose a combination of radiation therapy and a lumpectomy (surgical removal of the malignant growth and a minimum amount of surrounding tissue).

Radiographic techniques employed for mammographic examinations have changed drastically over the last decade, resulting in a significant decrease in glandular dose. Direct exposure examinations, which yield a high skin and glandular dose per projection (see Table 1-4), are obsolete. Both xeromammography and screen-film mammography techniques provide acceptable skin and glandular doses per projection (see Table 1-4). Screen-film mammography yields the lowest skin and glandular dose when compared with xeroradiography or direct exposure techniques (see Table 1-4).

Because breast cancer is the primary cause of cancer death in women, the authors support the mammography screening guidelines recommended by the American Cancer Society in 1984. These guidelines include yearly mammography "for asymptomatic women age 50 and over, and a baseline mammogram for those 35 to 39. Women 40 to 49 should have mammography every 1 to 2 years, depending on physical and mammographic findings as well as other risk factors. In addition a professional breast examination is recommended every three years for women 20 to 40, and every year for those over 40."*

---

*American Cancer Society: *Cancer facts and figures,* 1984.

Patient dose in computed tomography

As defined by Johnson and Rowberg in volume 3 of *Merrill's Atlas of Radiographic Positions and Radiologic Procedures* by Ballinger, "CT is the process of creating a cross-sectional tomographic plane (slice) of any part of the body. The image then is reconstructed by a computer using x-ray absorption measurements collected at multiple points about the periphery of the part being scanned." Although a discussion of CT equipment, function, and procedure is not within the scope of this text, patient dose resulting from exposure to ionizing radiation is relevant because CT is a frequently employed diagnostic x-ray imaging modality.

There are two patient dose concerns when performing CT scanning. One concern is the skin dose, and the other is the dose distribution during the scanning procedure. When compared with any routine radiographic projection of the adult cranium or a single anteroposterior projection of the abdomen, the entrance exposure received by the patient after a succession of adjacent scans is greater than the entrance exposure from an individual x-ray projection. However, when a patient undergoes an ordinary but complicated x-ray examination, many radiographs involving different projections are obtained. If the doses from this extensive radiographic series were added together, the sum would be comparable to the dose from a CT examination. There is still another consideration. CT examinations generally expose a smaller mass of tissue than that which would be exposed when an ordinary x-ray series is performed. The reason for this is that the CT x-ray beam is more tightly collimated than is the conventional radiographic beam. The entrance exposure from a CT examination may also be compared with the entrance exposure received during a routine fluoroscopic examination. In this instance, the entrance exposure received during a CT examination would be less than that received during a routine fluoroscopic procedure.

The dose distribution resulting from a CT scan is not the same as the dose distribution occurring in routine radiologic procedures. Because CT scanners use an x-ray beam that is tightly collimated, the amount of scatter radiation generated is lower than the scatter produced by the less tightly collimated radiographic beam. Because CT scanners collimate the x-ray beam so well, the mass of human tissue exposed to radiation falls off rapidly outside the plane of concern during the production of any given scan. Although only one slice is exposed and imaged at a time, there is some overlap of the margins of the x-ray beam when each single tomographic section is made. Also when adjacent slices are obtained, some radiation scatters from the slice being made into the adjacent slices (interslice scatter). Both of these contribute to dose increase and are why a succession of adjacent tomographic sections (slices) imparts a higher absorbed dose than would a single tomographic section.

Bushong* identifies average skin dose ranges from scans of the cranial region to be from 0.5 to 3 rad (5 to 30 mGy) and dose ranges for scans of the body to be from 1 to 6 rad (10 to 60 mGy).* Actual doses delivered during any CT scanning procedure depend on the type of scanner being used and the radiation technique selected.

PEDIATRIC CONSIDERATIONS

When considering the potential for biological damage from exposure to ionizing radiation, children are more vulnerable to both the late somatic effects and the genetic effects of radiation than are adults. Hence, children require special consideration when undergoing diagnostic radiologic studies. Appropriate radiation protection methods must be used for each procedure.

Because children have a greater life expectancy, they may easily survive long enough to develop a leukemia induced by radiation or develop a radiogenic malignancy such as lung or thyroid cancer. In fact, according to studies published by Beebe and others in 1978,** the risk of a radiation-induced leukemia in children after a substantial dose of ionizing radiation is about two times that of the adult. For low doses such as those encountered in diagnostic radiology, data are still inconclusive (see Chapter 6 for further information). With this consideration in mind, it is prudent to take every precaution to minimize exposure to all pediatric patients.

In general, smaller doses of ionizing radiation suffice to obtain useful images in pediatric radiologic procedures than are necessary for adult radiologic procedures. For example, an entrance exposure below 5 mR† will result from an AP projection of an infant's chest, whereas the same projection or a PA projection of an adult's chest will yield an entrance exposure ranging from 12 to 26 mR (see Table 1-3).

Patient motion is frequently a problem encountered in diagnostic pediatric radiography. Because of the limited ability of children to understand the radiologic procedure and, in most cases, their limited ability to cooperate, children are less likely to remain still during a radiographic

---

*Bushong SC: *Radiologic science for technologists: physics, biology, and protection,* ed 5, St Louis, 1993, Mosby, p 658.
**Beebe GW, Kato H, Land CE: Studies of the mortality of A-bomb survivors. 6. Mortality and radiation dose, 1950-1974, *Radiat Res* 75:138, 1978.
†National Council on Radiation Protection and Measurements (NCRP): Report No. 68, *Radiation protection in pediatric radiology,* Washington, DC, 1981, NCRP Publications, p 7.

or fluoroscopic exposure. To solve or at least minimize this problem, the radiographer must use effective immobilization techniques. For some examinations, such as chest radiography, special pediatric immobilization devices are available to hold the pediatric patient securely and safely in the required position, thus providing adequate immobilization. The employment of such techniques along with the use of appropriate radiographic or fluoroscopic exposure factors and proper processing techniques greatly reduces or eliminates the need for repeat examinations that increase patient dose.

Essentially, the same patient protection methods used to reduce the radiation exposure for adults may be employed to reduce the radiation exposure for pediatric patients. Hence, in general, the techniques discussed in this chapter may be applied to meet the needs of the infant or child.

SPECIAL PRECAUTIONS EMPLOYED IN MEDICAL RADIOGRAPHY TO PROTECT THE PREGNANT OR POTENTIALLY PREGNANT PATIENT

Because there is evidence that the developing embryo or fetus is especially radiation sensitive, special care is taken in medical radiography to prevent unnecessary exposure of the abdominal area of pregnant females. Unfortunately, most women are not aware that they are pregnant during the earliest stage of pregnancy so that there is concern over the exposure of the abdominal area of *potentially* pregnant (i.e., fertile) women. In 1970, the International Commission on Radiation Protection (ICRP)* proposed a "10-day rule." This rule is based on the low degree of probability that a woman would be pregnant during the first 10 days after the onset of menstruation and suggests that abdominal x-ray exams of fertile women be postponed until sometime during the first 10 days after the onset of the next menstruation if the results of the exam are not of importance in connection with an immediate illness. However, such scheduling is difficult in practice to achieve in many Radiology Departments where there is likely to be little sustained contact among the radiologist, the referring physician, and the patient. Because most fertile women are *not* pregnant at any given time, the 10-day rule can result in *unnecessary postponement* of exams for the *majority* of female patients. For the above reasons, the 10-day rule is not used in many large Radiology Departments. It is the official position of the American College of Radiology (ACR), the major professional organization of radiologists in the United States, that "abdominal radiological exams that have been requested

---

*International Commission on Radiation Protection: Publication no. 16, *Protection of the patient in x-ray diagnosis,* Oxford, England, 1970, Pergamon Press.

after *full* consideration of the clinical status of the patient including the possibility of pregnancy need *not* be postponed or selectively scheduled."†

In the event that a pregnant patient is inadvertently irradiated, a radiological physicist should perform the calculations necessary to determine fetal exposure. This may include the taking of measurements using phantoms to simulate the patient and the use of ion chambers to record exposure. The question sometimes arises: Should a therapeutic abortion be performed to prevent the birth of an infant because of radiation exposure during pregnancy? Studies of groups such as the atom bomb survivors of Hiroshima have shown that damage to the newborn is *unlikely* for doses *below* 20 rad. Most medical procedures would result in fetal exposures of less than 1 rad so that the risk of abnormality is small. The National Council on Radiation Protection and Measurements states that:

> This risk is considered to be negligible at 5 rad or less when compared to the other risks of pregnancy, and the risk of malformations is significantly increased above control levels only at doses above 15 rad. Therefore, the exposure of the fetus to radiation arising from diagnostic procedures would very rarely be cause, by itself, for terminating a pregnancy. If there are reasons, other than the possible radiation effects, to consider a therapeutic abortion, such reasons should be discussed with the patient by the attending physician, so that it is clear that the radiation exposure is not being used as an excuse for terminating the pregnancy.‡

If the physician feels it is in the *best interests* of a pregnant or potentially pregnant patient to undergo a radiologic examination, the examination *should be performed* without delay. Under such circumstances, special efforts should be made to *minimize* the dose of radiation received by the patient's lower abdomen and pelvic region. This can be accomplished by selecting technical exposure factors that are appropriate for the examination (i.e., by using the smallest exposure that will generate a diagnostically useful radiograph) and by adequately collimating the radiographic beam to include only the anatomical area of interest. When the patient's lower abdomen and pelvic region does not have to be included in the area to be irradiated, it should be protected with a lead apron (Fig. 7-21) so that a developing embryo or fetus does not receive unnecessary radiation exposure.

SUMMARY

This chapter has described the need for protecting the patient during diagnostic radiologic procedures and the various tools and techniques used there-

---

†Reynold FB: Prepared remarks for the October 20, 1976, American College of Radiology press conference.

‡National Council on Radiation Protection and Measurements (NCRP): Report #54, *Medical exposure of pregnant and potentially pregnant women*, Washington, DC, 1977, NCRP Publications.

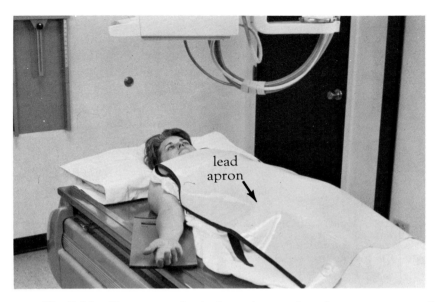

Fig. 7-21   To protect a developing embryo or fetus from unnecessary radiation exposure, place a lead apron over the female patient's lower abdomen and pelvic region when it does not have to be included in the area to be irradiated.

in. The reader should be able to explain the need for effective communication between the patient and the radiographer and discuss the significance of adequate immobilization of the patient. In addition, the reader should be able to identify the various beam-limiting devices, explain the function of filtration, discuss the reason for using gonadal shielding during radiologic procedures, identify the various types of shields available, describe half-value layer and give examples of HVLs for selective peak kilovoltages, and discuss how radiographic exposure factors can be adjusted to reduce patient dose. The various methods of reducing patient exposure during radiographic and fluoroscopic procedures have been described in detail. The reader should be capable of discussing this subject matter. The importance of a repeat analysis program has been described. The reader should be able to identify the consequences of repeat radiographs and the benefits of a repeat analysis program. Finally, special precautions to be employed in medical radiography to protect the pregnant or potentially pregnant patient have been explained. The reader should be able to discuss patient dose considerations and identify appropriate radiation protection measures for such patients.

REVIEW QUESTIONS

1. The number of repeat radiographs in a radiology department can be reduced by:
   a. effective communication between the patient and the radiographer
   b. eliminating voluntary patient motion through adequate immobilization
   c. careful and appropriate selection of radiation exposure factors by the radiographer
   d. all of the above

2. Which of the following is *not* a beam limitation device?
   a. filter
   b. aperture diaphragm
   c. cone
   d. collimator

3. Patient exposure resulting from off-focus radiation can be reduced by:
   a. placing the second pair of shutters in the collimator below the level of the light source and mirror
   b. placing the first pair of shutters in the collimator as close as possible to the tube window
   c. transmitting an electric signal through the collimator's first and second pair of shutters
   d. off-focus radiation in a collimator cannot be reduced

4. The radiographic beam should be collimated so that it is:
   a. slightly larger than the image receptor
   b. no larger than the image receptor
   c. twice as large as the image receptor
   d. four times as large as the image receptor

5. The function of filtration in diagnostic radiologic procedures is to:
   a. decrease beam hardness, thereby reducing patient skin dose
   b. increase beam hardness, thereby reducing patient skin dose
   c. eliminate short wavelength radiation to reduce patient dose
   d. increase beam hardness, thereby increasing patient skin dose

6. A fixed radiographic unit operating at 90 kVp would require:
   a. 1.0 mm aluminum-equivalent total filtration
   b. 1.5 mm aluminum-equivalent total filtration
   c. 2.0 mm aluminum-equivalent total filtration
   d. 2.5 mm aluminum-equivalent total filtration

7. The first step in providing gonadal protection for a patient during a radiographic exposure of the chest must be:
   a. place a lead shield over the reproductive organs
   b. increase total aluminum filtration to 5.0 mm
   c. properly collimate the radiographic beam to include only the area of clinical interest
   d. always use a grid cassette with a 16:1 ratio

8. Which of the following types of gonadal shielding would provide the *best* protection for a male patient during most radiologic procedures?
   a. flat contact shield containing 1 mm of lead
   b. shadow shield
   c. shaped contact shield containing 1 mm of lead
   d. none of the above

9. Which of the following combinations of exposure factors would reduce patient radiation dose during a radiographic examination?
   a. lower kVp, higher mAs, decreased filtration
   b. higher kVp, lower mAs, increased filtration
   c. higher kVp, higher mAs, decreased filtration
   d. lower kVp, lower mAs, increased filtration

10. Patient dose *decreases* when:
    a. high-speed radiographic film is used in combination with high-speed calcium tungstate intensifying screens
    b. rare-earth intensifying screens and appropriate radiographic film are used
    c. higher kVp techniques are used
    d. all of the above

11. Which of the following result in an *increase* in patient dose?
    a. using a radiographic grid
    b. using proper radiographic processing techniques
    c. using a rare-earth intensifying screen with appropriate radiographic film rather than using a high-speed calcium tungstate intensifying screen with appropriate film
    d. using the highest practicable kVp with the lowest possible mAs for each examination

12. To reduce the radiation exposure rate and thereby reduce patient dose when operating a mobile radiographic unit, the radiographer must use a *minimum* source-skin distance of:
    a. 6 inches (15 cm)
    b. 12 inches (30 cm)
    c. 15 inches (38 cm)
    d. 18 inches (45 cm)

13. Which of the following examinations yields the *highest* patient dose?
    a. multiple radiographs of the hand done with a properly collimated x-ray beam
    b. PA and lateral chest radiographs on an adult patient
    c. skull radiographs
    d. fluoroscopy of an adult patient's chest

14. When a fluoroscopic image is electronically amplified by an image intensification system, certain benefits result. These benefits are:
    a. increased image brightness
    b. saving of time for the radiologist
    c. patient dose reduction
    d. all of the above

15. Patient dose *decreases* and the life of the fluoroscopic tube *increases* when the radiologist uses the practice of:
    a. restricting the size of the fluoroscopic field to include only the area of clinical interest
    b. conventional fluoroscopy rather than image intensification
    c. intermittent fluoroscopy
    d. darkness adaptation

16. The function of a filter in diagnostic radiology is to:
    a. permit only alpha rays to reach the patient's skin
    b. remove alpha particles from the x-ray beam
    c. decrease the radiation dose to the patient's skin
    d. permit only beta particles to interact with the atoms of the patient's body

17. Federal government specifications recommend a *minimum* total aluminum-equivalent filtration of _____ for fluoroscopic units.
    a. 1.0 mm aluminum-equivalent
    b. 1.5 mm aluminum-equivalent
    c. 2.0 mm aluminum-equivalent
    d. 2.5 mm aluminum-equivalent

18. Image intensifier fluoroscopic systems require a source-table-top distance of at least _____ but prefer a distance of not less than _____ .
    a. 6 inches (15 cm), 12 inches (30 cm)
    b. 12 inches (30 cm), 15 inches (38 cm)
    c. 15 inches (38 cm), 18 inches (45 cm)
    d. 9 inches (23 cm), 12 inches (30 cm)

19. Current federal standards limit general purpose intensified fluoroscopic unit exposure rate to a maximum of:
    a. 5 R/min
    b. 10 R/min

       c. 15 R/min
       d. 20 R/min

20. During fluoroscopy, to decrease patient dose by one fourth:
    a. increase filtration from 1 mm aluminum to 3 mm aluminum
    b. increase filtration from 1 mm aluminum to 5 mm aluminum
    c. decrease filtration from 1 mm aluminum to ½ mm aluminum
    d. completely remove all aluminum filtration from the path of the x-ray beam

21. When the radiologist limits fluoroscopic field size to include only the area of
    clinical interest:
    a. exposure factors must be increased significantly to provide adequate compen-
       sation
    b. patient dose decreases significantly
    c. patient dose increases somewhat
    d. patient dose remains the same

22. Repeat radiographs result in:
    a. a double dose of radiation to the patient's skin and gonads
    b. no additional exposure for the patient
    c. ten times more exposure for the patient
    d. none of the above

23. To protect the patient's skin from exposure to electrons produced by photon inter-
    action with the collimator, the skin surface should be at least _____
    below the collimator.
    a. 6 cm
    b. 12 cm
    c. 15 cm
    d. 20 cm

24. Greater beam limitation is achieved when the cone or cylinder is _____
    and the diameter of the opening is _____ .
    a. shorter, smaller
    b. longer, bigger
    c. shorter, bigger
    d. longer, smaller

25. Which of the following is the *most* versatile type of x-ray beam limitation de-
    vice?
    a. cylinder
    b. collimator
    c. cone
    d. aperture diaphragm

26. Both alignment and length and width dimensions of the radiographic and light beams must correspond to within:
    a. 1% of the SID
    b. 2% of the SID
    c. 5% of the SID
    d. 10% of the SID

27. HVL may be defined as the thickness of a designated absorber required to:
    a. increase the intensity of the primary beam by 50% of its initial value
    b. increase the intensity of the primary beam by 25% of its initial value
    c. decrease the intensity of the primary beam by 50% of its initial value
    d. decrease the intensity of the primary beam by 25% of its initial value

28. Any radiograph that must be done more than once because of human or mechanical error in the process of producing the initial radiograph is termed a:
    a. blooper
    b. double exposure
    c. practice exposure
    d. repeat

29. The source-to-tabletop distance must not be less than _____ for fixed fluoroscopes and not less than _____ for mobile fluoroscopes to ensure that the entrance surface of the patient does not receive excessive exposure.
    a. 15 inches (38 cm), 12 inches (30 cm)
    b. 12 inches (30 cm), 6 inches (15 cm)
    c. 15 inches (38 cm), 9 inches (23 cm)
    d. 18 inches (45 cm), 15 inches (38 cm)

30. Which of the following are considered to be benefits of a repeat analysis program?
    1. increased awareness among staff and student radiographers of the need to produce optimal quality images
    2. radiographers become more careful in producing the radiographs because they are aware that the radiographs are being reviewed
    3. when problems or concerns are identified, in-service education programs can be designed for radiography personnel to cover the topic of concern
    a. 1 only
    b. 2 only
    c. 3 only
    d. 1, 2, and 3

31. A cumulative timing device times the x-ray exposure and sounds an audible alarm after the fluoroscope has been activated for:
    a. 1 minute
    b. 3 minutes

     c. 5 minutes
     d. 10 minutes

32. Skin dose is *most frequently* assessed by using:
     a. thermoluminescent dosimeters
     b. filtration equivalent to 4.0 mm aluminum in the path of the beam
     c. no filtration in the path of the beam
     d. extension cylinders

33. The genetically significant dose (GSD) for the population of the United States
    is about:
     a. 100 mrem
     b. 80 mrem
     c. 40 mrem
     d. 20 mrem

34. Three of the radiographic procedures listed below may be considered unneces-
    sary. Which procedure does *not* fall into this category?
     a. lumbar spine x-rays as part of a pre-employment physical
     b. cervical spine x-rays after neck trauma from a motor vehicle accident
     c. chest x-ray as part of a routine health check-up
     d. chest X-ray upon scheduled admission to the hospital for a patient who has
        no clinical indication of chest disease or other problems associated with the
        chest

35. Which radiographic technique employed for mammography yields the *lowest*
    skin and glandular dose?
     a. direct exposure
     b. screen-film
     c. xeroradiography
     d. none of the above

36. Interslice scatter during a CT scanning procedure results in:
     a. a uniform distribution of dose into all adjacent areas
     b. a poorly defined cross-sectional image of the anatomy
     c. an increase in patient dose
     d. a decrease in patient dose

37. Pediatric patients require special consideration and appropriate radiation protec-
    tion procedures because they are more vulnerable to:
     a. both the late somatic effects and the genetic effects of radiation
     b. only the late somatic effects of radiation
     c. only the genetic effects of radiation
     d. only the early somatic effects of radiation

38. In image intensification fluoroscopy, an x-ray beam half-value layer of 3 mm aluminum is considered acceptable when peak kilovoltage ranges from:
    a. 50 to 70
    b. 70 to 80
    c. 80 to 90
    d. 90 to 100

39. It is preferable that the radiologic examination of the lower abdomen or pelvis of a fertile woman be limited to the _____ whenever possible.
    a. earliest part of the menstrual cycle
    b. middle of the menstrual cycle
    c. end of the menstrual cycle
    d. time of the menstrual cycle when ovulation occurs

40. When a pregnant patient must undergo a radiographic examination, radiation exposure can be minimized by:
    a. selecting technical exposure factors that are appropriate for the part of the body to be radiographed
    b. opening the x-ray beam collimator as wide as possible to ensure adequate coverage of the image receptor
    c. adequately collimating the x-ray beam to include only the anatomical area of interest and shielding the lower abdomen and pelvis when this area does not need to be included in the area to be irradiated
    d. a and c

Bibliography

American Cancer Society: *Cancer facts and figures,* 1984.

Ballinger PW: *Merrill's atlas of radiographic positions and radiologic procedures,* ed 5, vol 1, St Louis, 1982, Mosby–Year Book.

Beebe GW et al: Studies of the mortality of A-bomb survivors. 6. Mortality and radiation dose, 1950–1974, *Radiat Res* 75:138, 1978.

Brown RF: Prepared remarks for the October 20, 1976, American College of Radiology press conference.

Bushong S: *Radiologic science for technologists: physics, biology, and protection,* ed 2, St Louis, 1980, Mosby–Year Book.

Bushong SC: In Ballinger PW, editor: *Merrill's atlas of radiographic positions and radiologic procedures,* ed 7, vol 1, St Louis, 1991, Mosby–Year Book, p 18.

Bushong SC: *Radiologic science for technologists: physics, biology, and protection,* ed 5, St Louis, 1993, Mosby–Year Book.

Christensen EE, Curry III TS, Dowdey JE: *An introduction to the physics of diagnostic radiology,* ed 2, Philadelphia, 1978, Lea & Febiger.

Cullinan JE, Cullinan AM: *Illustrated guide to x-ray technics,* ed 2, Philadelphia, 1980, JB Lippincott.

Curry III, TS, Dowdey JE, Murry Jr RC: *Christensen's introduction to the physics of diagnostic radiology,* ed 3, Philadelphia, 1984, Lea & Febiger.

Donohue DP: *An analysis of radiographic quality: lab manual and workbook,* Baltimore, 1980, University Park Press.

Donohue DP: *An analysis of radiographic quality: lab manual and workbook,* ed 2, Rockville, MD, 1984, Aspen.

Dorst JP et al: In Ballinger PW, editor: *Merrill's atlas of radiographic positions and radiologic procedures,* ed 7, vol 3, St Louis, 1991, Mosby–Year Book, p 1.

Eddy DM et al: The value of mammography

screening in women under age 50 years, *JAMA* 259(10):1512, 1988.

Frankel R: *Radiation protection for radiologic technologists,* New York, 1976, McGraw-Hill.

Hendee WR, editor: *Health effects of low-level radiation,* Norwalk, CT, 1984, Appleton-Century-Crofts.

International Commission on Radiation Protection: Publication no. 16, *Protection of the patient in x-ray diagnosis,* Oxford, England, 1970, Pergamon Press.

Jayaraman S et al: Analysis of radiation risk versus benefit in mammography, *Applied Radiology* Mar/Apr:45, 1986.

Johnson KC, Rowberg AH: In Ballinger PW, editor: *Merrill's atlas of radiographic positions and radiologic procedures,* ed 7, vol 3, St Louis, 1991, Mosby–Year Book, p 249.

Malott JC, Fodor III, J: *The art and science of medical radiography,* ed 7, St Louis, 1993, Mosby–Year Book.

National Council on Radiation Protection and Measurements (NCRP): Report #33, *Medical x-ray and gamma-ray protection for energies up to 10 MeV: equipment design and use,* Washington, DC, 1968, NCRP Publications.

National Council on Radiation Protection and Measurements (NCRP): Report #39, *Basic radiation protection criteria,* Washington, DC, 1971, NCRP Publications.

National Council on Radiation Protection and Measurements (NCRP): Report #54, *Medical exposure of pregnant and potentially pregnant women,* Washington, DC, 1977, NCRP Publications.

National Council on Radiation Protection and Measurements (NCRP): Report #68, *Radiation protection in pediatric radiology,* Washington, DC, 1981, NCRP Publications.

National Council on Radiation Protection and Measurements (NCRP): Report #91, *Recommendations on limits for exposure to ionizing radiation,* Bethesda, MD, 1987, NCRP Publications.

Noz ME, Maguire Jr GQ: *Radiation protection in the radiologic and health sciences,* Philadelphia, 1979, Lea & Febiger.

Noz ME, Maguire Jr GQ: *Radiation protection in radiologic and health sciences,* ed 2, Philadelphia, 1985, Lea & Febiger.

Olsen JO: In Ballinger PW, editor: *Merrill's atlas of radiographic positions and radiologic procedures,* ed

7, vol 3, St Louis, 1991, Mosby–Year Book, p 53.

Ritenour ER: *Radiation protection and biology, a self-instructional multimedia learning series, instructor manual,* Denver, 1985, Multi-Media Publishing.

Scheele RV, Wakley J: *Elements of radiation protection,* Springfield, IL, 1975, Charles C Thomas.

Selman J: *The fundamentals of x-ray and radium physics,* ed 6, Springfield, IL, 1978, Charles C Thomas.

Selman J: *The fundamentals of x-ray and radium physics,* ed 7, Springfield, IL, 1985, Charles C Thomas.

Statkiewicz MA: Communication skills for the radiologic technologist, *Radiol Technol* 54:449, 1983.

Thomas CL, editor: *Taber's cyclopedic medical dictionary,* ed 13, Philadelphia, 1973, FA Davis.

Travis EL: *Primer of medical radiobiology,* ed 2, Chicago, 1989, Year Book Medical Publishers.

Thompson TT: *Cahoon's formulating x-ray techniques,* ed 9, Durham, NC, 1979, Duke University Press.

Thompson TT: *A practical approach to modern imaging equipment,* ed 2, Boston, 1985, Little, Brown.

US Department of Health and Human Services (HHS), Public Health Service, Food and Drug Administration, Bureau of Radiological Health: *The correlated lecture laboratory series in diagnostic radiological physics,* HHS Publication FDA 81-8150. Rockville, MD, 1981, HHS.

US Department of Health, Education, and Welfare (HEW), Public Health Service, Food and Drug Administration, Bureau of Radiological Health: *Gonadal shielding in diagnostic radiology,* HEW Publication FDA 75-8024, Rockville, MD, June 1975, HEW.

US Department of Health, Education, and Welfare (HEW), Public Health Service, Food and Drug Administration, Bureau of Radiological Health: *Analysis of retakes: understanding, managing, and using an analysis of retakes program for quality assurance,* HEW Publication FDA 79-8097, Rockville, MD, Aug 1979, HEW.

US Department of Health, Education, and Welfare (HEW), Public Health Service, Food and Drug Administration, Bureau of Radiological Health: *Quality assurance programs for diagnostic radiology facilities,* HEW Publication FDA 80-80-1110, Rockville, MD, Feb 1980, HEW.

US Department of Health, Education, and Welfare (HEW), Public Health Service, Food and Drug Administration, Bureau of Radiological Health: *The selection of patients for x-ray examinations,* HEW Publication FDA 80-8104, Rockville, MD, Jan 1980, HEW.

US Government Printing Office: *Pre-surgical chest x-ray screening examinations,* FDA Publication 86-8265, Superintendent of Documents, Washington, DC 20402.

Webster EW et al: AAPM Report No 18, *A primer on low-level ionizing radiation and its biological effects,* New York, 1986, American Institute of Physics (published for the American Association of Physicists in Medicine; AAPM).

Protecting Occupationally Exposed Personnel During Diagnostic Radiologic Procedures

OBJECTIVES

Upon completion of this chapter, the reader will be able to:

- state the annual effective dose equivalent limit for whole-body occupational exposure of diagnostic radiology personnel
- explain why occupational exposure of diagnostic radiology personnel must be limited
- identify the type of x-radiation that poses the greatest occupational hazard in diagnostic radiology
- explain how various methods and techniques that reduce patient exposure during a diagnostic examination also reduce exposure for the radiographer and other diagnostic personnel
- describe the construction of protective structural shielding and identify the factors that govern the selection of appropriate construction materials
- state the effective absorbed dose equivalent limit in millirems per week for controlled and uncontrolled areas
- explain how distance reduces radiation exposure
- state and explain the inverse square law
- describe the protective garments that can be worn to reduce whole-

body exposure and identify the circumstances in which such garments would be worn

- identify persons and methods that can provide patient restraint during a radiologic procedure
- explain the various methods and devices that can be used to reduce exposure for personnel during a fluoroscopic examination
- explain the various methods and devices that can be used to reduce the radiographer's exposure during a mobile radiographic examination

Federal government standards permit diagnostic radiology personnel to receive an "annual effective dose equivalent limit of 50 mSv (5 rem)"* for whole-body occupational exposure during routine operations. This upper boundary dose equivalent limit is larger than the annual effective dose equivalent limit allowed for individual members of the general population not occupationally exposed. That limit is 1 mSv (0.1 rem) for continuous (or frequent) exposure from man-made sources other than medical† and 5 mSv (0.5 rem) for infrequent annual exposure.‡ The 1 mSv (0.1 rem) annual effective dose equivalent limit "recommendation is designed to limit the exposure of members of the public to reasonable levels of risk comparable with risks from other common sources, i.e., about 10^{-5} annually"‡ (10^{-5} annually means an excess cancer risk of one chance in a hundred thousand per year). The 5 mSv (0.5 rem) maximum annual effective dose limit recommendation "is made because annual exposures in excess of this limit, to a small group of people, need not be regarded as especially hazardous, provided they do not occur often to the same groups."‡ Both of these limits "will keep the dose equivalent to those organs and tissues that are annually considered in the effective dose equivalent system *below* levels of concern for nonstochastic effects."‡

Valid reasons exist for allowance of a larger absorbed dose equivalent for radiation workers. Among the most important of these reasons is that the work force in radiation-related jobs is small when compared to the population as a whole. Thus, the amount of radiation that this work force receives can be larger than the amount that the general public receives without alter-

---

*National Council on Radiation Protection and Measurements (NCRP): NCRP Report #91, *Recommendations on limits for exposure to ionizing radiation*, Bethesda, MD, 1987, NCRP Publications, p 24.
†NCRP Report #91, pp 37, 38.
‡NCRP Report #91, p 38.

ing the genetically significant dose (GSD), the average annual gonadal absorbed dose equivalent to members of the population who are of childbearing age (see Chapter 7 for discussion of GSD). This means that the extra amount of radiation absorbed by the radiation work force does not increase significantly the total number of deleterious mutations in the United States.

Although the radiographer and other diagnostic radiology personnel may absorb more radiation, the absorbed dose equivalent received must be minimized whenever possible. This chapter gives the reader an overview of methods that can be employed to reduce occupational exposure during diagnostic radiologic procedures.

There is a further protection principle, beyond the effective absorbed dose equivalent limit system, known as the ALARA principle. Simply stated and as defined in Chapter 4, the ALARA concept holds that occupational exposure of the radiographer and other occupationally exposed persons should be kept As Low As Reasonably Achievable. This implies that actual absorbed dose equivalent values should be kept *well below* their allowable maximum limits. The *best* way for a radiologist and a radiographer to do this is to employ proper radiation control procedures. An example of such a procedure is the accurate placement and collimation of the radiographic beam (Fig. 8-1). Because employment of such procedures ensures a high degree of

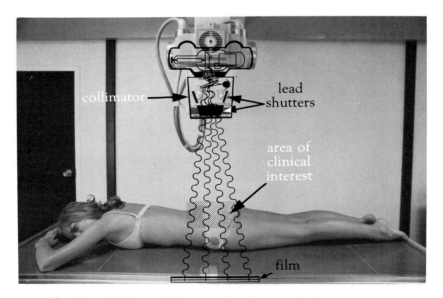

Fig. 8-1   Radiographic beam collimation (restricting the X-ray beam to the area of clinical interest) limits the production of scattered radiation. This radiation control procedure helps to keep the radiographer's occupational exposure as low as reasonably achievable.

safety from most radiation exposures, radiography is *not* considered a hazardous profession. In fact, as stated in Chapter 4, the total risk for diagnostic radiology personnel may be compared with the total risk for persons employed in other "safe" industries such as manufacturing, trade, service, and government. These "safe" industries have "an associated annual fatality accident rate of 1 or less per 10,000 workers, i.e. an average annual risk of 10^{-4}."* The annual risk for radiation workers is unlikely to exceed this rate.

Methods and techniques that reduce patient exposure also reduce exposure for the radiographer and other occupationally exposed persons. For example, repeat examinations should be avoided whenever possible to eliminate additional exposure. Other such considerations are identified in this chapter.

During a diagnostic examination, the patient becomes a source of scattered radiation as a consequence of the Compton interaction process (see Chapter 2). At a 90-degree angle to the primary x-ray beam, at a distance of 1 meter (3 feet), the scattered x-ray intensity is generally approximately 1/1000 of the intensity of the primary x-ray beam.

Because scattered radiation poses the *greatest* occupational hazard in diagnostic radiology, the use of any device or technique that minimizes the amount of scattered radiation produced decreases occupational exposure for diagnostic radiology personnel. The use of beam limitation devices such as the collimator decreases the size of the radiographic beam so that its margins do *not* extend beyond the image receptor (radiographic film). This reduction in beam size results in a decrease in the number of x-ray photons available to undergo Compton scatter. Because scatter is reduced, the radiographer's exposure decreases.

When a radiographic beam is properly filtered, nonuseful low-energy photons are removed from the primary beam. Without proper filtration, a relatively high percentage of the normally filtered low-energy photons would interact with the tissues of the patient's body. A portion of these photons will undergo Compton scatter. The radiologist's and radiographer's absorbed dose equivalent could therefore increase as a result of exposure to this excess scattered radiation. Most of these low-energy photons, however, will be absorbed in the patient, contributing nothing to the radiographic image but, rather, increasing the absorbed dose to the patient. Thus filtration primarily benefits the patient.

Protective lead aprons (Fig. 8-2, *A*) and shielded barriers (Fig. 8-2, *B*) function as gonadal shields for diagnostic radiology personnel. These devices protect them from scattered radiation.

Exposure factors control the quantity of scattered radiation produced,

---

*NCRP Report #91, p 8.

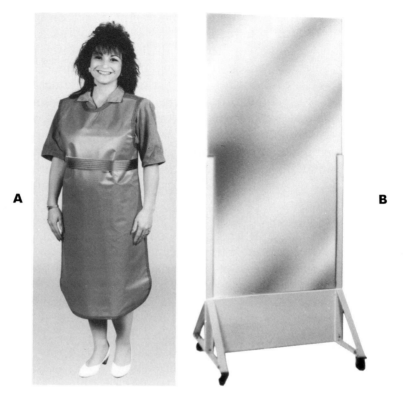

Fig. 8-2   *A,* Lead apron protects occupationally exposed personnel from scattered radiation. *B,* Clear lead mobile x-ray barrier of 0.5 or 1.0 mm lead equivalence provides protection from scattered radiation. It may be used during special procedures, in the operating room and in cardiac cath units.
(Courtesy Nuclear Associates, Carle Place, N.Y.)

although this effect is not very large. Higher peak kilovoltage techniques increase the mean energy of the photons comprising the radiographic beam and also require lower photon beam intensity (i.e., lower milliamperage). As the average energy of the beam increases, backscatter decreases and forward scatter increases. Hence, less scatter radiation is available to reach the imaging personnel and their absorbed dose equivalent is reduced.

When high-speed image receptor systems are used, lower radiographic exposures (less milliamperage) are required, which result in fewer x-ray photons being available to produce Compton scatter. Because less scatter exits from the object being radiographed, personnel exposure is decreased.

Finally, as was discussed in Chapter 7, the employment of proper radiographic processing techniques leads to a decrease in the number of repeat examinations required, with a resultant exposure reduction to the radiographer.

PROTECTIVE STRUCTURAL SHIELDING

Protective barriers provide radiation shielding for both Radiology Department personnel and the general public. Sheets of lead of appropriate thickness placed in the walls of the radiographic or fluoroscopic room are generally employed to provide proper structural shielding.

Exact shielding requirements for a particular radiologic facility should be determined by a qualified medical physicist. Radiographers need to understand the concept of shielding but are not responsible for determining barrier thickness.

Primary protective barrier

The primary beam is made up of the x-ray photons that follow straight-line paths between all sets of collimator shutters. Primary protective barriers are located perpendicular to the line of travel of the primary x-ray beam (Fig. 8-3). If the peak energy of the beam is 140 kVp, the primary protective barrier in a typical installation consists of $\frac{1}{16}$ inch lead and extends 7 feet (2.1 m) upward from the floor of the x-ray room when the x-ray tube is 5 to 7 feet from the wall in question.

Secondary protective barrier

Secondary radiation consists of radiation that has been deflected from the primary beam. Leakage from the tube housing (photons that pass through the housing when a defect occurs in the lead shielding around the tube) and scatter (primarily from the patient) make up the secondary radiation. A secondary protective barrier provides protection from secondary radiation (leakage and scattered radiation) only and, as such, is located parallel to the direction of travel of the x-ray beam (Fig. 8-3). This barrier should overlap the primary protective barrier by about $\frac{1}{2}$ inch and must extend to the ceiling. In a typical installation, the secondary barrier consists of $\frac{1}{32}$ inch lead.

X-ray rooms housing fixed radiographic equipment contain a shielded control booth (or fixed protective barrier) for the protection of the radiographer. Since this booth intercepts leakage and scattered radiation *only*, it may be regarded as a secondary protective barrier. To ensure maximum protection during radiographic exposures, it is imperative that personnel remain completely behind the barrier. The radiographer may observe the patient through the lead glass window in the booth (Fig. 8-4). This window typically consists of 1.5 mm lead equivalent. To further ensure radiation safety,

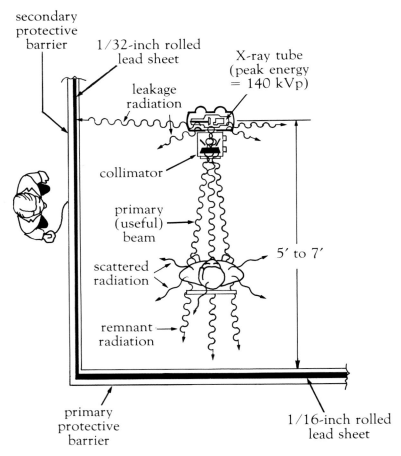

Fig. 8-3   Protective barriers are lined with lead to protect personnel and the general public from radiation. The primary protective barrier is located perpendicular to the line of travel of the primary (useful) x-ray beam. The secondary protective barrier runs parallel to the primary x-ray beam and protects diagnostic radiology personnel from secondary (leakage and scattered) radiation. The walls which are not in the direct line of travel of the primary beam are called *secondary protective barriers,* since they are designed to shield against secondary (leakage and scattered) radiation.

the exposure cord *must* be short enough so that the exposure switch can be operated *only* when the radiographer is completely behind the control booth barrier.

Clear lead-plastic material impregnated with approximately 30% lead by weight can be fashioned into an effective secondary protective barrier such as the control booth (Fig. 8-5). This creates a modern appearance of

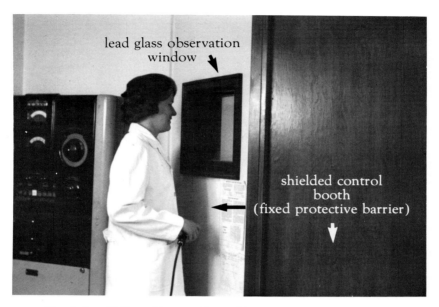

lead glass observation window

shielded control booth (fixed protective barrier)

Fig. 8-4   While making a radiographic exposure with a fixed radiographic unit, the radiographer must remain completely within the shielded control booth (behind the fixed protective barrier) to ensure his or her own safety. The radiographer can observe the patient through the lead glass observation window in the control booth.

the facility and permits a panoramic view whereby diagnostic radiology personnel and patient may view each other. These modular x-ray barriers are shatter-resistant, can extend 7 feet upward from the floor, and be obtained in a lead equivalency from 0.3 to 2 mm.

Clear lead-plastic protective barriers can also be used as overhead x-ray barriers (Fig. 8-6) to provide both an open view and effective protection during special procedures and cardiac catheterization. This shielding ensures 0.5 mm lead equivalency protection.

Protective barrier thickness considerations

Several factors must be considered when determining the thickness requirements for protective barriers. These factors include: distance (d), occupancy (T), workload (W), and use (U).

Distance

One thing that determines the thickness requirements of a barrier is the distance (d) (expressed in meters) from the x-ray source to the barrier; the *greater* the distance between source and barrier, the *less* the exposure rate to

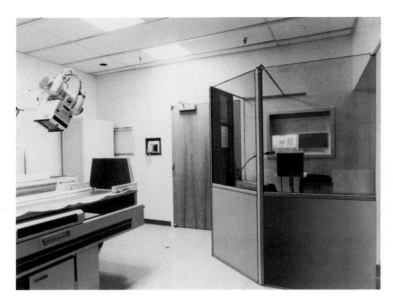

Fig. 8-5 Clear lead-plastic secondary protective barrier impregnated with approximately 30% lead provides a modern appearance of the facility.
(Courtesy Nuclear Associates, Carle Place, N.Y.)

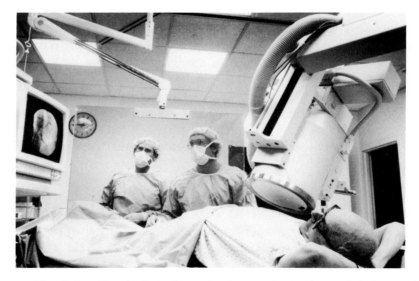

Fig. 8-6 Clear lead-plastic overhead protective barrier used during special procedures and cardiac catheterization.
(Courtesy Nuclear Associates, Carle Place, N.Y.)

the barrier and the *less* thick the lead lining of the barrier need be. A medical physicist evaluates the layout of the planned x-ray room, determines the distances from the x-ray source to potentially occupied areas, and then uses the inverse square law to determine the exposure rates at those areas.

Occupancy

Occupancy within a hospital is divided into two types for the purpose of radiation protection: *uncontrolled* and *controlled*. *Uncontrolled areas* are those areas in which members of the general public may be found. Examples of uncontrolled areas are waiting rooms, stairways, hallways, the exterior of the hospital (i.e., streets, parking lots), and toilets with general hospital access. The term *general public* may be somewhat misleading, because it actually refers to individuals who are not trained to work with radiation. Thus, areas frequented by hospital employees other than those in radiology are usually considered "general public" areas and are therefore considered uncontrolled. The term *controlled areas* refers to areas occupied by workers who have been trained in radiation safety procedures and who wear radiation monitoring devices.

The occupancy factor (T) is used to indicate the fraction of time that an area of the hospital may be occupied by a given individual. The occupancy factor for uncontrolled areas can take on different values according to the usual purpose of the area. For example, hallways are assigned an occupancy factor of $\frac{1}{4}$; stairways, general access toilets, and unattended elevators are assigned an occupancy factor of $\frac{1}{16}$. Occupancy factors are designed to overestimate the fraction of time that a given individual might actually spend in an area so that, when the shielding is designed, it will more than ensure that exposure will be kept low. For controlled areas, the occupancy factor is always assumed to be equal to 1. This would imply that a given worker (or "occupationally exposed" individual) is always present, if not in a particular controlled area then in some other controlled area.

The shielding for uncontrolled areas is designed to maintain absorbed dose-equivalent to occupants of those areas at less than the maximum annual effective dose equivalent limit for occasional (infrequent) exposure of the general public, that is, less than 5 mSv (0.5 rem) in a year. Shielding for controlled areas is designed to maintain absorbed dose equivalent to occupants of controlled areas at less than 50 mSv (5 rem) in a year. For shielding design purposes, it is more convenient to determine the maximum absorbed dose equivalent limit for a week than for an entire year. If an occupationally exposed worker is assumed to be present for 50 weeks per year (because of holidays, illness, and vacation the figure 50 weeks is taken instead of 52 weeks), then the weekly maximum absorbed dose equivalent limit becomes

50 mSv (5 rem) per year divided by 50 weeks/yr or 1 mSv (0.1 rem) per week. This is equivalent to 100 mrem/wk. The weekly maximum absorbed dose equivalent limit for noncontrolled areas would then translate to 10 mrem per week. An additional factor of 5 (for a margin of safety) is often used, bringing the design limit for uncontrolled areas down to 2 mrem per week. Realizing that rem and roentgen (R) are equivalent for diagnostic x-rays (see "quality factor"), the limits are often expressed as 100 mR/wk for controlled areas and 2 mR/wk for uncontrolled areas.

Because controlled areas have a higher maximum absorbed dose equivalent limit than uncontrolled areas, they would normally require less shielding, all other factors being the same. However, current trends in shielding design follow the ALARA concept. Thus, shielding for controlled areas is being designed so that expected exposures do *not* exceed 10 mR/wk when doing so would *not* significantly increase the cost of the installation.

Workload

The maximum voltage and milliamperage (mA) of the x-ray generator and the amount of x-ray activity (number of x-ray exams performed per week) are two more factors that determine the shielding thickness requirements for an x-ray room. More shielding is required in an x-ray room where a larger number of x-ray examinations is performed. The workload (W) is measured in milliampere-minutes per week (mA min/wk or tube current in milliamperes and time of exposure in minutes per week). When the number of x-ray examinations performed per day in a specific x-ray room is increased, workload values in milliampere-minutes per week will be higher. Such an x-ray room requires thicker shielding to maintain within former levels the cumulative absorbed dose equivalent to those occupying areas adjacent to the room for any lengthy period of time. When a higher peak kilovoltage is used for the majority of exams in a particular room, the workload is smaller because fewer milliampere-seconds (mAs) are required. In this case, the greater penetration of the higher energy x-rays might not, however, be compensated by the lower workload and so the shielding may have to be increased.

Workloads are usually meant to be *overestimates* of the activity in a room so that shielding determined by the estimated workload will be *more* than adequate to ensure the protection of personnel and the public.

Use or beam direction factor

The use factor (U) or beam direction factor indicates the proportional amount of time during which the x-ray beam is energized or directed toward a particular barrier. Because the primary x-ray beam is directed toward the floor most of the time, the floor is given a use factor of 1, whereas primary wall barriers are given a use factor of ¼. Because leakage and scattered radiation are present during all diagnostic examinations when the x-ray tube is energized, secondary barriers are given a use factor of 1. The ceiling is most often considered to be a secondary barrier for radiographic procedures.

DIAGNOSTIC-TYPE PROTECTIVE TUBE HOUSING

A lead-lined metal diagnostic-type protective tube housing (Fig. 8-7) is required to protect both the radiographer and the patient from off-focus or leakage radiation by restricting the emission of x-rays to the area of the useful or primary beam (those x-rays emitted through the x-ray tube window or port).

The housing that encloses the x-ray tube must be constructed so that leakage radiation measured at a distance of 1 m (3 feet) from the x-ray source does *not* exceed 100 mR/hr (2.58×10^{-5} C/kg/hr) when the tube is operated continuously at its highest current for its full potential (voltage). Although the x-ray tube housing is designed to protect the operator from the hazard of electric shock, the radiographer must handle this piece of equipment and its adjoining part, the collimator, carefully and cautiously. When manipulating the tube housing for a radiographic examination, the ra-

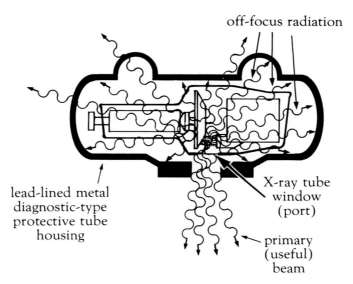

Fig. 8-7 A lead-lined metal diagnostic-type protective tube housing protects the radiographer and the patient from off-focus or leakage radiation by restricting x-ray emission to the area of the primary (useful) beam.

diographer should *always avoid* handling or severely bending the high tension cables that connect to the positive and negative terminals of the x-ray tube. *No one* should touch the tube housing or high tension cables while a radiographic exposure is in progress.

PROTECTION DURING FLUOROSCOPIC PROCEDURES

Many of the methods and devices that reduce the radiographer's exposure when operating fixed radiographic equipment also reduce the dose received by the radiographer and the radiologist during a fluoroscopic procedure. These include: proper beam collimation, use of filtration, gonadal shielding, control of exposure factors, the use of high-speed image receptor systems, proper radiographic processing, adequate structural shielding, appropriate source-to-tabletop distance, use of a cumulative timing device, and housing of the x-ray tube in a diagnostic-type protective encasement. Some additional requirements are included in the federal government specifications for the use of fluoroscopic equipment to ensure adequate protection for the radiographer and the radiologist.

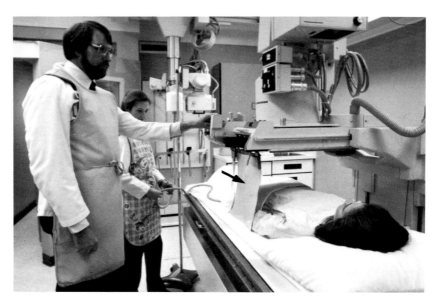

Fig. 8-8   Scattered radiation produced during a fluoroscopic examination can be absorbed by a protective sliding panel with a minimum of 0.25 mm lead equivalent placed between the fluoroscopist and the patient.

Fluoroscopic exposure switch

The fluoroscopic exposure switch (the foot pedal) must be the dead-man type; only continuous pressure applied by the operator (usually a radiologist) can keep such a switch closed and the fluoroscopic tube emitting x-radiation. This means that the exposure terminates if the person operating the switch becomes incapacitated (i.e., suffers a heart attack).

Protective drape or sliding panel

A protective drape or sliding panel with a *minimum* of 0.25 mm lead equivalent should be positioned between the fluoroscopist and the patient to intercept scattered radiation (Fig. 8-8).

Bucky slot shielding device

A Bucky slot shielding device (Fig. 8-9) of *at least* 0.25 mm lead equivalent should automatically cover the Bucky slot opening during a fluoroscopic examination when the Bucky tray is positioned at the foot end of the fluoroscopic table. This shielding device provides the radiologist and radiographer with protection at gonadal level.

Fluoroscopy exposure monitor

Occupational exposure during fluoroscopic procedures can be reduced significantly through the use of a fluoroscopy exposure monitor (Fig. 8-10), which "provides an instantaneous audible indication of the intensity of sec-

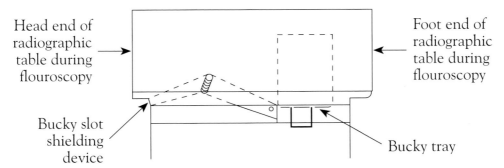

Fig. 8-9 To provide protection at gonadal level for the fluoroscopist, the Bucky slot shielding device should be at least 0.25 mm lead equivalent. (Modified from Ritenour ER: *Radiation protection and biology: a self-instructional multimedia learning series, Instructor's manual,* Denver, 1985, Multi-Media Publishing, pp. 5-12.)

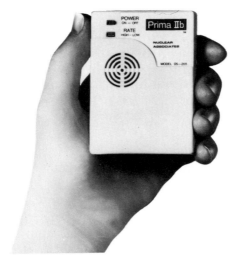
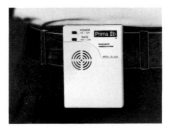
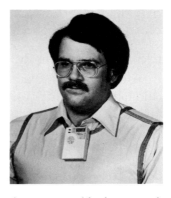

Fig. 8-10 Fluoroscopy exposure monitor can be worn outside the protective apron at collar or waist level.
(Courtesy Nuclear Associates, Carle Place, N.Y.)

ondary radiation."* This device emits "a soft chirping signal, whose frequency varies in direct proportion to the exposure rate."* Personnel using this monitor can select a position to stand relative to the source of radiation, thereby achieving the *greatest* protection. The device should be clipped to the *outside* of the lead apron at collar or waist level.

Rotational scheduling of personnel

Diagnostic radiology personnel receive the *highest* occupational exposure during fluoroscopy, mobile radiography, and special procedures. This exposure can be decreased by scheduling personnel to spend *less* time in these higher radiation areas. To accomplish this, radiographers may be assigned to clinical areas in a rotational pattern. This type of scheduling uses the cardinal principle of *time* as a means of radiation protection.

---

*Catalog G-5, *Instruments and accessories for improved imaging and safety in diagnostic radiology, CT and MRI,* 1988, Victoreen, p 51.

PROTECTION DURING MOBILE RADIOGRAPHIC EXAMINATIONS

Mobile radiographic equipment requires special radiation protection considerations for the radiographer. Suitable protective garments (lead aprons and gloves) *should* be worn by the radiographer whenever structural or mobile protective shielding is unavailable.

The cord leading to the exposure switch *should* be long enough to permit the radiographer to stand at least 2 m (approximately 6 feet or 72 inches) from the patient, the x-ray tube, and the useful beam. This permits the radiographer to use the inverse square effect of distance to reduce exposure.

The radiographer *should* stand at right angles (90 degrees) to the scattering object; when the protection factors of distance and shielding have been accounted for, this is where the least amount of scattered radiation will be received (Fig. 8-11). However, it is important to remember that the factors of distance and shielding have much more influence on the reduction of the exposure of the technologist. Therefore distance and shielding should be taken care of first.

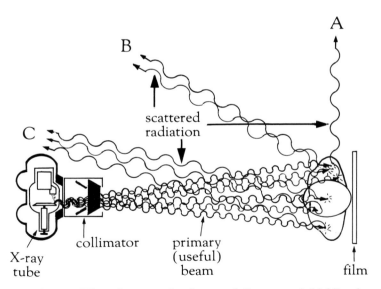

Fig. 8-11 When the protective factors of distance and shielding have been accounted for, the radiographer will receive the least amount of scattered radiation by standing at right angles (90°) to the scattering object (the patient) [in position A]. The most scattered radiation would be received at point C because of backscatter coming from the patient. (Intensity or quantity of X-ray exposure at any given point is indicated in this picture by the number of scattered x-rays reaching that point.)

DISTANCE

Distance is the *most effective* means of protection from ionizing radiation. Radiographers receive *less* radiation exposure by standing farther away from a source of radiation. The inverse square law expresses the relationship between distance and intensity (quantity) of radiation. The law states: *The intensity of the radiation is inversely proportional to the square of the distance.* This means that, as the distance between the radiation source and a measurement point increases, the quantity of radiation measured at that point decreases by the square of its distance from the source (Fig. 8-12). This decrease in radiation intensity occurs because the area with the same flux of x-rays at the original location now has to cover at the new location has increased by the square of the distance. For example, when the distance from the x-ray target, a point source of radiation, is doubled, the radiation at the new location spans an area four times larger than the original area. However, because the same amount of radiation exists to cover this larger area, the intensity at the new distance consequently decreases by a factor of four. Figure 8-13 illustrates this concept.

The inverse square law may be stated in the form of a formula:

$$\frac{I_1}{I_2} = \frac{(D_2)^2}{(D_1)^2}$$

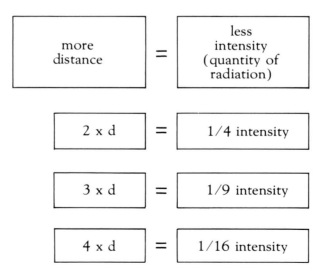

Fig. 8-12   As the distance between the source of radiation and any given measurement point increases, radiation intensity (quantity) measured at that point decreases by the square of its distance.

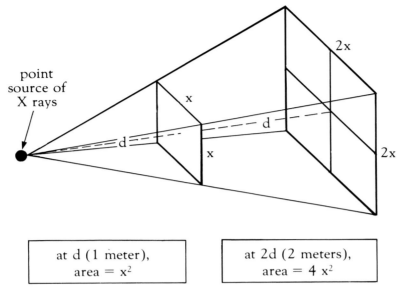

at d (1 meter),
area $= x^2$

at 2d (2 meters),
area $= 4 x^2$

Fig. 8-13   When the distance from a point source of radiation is doubled, the radiation at the new location spans an area four times larger than the original area. However, the intensity at the new distance is only one fourth the original intensity.

where I_1 expresses the exposure (intensity) at the original distance, I_2 expresses the exposure (intensity) at the new distance, D_1 expresses the original distance from the source of radiation, and D_2 expresses the new distance from the source of radiation.

EXAMPLE: If a radiographer stands 1 m (3 feet) away from an x-ray tube and receives an exposure of 2 mR/hr, what will the exposure be if the same radiographer moves to a position located 2 m (6 feet) from the x-ray tube?

ANSWER: $\dfrac{I_1}{I_2} = \dfrac{(D_2)^2}{(D_1)^2}$

$\dfrac{2}{x} = \dfrac{(2)^2}{(1)^2}$

$\dfrac{2}{x} \diagdown \dfrac{4}{1}$ (cross multiply)

$4x = 2$

$x = 0.5$ mR/hr

The inverse square law *should* be applied, by increasing one's distance from a source of exposure, *whenever possible* to reduce the radiographer's exposure from sources of x-radiation. (This law may also be applied to sources of gamma and neutron radiation.)

The inverse square law also implies that *if* a radiographer should move closer to a source of radiation, then the radiation exposure to the radiographer will dramatically increase. For example, if the radiographer stands 2 feet away from an x-ray source instead of 6 feet, then according to the inverse square law, the radiographer's radiation exposure will increase by a factor of nine.

PROTECTIVE DEVICES

Protective lead aprons and gloves (Fig. 8-14) *should* be used whenever the radiographer *cannot* remain behind a protective lead barrier during an exposure. If the peak energy of the x-ray beam is 100 kVp, a protective lead (Pb) apron must be equivalent to a 0.25 mm thickness of lead. A lead apron of 0.5 or 1 mm lead equivalent would afford greater protection. All three of these thicknesses are available for protective apparel. However, the 0.5 mm lead equivalent is the *most widely* used thickness in diagnostic radiology.

During fluoroscopic examinations, the radiographer should *always* wear

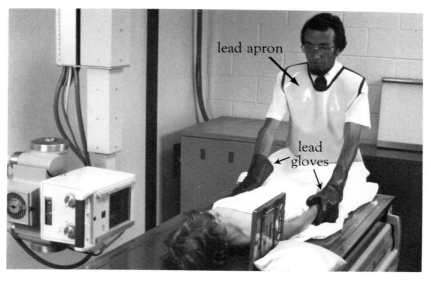

Fig. 8-14   Lead apron and gloves protect the radiographer from scattered radiation.

a protective apron. Protective lead gloves of a *minimum* of 0.25 mm lead equivalent should be worn whenever the hands must be protected from the beam.

Because there is usually no protective barrier (i.e., control booth or moveable shield) present, lead aprons *must* be worn by radiographers during fluoroscopic and mobile radiographic procedures. For the latter the 6 foot long exposure cord, when fully extended, affords a significantly reduced exposure level because of the inverse square law.

A neck and thyroid shield of 0.5 mm lead equivalent (Fig. 8-15) can protect the thyroid area of occupationally exposed people during general fluoroscopy and x-ray special procedures.

Scatter radiation to the lens of the eyes of diagnostic radiology personnel can be substantially reduced by wearing protective eyeglasses (Fig. 8-16, *A*) with optically clear lenses that contain a minimum lead equivalent protection of 0.35 mm. Side shields on the protective glasses (Fig. 8-16, *B*) are also available for procedures that require turning of the head. A wrap-

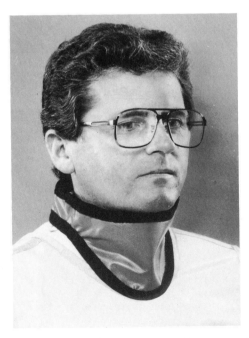

Fig. 8-15 The neck and thyroid gland can be protected from radiation exposure through the use of a 0.5 mm lead equivalent protective shield.
(Courtesy Nuclear Associates, Carle Place, N.Y.)

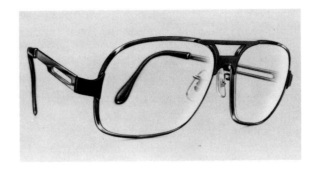

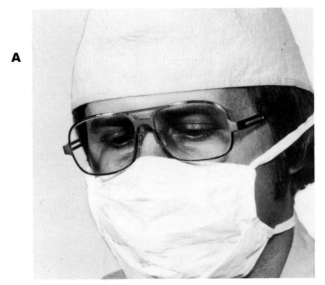

A

Fig. 8-16   *A,* Protective eyeglasses provide protection for the lens of the eyes during general fluoroscopy and special procedures.

around frame containing optically clear lenses with a 0.5 mm lead equivalency (Fig. 8-16, *C*) is also available.

PATIENT RESTRAINT

Radiographers should *never* stand in the primary (useful) beam to restrain a patient during a radiographic exposure (Fig. 8-17, *A*). Other nonoccupational persons, wearing appropriate apparel, or mechanical restraining devices should be used to perform this function when required.

Patient holding may be necessary when an ill or injured person is un-

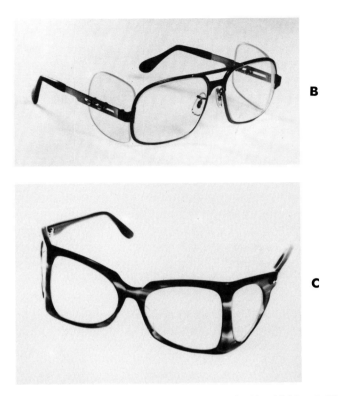

Fig. 8-16, cont'd. *B,* Protective eyeglasses with side shields. *C,* Wrap-around frame containing optically-clear lenses with 0.5 mm lead equivalency. (Courtesy Nuclear Associates, Carle Place, N.Y.)

able to support himself or herself. For example, a weak elderly patient may be unable to stand alone and raise his arms above his head for a lateral chest x-ray. In this situation, another person may need to hold the patient in position during the exposure. A mechanical restraining device may be used to hold an infant in the proper upright position for chest radiographs. If such a device is not available, appropriate nonoccupational assistants would be needed to hold the child during the exposure. When nonoccupational persons such as nurses, orderlies, relatives, or friends assist in holding the patient during an exposure, suitable protective garments (lead aprons and gloves) should be worn by each person participating in the examination (Fig. 8-17 *B*). This ensures maximum protection from exposure. Care should be taken by the radiographer so that nonoccupational individuals *do not* stand in the useful beam while holding the patient during the exposure. Pregnant females should *never* be permitted to assist in holding a patient

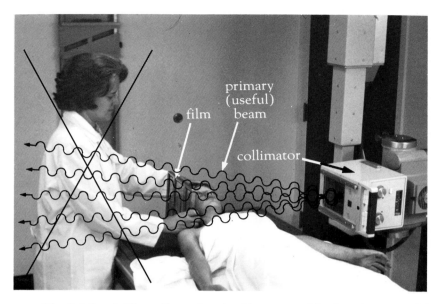

Fig. 8-17   *A,* The radiographer should *never* stand in the primary (useful) beam to restrain the patient.

during an exposure, because this could result in exposure of and possible damage to the embryo or fetus.

PROTECTION OF PERSONNEL WHEN PATIENTS CONTAIN A RADIOACTIVE MATERIAL

Although radiation protection as practiced for patients receiving radiation therapy treatments or undergoing nuclear medicine procedures is *not* within the scope of this text, it frequently occurs that such patients also receive concurrent diagnostic radiographic examinations. For example, a patient who has been therapeutically implanted with the isotope iridium−192 (HVL = 3 mm lead) to treat the patient's breast cancer, will require diagnostic radiographs to localize the placement of the radioactive sources. In this case, for the radiographer performing the diagnostic examination, distance from the implant and minimization of exposure time provide the *best* means of radiation protection. The standard 0.5 mm lead equivalent apron normally used for personnel shielding in diagnostic radiologic procedures offers *little* protection against the relatively high-energy gamma-ray emissions from iridium−192 (effective energy 380 keV). In fact, the wearing of this lead apron

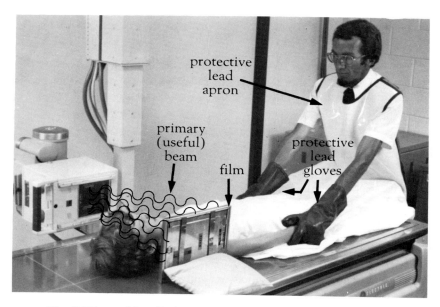

Fig. 8-17, cont'd. *B,* A nonoccupational person restraining a patient during a radiographic exposure should wear adequate protective apparel and stand outside of the primary beam.

could actually lead to an *increased* absorbed dose to the radiographer because of a *false* sense of security.

There are many isotopes used in nuclear medicine procedures for diagnostic purposes that have energies that overlap the diagnostic x-ray energy range. Patients containing the isotope technetium-99m (140 keV gamma-ray energy), especially as used for bone scans, are sources of exposure for technologists and other medical personnel. In this instance, a lead apron containing 0.5 mm lead equivalent would offer *significant* radiation protection. Even with the protection offered by the lead apron, time of exposure and distance from the source of radiation remain important safety factors.

SUMMARY

In this chapter the various methods of protecting personnel from exposure to ionizing radiation during diagnostic radiologic procedures were described. The reader should be able to explain why occupational exposure must be limited and how this can be accomplished.

REVIEW QUESTIONS

1. Because occupational exposure of the radiographer can be kept "as low as reasonably achievable" through individual monitoring and other protective measures and devices, and because exposure from radiation-related jobs will *not* alter the _____, radiation workers may receive more whole-body exposure than members of the general population.
   a. mean glandular dose
   b. genetically significant dose
   c. mean marrow dose
   d. tissue tolerance

2. Whenever scattered radiation decreases, the radiographer's exposure:
   a. decreases
   b. increases slightly
   c. remains the same
   d. increases 100 times

3. Of the devices listed below, which one eliminates low-energy photons within the collimator to decrease the scattered radiation potential?
      1. collimator light source
      2. electronic sensors
      3. aluminum filtration
   a. 1 only
   b. 2 only
   c. 3 only
   d. 1, 2, and 3

4. If the peak energy of the x-ray beam is 140 kVp, the primary protective barrier should consist of _____ and extend _____ upward from the floor of the x-ray room when the tube is 5 to 7 feet from the wall in question.
   a. $\frac{1}{32}$ inch lead, 10 feet
   b. $\frac{1}{32}$ inch lead, 7 feet
   c. $\frac{1}{16}$ inch lead, 10 feet
   d. $\frac{1}{16}$ inch lead, 7 feet

5. Of the following factors, which would be considered when determining thickness requirements for protective barriers?
      1. distance and the occupancy factor
      2. workload
      3. use factor
   a. 1 only
   b. 2 only
   c. 3 only
   d. 1, 2, and 3

6. When considering total risk, radiography may be compared with the total risk associated with:
   a. extremely hazardous industries
   b. other "safe" industries
   c. a nuclear war
   d. a radiation accident like the Chernobyl nuclear power station disaster

7. The cord leading to the exposure switch of a mobile radiographic unit should be long enough to permit the radiographer to stand *at least* _____ from the patient, the x-ray tube, and the useful beam to reduce occupational exposure.
   a. 1 m (3 feet)
   b. 2 m (6 feet)
   c. 3 m (9 feet)
   d. 5 m (15 feet)

8. When performing a mobile radiographic examination, if the protection factors of distance and shielding are equal, the radiographer should stand at _____ to the scattering object.
   a. a 30° angle
   b. a 45° angle
   c. a right angle
   d. a 75° angle

9. If a radiographer stands 6 m away from an x-ray tube and receives an exposure of 4 mR/hr, what will the exposure be if the same radiographer moves to stand at a position located 12 m from the x-ray tube?
   a. 1 mR/hr
   b. 2 mR/hr
   c. 3 mR/hr
   d. 4 mR/hr

10. If the peak energy of the x-ray beam is 100 kVp, a protective lead apron *must* be the equivalent of:
    a. a 0.25 mm thickness of lead
    b. a 0.5 mm thickness of lead
    c. a 1.0 mm thickness of lead
    d. a 1.5 mm thickness of lead

11. Which of the following statements is true?
    a. Radiographers may stand in the useful beam to restrain a patient during a difficult radiologic procedure provided that a protective apron is worn.
    b. Nurses, orderlies, relatives, or friends may stand in the useful beam to restrain a patient during a difficult radiologic procedure provided that a protective apron is worn.

c. Pregnant females may stand in the useful beam to restrain a patient during a difficult radiologic procedure provided that a protective apron is worn.

d. Radiographers should never stand in the useful beam to restrain a patient during a radiographic exposure.

12. Which of the following is the *most effective* means of protection from ionizing radiation normally available to the radiographer?
   a. decrease the amount of time spent near a source of radiation
   b. use protective shielding garments
   c. place as much distance as possible between one's self and the source of radiation
   d. remain behind a mobile protective shield during an exposure

13. If the intensity of the x-ray beam is inversely proportional to the square of the distance, when the distance from a point source of radiation is tripled, the intensity:
   a. increases by a factor of 3 at the new distance
   b. increases by a factor of 9 at the new distance
   c. decreases by a factor of 9 at the new distance
   d. decreases by a factor of 3 at the new distance

14. A Bucky slot shielding device of at least _____ should automatically cover the Bucky slot opening during a fluoroscopic examination when the Bucky tray is positioned at the foot end of the fluoroscopic table.
   a. 0.25 mm aluminum equivalent
   b. 0.25 mm lead equivalent
   c. 0.5 mm aluminum equivalent
   d. 0.5 mm lead equivalent

15. Protective shielding for a controlled area must ensure that the exposure rate remains below _____ mR/wk.
   a. 1000
   b. 100
   c. 2
   d. 10

16. The proportional amount of time during which the x-ray beam is energized or directed toward a particular barrier is called the:
   a. occupancy factor
   b. workload factor
   c. distance factor
   d. use factor

17. A diagnostic-type protective tube housing must be constructed so that leakage radiation measured at a distance of 1 m from the x-ray source does *not* exceed

_____ when the tube is operated continuously at its highest current for its full potential.
a. 500 mR/hr
b. 300 mR/hr
c. 100 mR/hr
d. 50 mR/hr

18. Which of the following methods and devices reduce the radiographer's exposure during a fluoroscopic examination?
    1. proper beam collimation
    2. control of exposure factors
    3. gonadal shielding of the patient
a. 1 only
b. 2 only
c. 3 only
d. 1 and 2

19. Which of the following adjustments in exposure techniques decrease the production of scattered radiation?
a. decrease kVp and increase mAs in compensation
b. decrease kVp and decrease mAs
c. increase kVp and decrease mAs in compensation
d. increase kVp and increase mAs

20. A protective drape or sliding panel of a minimum thickness of 0.25 mm lead equivalent should be positioned between the fluoroscopist and the patient to intercept:
a. primary radiation
b. scattered radiation
c. remnant radiation
d. useful radiation

21. A dead-man type fluoroscopic exposure switch _____ the exposure if the person operating the switch becomes incapacitated.
a. continues
b. prolongs
c. starts
d. terminates

22. Units of milliampere-minutes per week are used to determine the _____ for a specific x-ray room.
a. workload
b. use factor
c. occupancy factor
d. distance factor

23. The lead glass window of the shielded control booth in a fixed radiographic installation typically consists of:
    a. 0.25 mm lead equivalent
    b. 0.5 mm lead equivalent
    c. 1.0 mm lead equivalent
    d. 1.5 mm lead equivalent

24. Which of the following equivalents for protective gloves would provide the radiographer with the *most* protection from ionizing radiation?
    a. 0.25 mm lead equivalent
    b. 0.1 mm lead equivalent
    c. 0.3 mm lead equivalent
    d. 0.5 mm lead equivalent

25. Diagnostic radiology personnel may receive an annual effective dose equivalent limit of _____ for whole-body occupational exposure during routine operations.
    a. 1 mSv (0.1 rem)
    b. 5 mSv (0.5 rem)
    c. 25 mSv (2.5 rem)
    d. 50 mSv (5 rem)

26. Members of the general public *not* occupationally exposed have an annual effective dose equivalent limit of _____ for continuous (or frequent) exposure and a maximum annual effective dose equivalent limit of _____ for infrequent annual exposure.
    a. 50 mSv (5 rem), 25 mSv (2.5 rem)
    b. 1 mSv (0.1 rem), 5 mSv (0.5 rem)
    c. 3 mSv (0.3 rem), 5 mSv (0.5 rem)
    d. 5 mSv (0.5 rem), 3 mSv (0.3 rem)

27. Which part(s) of a diagnostic x-ray unit should a radiographer avoid touching while a radiographic exposure is in progress?
    a. control panel
    b. exposure switch
    c. kilovoltage control on the control panel only
    d. tube housing, collimator, and high tension cables

28. The ALARA concept holds that occupational exposure of the radiographer should:
    a. not exceed maximum annual effective dose equivalent established for members of the general public
    b. be as high as necessary to allow for radiographers to hold patients during diagnostic radiographic procedures
    c. be kept "as low as reasonably achievable"

d. be as high as necessary to allow radiographers to hold patients during diagnostic fluoroscopic procedures

29. Use factor (U) is another term for:
    a. workload factor
    b. occupancy factor in controlled and uncontrolled areas
    c. beam direction factor
    d. protective barrier thickness consideration factor

30. During which of the following radiologic examinations should radiographers wear a thyroid shield?
    a. fluoroscopy and x-ray special procedures
    b. mobile radiographic procedures
    c. general diagnostic radiographic procedures
    d. computed tomographic procedures

Bibliography

Ballinger PW: *Merrill's atlas of radiographic positions and radiologic procedures*, ed 5, vol 1, St Louis, 1982, Mosby–Year Book.

Bushong SC: *Radiologic science for technologists: physics, biology, and protection*, ed 2, St Louis, 1980, Mosby–Year Book.

Bushong SC: In Ballinger PW, editor: *Merrill's atlas of radiographic positions and radiographic procedures*, ed 7, vol 1, St Louis, 1991, Mosby–Year Book, p 18.

Bushong SC: *Radiologic science for technologists: physics, biology and protection*, ed 5, St Louis, 1993, Mosby–Year Book.

Christensen EE, Curry III TS, Dowdey JE: *An introduction to the physics of diagnostic radiology*, ed 2, Philadelphia, 1978, Lea & Febiger.

Curry III TS, Dowdey JE, Murry Jr RC: *Christensen's introduction to the physics of diagnostic radiology*, ed 3, Philadelphia, 1984, Lea & Febiger.

Donohue DP: *An analysis of radiographic quality: lab manual and workbook*, Baltimore, 1980, University Park Press.

Donohue DP: *An analysis of radiographic quality: lab manual and workbook*, ed 2, Rockville, MD, 1984, Aspen.

Frankel R: *Radiation protection for radiologic technologists*, New York, 1976, McGraw-Hill.

Malott JC, Fodor III J: *The art and science of medical radiography*, ed 7, St Louis, 1993, Mosby–Year Book.

National Council on Radiation Protection and Measurements (NCRP): Report #33, *Medical x-ray and gamma-ray protection for energies up to 10 MeV: equipment design and use*, Washington, DC, 1968, NCRP Publications.

National Council on Radiation Protection and Measurements (NCRP): Report #49, *Structural shielding design and evaluation for medical use of x-ray and gamma rays with energies up to 10 MeV*, Washington, DC, 1976, NCRP Publications.

National Council on Radiation Protection and Measurements (NCRP): Report #91, *Recommendations on limits for exposure to ionizing radiation*, Bethesda, MD, 1987, NCRP Publications.

Ritenour ER: *Radiation protection and biology: a self-instructional multimedia learning series, Instructor's manual*, Denver, 1985, Multi-Media Publishing.

Scheele RV, Wakley J: *Elements of radiation protection*, Springfield, IL, 1975, Charles C Thomas.

Selman J: *The fundamentals of x-ray and radium physics*, ed 6, Springfield, IL, 1978, Charles C Thomas.

Selman J: *The fundamentals of x-ray and radium physics*, ed 7, Springfield, IL, 1985, Charles C Thomas.

Radiation Monitoring

OBJECTIVES

Upon completion of this chapter, the reader will be able to:

- state the reason why a radiation worker should wear a personnel monitoring device
- explain the function of a personnel monitoring device
- identify the appropriate location on the body of diagnostic radiology personnel where the personnel monitoring device should be placed during:
  a) routine radiographic procedures
  b) fluoroscopic procedures
  c) mobile radiographic procedures
  d) special radiographic procedures
- list the characteristics of a personnel monitoring device
- describe the various components of the film badge and explain the use of the device as a personnel monitor
- describe the pocket ionization chamber and explain the use of the device as a personnel monitor
- describe the thermoluminescent dosimeter and explain the use of the device as a personnel monitor
- explain the function of radiation survey instruments
- list four gas-filled radiation survey instruments
- explain the requirements for radiation survey instruments
- explain the function of the:
  a) ionization chamber-type survey meter
  b) proportional counter
  c) Geiger-Müller detector
  d) Victoreen condenser R-meter

To ensure that occupational radiation exposure levels are kept well *below* the annual dose equivalent limit, some means of monitoring personnel exposure must be employed. The radiographer and other occupationally exposed persons *must* be aware of the various personnel and area radiation exposure monitoring devices and their functions. This chapter provides an overview of personnel and area monitoring.

PERSONNEL MONITORING

Monitoring of radiation exposures to any person occupationally exposed on a regular basis to ionizing radiation is recommended. This exposure monitoring of personnel is required whenever such workers are likely to run the risk of receiving one fourth or more of the annual absorbed dose equivalent limit of 50 mSv (5 rem) in any one year. In keeping with the ALARA concept, most institutions issue personnel monitoring devices when personnel might possibly receive about 1% of the annual dose equivalent limit in any month or approximately 0.0005 Sv (0.5 mSv) or 0.05 rem (50 mrem).

The monitoring device provides some indication of the working habits and working conditions of diagnostic radiology personnel. By measuring the quantity of ionizing radiation to which it has been exposed over a period of time, it indicates occupational exposure. This device, however, does *not* protect the wearer from exposure.

Because the personnel monitoring device records only the exposure received in the area in which it is worn, it should be anatomically located so that it will provide an indication of the exposure received by the body trunk of occupationally exposed persons. During routine radiographic procedures, it is acceptable to wear a film badge monitoring device (Fig. 9-1, *A*) attached to the clothing on the front of the body at waist level or at chest level (Fig. 9-1, *B*) outside of the apron facing forward.

Fluoroscopy, special radiographic procedures, and mobile radiography produce the *highest* occupational radiation exposure for diagnostic radiology personnel. When a protective apron is worn during fluoroscopic procedures, special radiographic procedures, or a mobile radiographic examination, the monitor should be worn outside of the protective apron at collar level because the unprotected head, neck, and eye lenses receive 10 to 20 times more exposure than the protected body trunk. With the monitoring device located at collar level, a reading of the approximate absorbed dose equivalent to the thyroid gland and eyes of the occupationally exposed person can be obtained.

If the lead apron's shielding integrity is not compromised, a film badge reading outside the apron that is within acceptable limits ensures a lower reading under the apron.

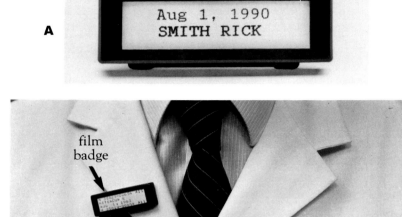

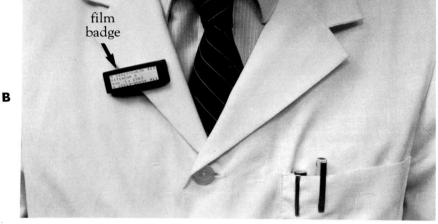

Fig. 9-1   *A,* Film badge monitoring device used in personnel monitoring. *B,* The film badge monitoring device should be worn on the body front at waist level or at chest level during routine radiographic procedures.
(*B* Courtesy Landauer, Inc., Glenwood, Ill.)

During fluoroscopic procedures, special radiographic procedures, or a mobile radiographic examination, some institutions may prefer to have diagnostic radiology personnel wear two separate film badge monitoring devices, one located under the protective apparel at waist level and the other outside the protective apparel at collar level to monitor the approximate absorbed dose equivalent to the thyroid gland and eyes. If two separate film badge monitoring devices are worn, each badge should be color coded to avoid mix-up of the monitoring devices.

The use of a second film badge monitoring device is essential in certain clinical situations. An additional monitoring device should be worn by pregnant occupationally exposed persons to monitor the abdomen during gestation. Another circumstance that necessitates the use of an additional monitoring device is performing a special radiographic procedure that requires

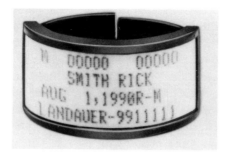

Fig. 9-2   Extremity monitoring device (TLD ring badge) can be used to monitor the absorbed dose equivalent to the hands.
(Courtesy Landauer, Inc., Glenwood, Ill.)

the hands to be near the primary x-ray beam. In this situation, an extremity monitoring device (Fig. 9-2) may be worn by personnel to monitor the absorbed dose equivalent to the hands.

A record of exposure recorded by personnel monitoring devices should become part of the employment record of all diagnostic radiology personnel. Table 9-1 gives occupational exposure values (gathered from film badge readings) for a typical year. The values represent the effective absorbed dose equivalent to the whole body.

CHARACTERISTICS OF PERSONNEL MONITORING DEVICES

A personnel monitoring device must be lightweight and easy to carry. It should be made of materials durable enough to tolerate normal daily use. The device must be able to detect and record small and large exposures in a consistent, reliable manner. Outside influences such as heat, humidity, and mechanical shock should not affect the performance of the instrument. Because many personnel may be required to wear a personnel radiation monitor, the device should be reasonably low in cost. This permits institutions to accommodate large numbers of personnel in a cost-effective manner.

TYPES OF PERSONNEL MONITORING DEVICES

Three types of personnel monitoring devices can be used to measure individual exposure to ionizing radiation: film badges, pocket ionization chambers, and thermoluminescent dosimeters.

Table 9-1 Occupational Exposure Values for a Typical Year

Occupational category	Number of workers (thousands)		Average annual effective dose equivalent (mSv)*		Collective effective dose equivalent (person-Sv)†
	All	Exposed	All	Exposed	
Medicine	584	277	0.7	1.5	410
Industry	305	156	1.2	2.4	380
Nuclear fuel cycle	151	91	3.6	6.0	540
Government	204	105	0.6	1.2	120
Miscellaneous	76	31	0.7	1.6	50
Other workers	115	107	1.7	1.8	200
Others (e.g., visitors)	155	42	0.25	0.9	40
ROUNDED SUBTOTAL	1590	810	1.1	2.1	1700
Additional					
Industrial‡	6.9	2.1	1.56	5.2	11‖
Uranium mining§	—	10	—	1.15	12¶
Well loggers	8.7	7.3	3.50	4.2	30#
DOE contractors	—	81	—	1.8	160**
USPHS	4.6	0.7	0.07	0.47	0.3**
ROUNDED TOTAL	1610+	911	1.24	2.2	2000

*1 mSv = 100 mrem.
†1 person-Sv = 100 person-rem.
‡Ten states only.
§External effective dose equivalent based on sample of 47 open pit miners. Population exposed based on underground mining population.
‖1970 to 1975.
¶1975 to 1976.
#1979.
**1983.
From: NCRP Report #93, p 19, Table 8.1.

Film badges

Film badges (Fig. 9-3) are the *most widely* used and economical type of personnel monitoring device. These devices record radiation exposure accumulated at a low rate over a long period of time.

The film badge consists of three parts: a durable, lightweight plastic film holder, an assortment of metal filters, and a film packet. The plastic film holder should be made of a plastic material of a low atomic number to filter low energy x-radiation (most plastic film holders can also filter low-energy gamma and beta radiation). Contained in the plastic holder are metal filters

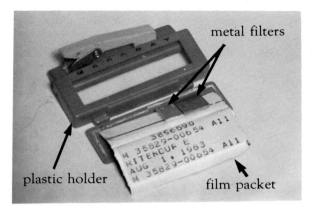

Fig. 9-3   Disassembled film badge, demonstrating badge components: plastic holder, metal filters, and film packet.
(Courtesy Landauer, Inc., Glenwood, Ill.)

of aluminum or copper. These filters allow the measurement of the approximate energy of the radiation reaching the monitoring device. Penetrating radiations cast a faint shadow of the filters on the processed monitoring film, whereas soft radiations cast a more pronounced image of the filters. The density of the image cast by the filters permits the energy of the radiation to be estimated. In addition, the direction from which the radiation reached the film (from front to back or from back to front) can be estimated from the filter shadows imaged on the processed monitoring film. The filters may also be used to determine whether the exposure was due to excessive amounts of scattered radiation or to a single exposure from a primary beam. Excessive exposure to scatter, such as would result from poor working habits (i.e., radiographer standing too close to a patient during an exposure) or poor facility design, would result in a relatively fuzzy image of the filters because the film badge would have been irradiated from many different angles. A single exposure from a primary beam, such as would result if a radiographer inadvertently left the film badge on a table during an exposure (the badge may have fallen off while the radiographer was positioning the patient and gone unnoticed), would result in a sharply defined image.

The radiographic film packet contains a special radiation-dosimetry film similar to dental film. This film is sensitive to doses ranging from as low as 0.0001 Sv or 0.1 mSv (10 mrem) to as high as 5 Sv or 5000 mSv (500 rem). The outside of the film packet forms a light-free envelope for the dosimetry film. Inside the envelope a sheet of lead foil backs the film to absorb scatter radiation coming from behind the monitoring device. When radiation

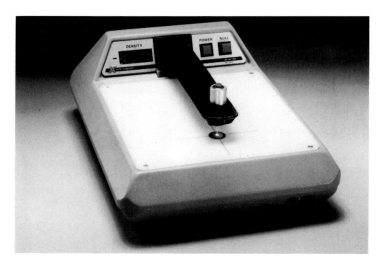

Fig. 9-4   The densitometer, an instrument which measures occupational exposure by comparing densities of exposed film badge (dosimetry) films. (Courtesy X-rite Inc., Grandville, Mich.)

interacts with the film in the badge, it causes the film to darken once it is developed. After processing, the density of the image of the filters recorded on the dosimetry film is proportional to the amount of radiation received and the energy of the radiation. An instrument called a densitometer (Fig. 9-4) is used to measure this density. It measures the intensity of light transmitted through a given area of the dosimetry film and compares it with the intensity of light incident on the one side of the film. The amount of radiation the film was exposed to is determined by locating the exposure value of a control film of a similar density on a characteristic curve (Fig. 9-5). For example, in the characteristic curve in Fig. 9-5, if the density of the dosimetry film is determined to be 0.5, the film badge has received slightly more than 0.0001 Sv, or 0.1 mSv (10 mrem).

The monitoring company that supplies an institution with film badges provides a "control badge" with each batch of badges. This control badge serves as a base for comparing the rest of the film badge batch after they have been returned to the monitoring company for processing. Because the control badge has been kept in a radiation-free area of a given radiological facility, its density reading should be zero. If after processing a reading above zero is indicated, the batch of badges may have been exposed while in transit to or from the institution. To ensure that false readings are *not* reported, the control badge reading is reported to the institution. This reading must be

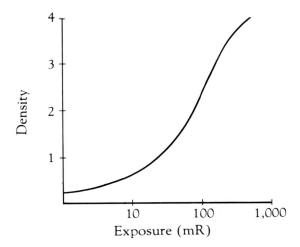

Fig. 9-5   Typical characteristic curve.

subtracted from each of the remaining film badges in the batch to ensure accuracy in exposure reporting.

Results from personnel monitoring programs must be recorded accurately and maintained for review to meet state and federal regulations. To comply with such requirements, institutions frequently use established dosimetry services. These monitoring services process film badges and other types of personnel monitors and prepare a written report (Fig. 9-6, *A*) for the health care facility. This report lists the deep* and shallow† occupational exposure of each person in that institution as measured by the exposed monitors. Information on the report is arranged in a series of columns. These columns include the following:

1. Personal data listing each participant's identification number (the same number as on the front of each person's film badge packet or other personnel monitor), name, Social Security number, birth date, and sex.
2. Type of dosimeter: "G" representing a film badge used to monitor x, gamma, and beta radiation; "U" representing a finger badge used to monitor similar types of radiation.

---

*Deep dose is defined, for example, by Landauer, Inc., of Glenwood, IL, as the absorbed dose equivalent from all types of radiation at a depth of 1 cm in soft tissue. This number is regarded as the absorbed dose equivalent to the whole body.

†Shallow dose is defined, for example, by Landauer, Inc., of Glenwood, IL, as the absorbed dose equivalent from all radiations at approximately 0.007 cm depth in soft tissue. This dose is considered by Landauer as "equivalent to the dose to the skin of the whole body."

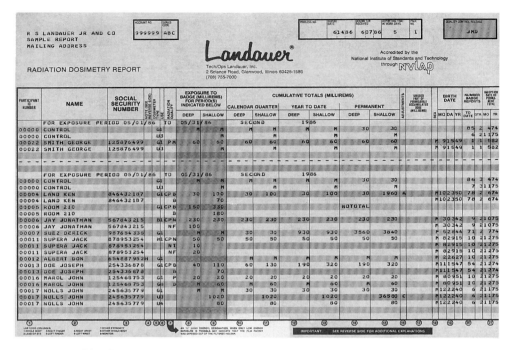

Fig. 9-6 *A,* Personnel film badge report provided by a monitoring company states the individual deep and shallow occupational exposure of each person in a particular institution as measured by the exposed film badges.

3. Radiation quality (e.g., x-ray exposure, beta particle exposure, neutron exposure, or combined radiation exposure).

4. Absorbed dose equivalent data, including current deep and shallow recorded absorbed dose equivalents (millirems) for the time indicated on the report (e.g., 05/01/86 to 05/31/86).

5. Cumulative absorbed dose equivalents for deep and shallow radiation exposures for the calendar quarter (3 months), for the year to date, and for lifetime radiation.

The cumulative columns provide a continuous audit of actual absorbed radiation dose equivalent. These totals can be compared with allowable values established by regulatory agencies. Whenever the letter "M" appears under the current monitoring period or in the cumulative columns, it signifies that an absorbed dose equivalent below the minimum measurable quantity of radiation has been recorded during that time. According to Landauer, Inc., for x-rays and gamma rays M can represent a value up to 10 mrem, for energetic beta particles a value up to 40 mrem, for fast neutrons up to 20 mrem, and up to 10 mrem for thermal neutrons.

CURRENT OCCUPATIONAL RADIATION EXPOSURE

Prepared by

Landauer®

Accredited by the
National Institute of Standards and Technology
through NVLAP

Landauer, Inc.
2 Science Road   Glenwood, Illinois 60425-1586
Telephone: (708) 755-7000 Facsimile: (708) 755-7016

ACCOUNT NO.	SERIES CODE	PARTICIPANT NO.	PREPARATION DATE	MO. DAY YR.	TERMINATION REPORT	FIRST REPORT FOR MONITORED INDIVIDUAL (to be completed by customer)
257	A	01184		8/15/91		

IDENTIFICATION

1. NAME (LAST, FIRST AND MIDDLE)	2. SOCIAL SECURITY NUMBER	3. SEX	4. DATE OF BIRTH MO. DAY YEAR
DOE MARY	- -	F	4 / 13 / 59

5. NAME OF LICENSEE OR REGISTRANT	6. EMPLOYER - IF DIFFERENT FROM LICENSEE (COMPLETED BY CUSTOMER)
LANDAUER, INC.	

7. CITY OR STATE REGISTRATION NUMBER	8. NRC, AGREEMENT STATE, OR STATE LICENSE
4677	

OCCUPATIONAL EXPOSURE (EXTERNAL)

9. DOSE RECORD FOR **4**

CODE:
TOTAL BODY (DEEP) - 1   RIGHT WRIST - 5
SKIN OF TOTAL BODY (SHALLOW) - 2   LEFT WRIST - 6
RIGHT HAND - 3   OTHER EXTREMITY - 7
LEFT HAND - 4   OTHER TOTAL BODY - 8

10. METHOD OF MONITORING **4**

CODE:
FILM/TLD BADGE - 1   SOLID STATE - 4
POCKET CHAMBER - 2   OTHER - 5
CALCULATIONS - 3

11. PERIOD OF EXPOSURE FROM MO. DAY YR.	TO MO. DAY YR.	12. X OR GAMMA DOSE FOR THE PERIOD (REM) DECIMAL	13. BETA DOSE FOR THE PERIOD (REM) DECIMAL	14. NEUTRON DOSE FOR THE PERIOD (REM) DECIMAL	15. TOTAL DOSE FOR THE PERIOD (REM) DECIMAL	16. TOTAL LIFETIME ACCUMULATED DOSE (REM) DECIMAL	17. PERMISSIBLE ACC. DOSE 5(N-18)(REM)	18. UNUSED PART OF PERMISSIBLE ACC. DOSE IN (REM) DECIMAL	19. NUMBER OF BADGES REPORTED
1/01/91	3/31/91				M	M			3
4/01/91	6/30/91				M	M			2
	YEARLY TOTAL—				M				

20. INCEPTION DATE OF SERVICE WITH TECH / OPS LANDAUER, INC. 10/86

21. PREVIOUSLY SUPPLIED TOTAL OCCUPATIONAL EXTERNAL RADIATION EXPOSURE HISTORY INCLUDED IN COLUMN 16. DECIMAL

SKIN DOSE EXPOSURE INCLUDES SUM OF X OR GAMMA, BETA AND NEUTRON EXPOSURE. "M" INDICATES EXPOSURE LESS THAN 10 MR.

ESTIMATE OF INTERNAL EXPOSURE (TO BE COMPLETED BY CUSTOMER)

22. PERIOD OF EXPOSURE FROM MO. DAY YR.	TO MO. DAY YR.	23. NUCLIDE(S)	24. CRITICAL ORGAN(S)	25. ESTIMATE OF EXPOSURE

CERTAIN REGULATORY AGENCIES REQUIRE THE REPORTING OF ADDITIONAL INFORMATION. THE FOLLOWING SPACE IS PROVIDED FOR YOUR CONVENIENCE IN ADDING THIS DETAIL.

26. OCCUPATIONAL CLASSIFICATION	CODE NO.	27. SOURCE OF EXPOSURE	CODE NO.	28.	CODE NO.	29.	CODE NO.
PHYSICIAN - 1 TECHNICIAN DIRECTED BY - 2 PHYSICIAN OTHER - 3		X-RAY - 1 RADIOACTIVE MATERIALS - 2 BOTH - 3		RMA - 1 - 1 RMA - 2 - 2			

This form is for use in place of certain reports required by OSHA, NRC licensees and by state regulations (29CFR1910.96 n, 10CFR19.13 and 10CFR20.401 - 20.409) or for the maintenance of individual personal radiation exposure files and satisfies regulations that require reporting of exposure to employees. It contains the requisite information for NRC FORM - 5, California RH - 2365, Illinois RMA - 1, Nebraska NRH - 2, New Hampshire RCA - 7, Tennessee RHS 8-2, TEXAS TRCR 22.13A, and other similar forms.

This report is furnished to you under the provisions of the Nuclear Regulatory Commission regulation 10 CFR part 19. You should preserve this report for further reference.

Fig. 9-6, cont'd. *B,* Report showing a summary of occupational exposure.
(Courtesy Landauer, Inc., Glenwood, Ill.)

When a radiation worker changes employment, the data pertinent to accumulated permanent absorbed dose equivalent must be conveyed to the new employer so that this information can be placed on file. Figure 9-6, *B,* provides an example of an appropriate summary of occupational exposure report. A copy of such a report should be received by the radiation worker upon termination of employment.

The main advantage of the film badge is that the film itself, which is maintained by the monitoring company, constitutes a *permanent legal* record of personnel exposure. In many institutions that have a well-structured radiation safety program, personnel monitoring reports are received and reviewed by a radiation safety officer. Film badge readings that exceed a trigger level decided on by the institution are investigated to ascertain the cause of that reading. Such a process should be an integral component of the institution's radiation safety programs. This practice is compatible with the policy known as "ALARA"; i.e., keeping radiation exposures to personnel "as low as is reasonably achievable."

The film badge also has other benefits. This monitoring device is reasonably economical, costing only a few dollars per unit per month. The film badge can be used to monitor x-, gamma, and all but very low energy beta radiation in a reliable manner. And it can discriminate between the types of radiation and the energies of each of these radiations.

Another advantage of the film badge is that it has mechanical integrity. For example, the dosimetry film will not be damaged if the badge is accidently dropped.

The film badge does have some objectional characteristics. It is *not* an effective monitoring device unless it is worn. Temperature and humidity cause fogging of the dosimetry film over long periods of time; this effect increases with the length of time that the badge is worn and potentially can result in a seriously inaccurate high exposure reading. Manufacturers recommend 1 month as the maximum period of time that a film badge should be worn for personnel monitoring.

Other types of personnel monitoring devices are *more sensitive* to ionizing radiation and are therefore *more effective* monitors in some situations. The film badge is *most sensitive* to photons having an energy of 50 keV; above and below this energy range, dosimetry film sensitivity decreases.

Film badge dosimetry film must be shipped to the monitoring company for processing and exposure determination. Because this takes time, a radiation worker's exposure cannot be determined on the day of occurrence.

Pocket ionization chambers (pocket dosimeters)

Pocket ionization chambers (pocket dosimeters) (Fig. 9-7) are the most sensitive personnel monitoring devices. However, the use of these monitors in

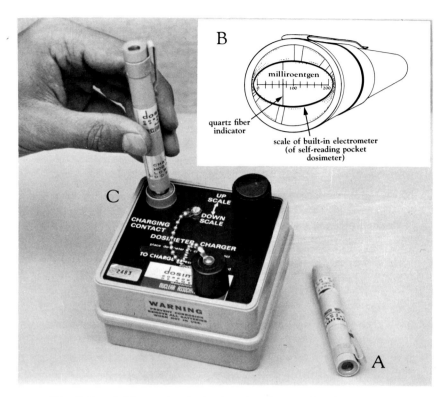

Fig. 9-7 *A,* The pocket ionization chamber (pocket dosimeter), the most sensitive personnel monitoring device, looks like a fountain pen from the outside but contains an ionization chamber which measures radiation exposure. *B,* The quartz fiber indicator of the built-in electrometer of the self-reading pocket dosimeter generally used in radiology indicates exposures of from 0 to 5.2×10^{-5} C/kg (0 to 200 mR). Before use, each pocket dosimeter must be charged to a predetermined voltage by a special charging unit *(C)* so that the charges of the positive and negative electrodes will be balanced and the quartz fiber indicator reads zero (0).
(Courtesy Dosimeter Corporation of America, Cincinnati, Ohio)

diagnostic radiology is infrequent. The pocket dosimeter looks like an ordinary fountain pen externally but contains a thimble ionization chamber.

There are two types of pocket ionization chambers: the self-reading type, which contains a built-in electrometer (a device that measures electrical charge), and the non-self-reading type, which requires a special accessory electrometer to read the device and which has been, for the most part, replaced by the self-reading type. The operating principle of both self-reading and non–self-reading pocket dosimeters is similar to that of the gold leaf electroscope, which detects the presence and sign of an electric charge.

The pocket ionization chamber contains two electrodes, one positively charged (the central electrode) and one negatively charged (the outer electrode). A quartz fiber can form part of the positive electrode and function as the indicator of the reading scale; in such a system, the quartz fiber casts a shadow onto a scale such that the amount of charge on the positively charged electrode determines the position of the shadow along the scale and is equivalent to the scale reading at that position. When the charged electrodes in the device are exposed to ionizing radiation, the air surrounding the central electrode $(+)$ becomes ionized and discharges the mechanism in direct proportion to the amount of radiation to which it has been exposed.

A special charging unit is required for pocket ionization chambers. Each dosimeter must be charged to a predetermined voltage before use so that the quartz fiber indicator of the reading scale indicates zero (0). As the dosimeter is exposed to ionizing radiation, it discharges and the fiber indicator indicates the exposure in milliroentgen. Pocket chambers generally used in radiology are sensitive to exposures ranging from 0 to 5.2×10^{-5} C/kg (0 to 200 mR).

There are some advantages to the use of pocket ionization chambers. Self-reading chambers provide an immediate exposure readout for radiation workers who work in high exposure areas; such persons can read the dosimeter on site and become aware of the dose received at the completion of a given assignment. The non–self-reading chambers are used in lower exposure areas. When immediate exposure readout is not necessary, the monitoring devices may be collected and read and the readings recorded each day by a radiation safety officer.

Pocket ionization chambers are compact units that are easy to carry and convenient to use. These instruments are reasonably accurate and sensitive. They are ideal monitoring devices for procedures that last for relatively short periods of time.

There are some disadvantages associated with the use of pocket ionization chambers. They are fairly expensive, costing $100.00 or more per unit. Care must be taken when obtaining pocket dosimeter readings; if the procedure is not carefully conducted, the readouts or results can be lost. If not read each day, the dosimeter may give an inaccurate reading because the electric charge tends to escape with time; a false high reading might be obtained from a dosimeter read too late. Pocket dosimeters can also discharge if subjected to some type of mechanical shock, which again would result in a false high reading. Because no permanent, legal record of exposure is provided with pocket dosimeters, institutions desiring a record of personnel exposure recorded with pocket dosimeters must delegate someone to keep such a record. This task should be the responsibility of a radiation safety officer.

However, these readings must be recorded accurately the first time because the electric charge tends to escape with time and the chambers are recharged for reuse soon after each use.

Thermoluminescent dosimeters

The exterior of the thermoluminescent dosimeter (TLD) badge (Fig. 9-8) looks similar to that of the film badge. However, the interior of this monitoring mechanism differs completely. This light-free device most often contains a crystalline form (powder or small chips) of lithium fluoride, which functions as the sensing material of the TLD.

Ionizing radiation causes the lithium fluoride crystals in the TLD to undergo changes in some of their physical properties. When irradiated, some of the electrons in the crystalline lattice structure absorb energy and are "excited" to higher energy levels or bands. The presence of impurities in the crystal causes these electrons to become trapped within these bands. When the lithium fluoride crystals are passed through a special heating process, these trapped electrons receive enough energy to rise above their present locations into a region called the conduction band. From here, the electrons can return to their original or normal state with the emission of energy in

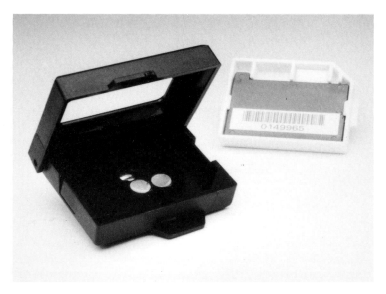

Fig. 9-8   Thermoluminescent dosimeter (TLD) badge containing the sensing material, lithium fluoride.
(Courtesy Landauer, Inc., Glenwood, Ill.)

the form of visible light. The intensity of the light is proportional to the amount of radiation that interacted with the crystals. A device called a *TLD analyzer* (Fig. 9-9) measures the amount of ionizing radiation to which a TLD badge has been exposed by first heating the crystals to free the trapped, highly energized electrons and then recording the amount of light emitted by the crystals (which is proportional to the TLD badge exposure).

The thermoluminescent dosimeter has several advantages over the film badge. The lithium fluoride crystals interact with ionizing radiation as human tissue does;* hence this monitor determines dose more accurately. Exposure as low as 1.3×10^{-6} C/kg (5 mR) can be measured with precision. Humidity, pressure, and normal temperature changes do not affect the TLD. Unlike the film in the film badge, which can fog if worn for more than 1

---

*The effective atomic number of lithium fluoride is equal to 8.2, which is similar to that of soft tissue (7.4).

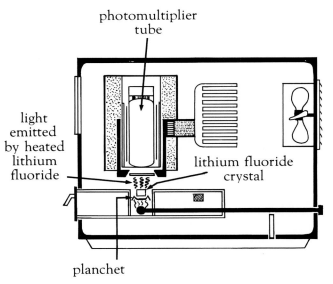

Fig. 9-9   Diagram of a typical analyzer. The analyzer measures the amount of ionizing radiation to which a badge has been exposed by heating the irradiated lithium fluoride crystals of the exposed badge with linearly rising temperatures using hot gas steam. This represents a departure from the previously used heating method, which relied upon physical contact between the crystals and a heated plate. The new method is a technical improvement, since any need for contact readjustments is eliminated.
(Courtesy Solon Technologies, Inc., Solon, Ohio)

month, the TLD may be worn for as long as 3 months. After the TLD reading has been obtained, the crystals can be reused. This makes the device somewhat cost-effective, even though the initial cost is high (approximately twice the cost of a film badge service).

TLDs have some disadvantages other than their initial high cost. A TLD can only be read once. The readout process destroys the stored information; the TLD may be reused, but once the crystal is heated the record of any previous exposure is gone. The necessity of using calibrated dosimeters (which must be prepared and read with each group of these monitoring devices when they are processed) with TLDs is also a disadvantage.

Table 9-2 provides a summary of the advantages and disadvantages of the personnel monitoring devices covered in this chapter.

RADIATION SURVEY INSTRUMENTS FOR AREA MONITORING

Radiation survey instruments are area monitoring devices that detect and/or measure radiation. The detection system indicates the presence or absence of radiation, whereas the dosimeter system measures radiation intensity.

When in contact with ionizing radiation, survey instruments respond to the charged particles that are produced as radiation interacts with and ionizes the gas (usually air) in the detector. These instruments measure either the total quantity of electrical charge resulting from the ionization of the gas or the rate at which the electrical charge is produced. The ionization chamber-type survey meter (cutie pie), the proportional counter, and the Geiger-Müller (G-M) detector are three different gas-filled radiation detectors that serve as field survey instruments that detect the presence of radiation and, when properly calibrated, give a reasonably accurate measurement of the exposure. The Victoreen condenser R-meter also uses a gas-filled ionization chamber but is capable of making a more accurate measurement of exposure and is not routinely used for surveys. Instead, historically, it has been used to calibrate x-ray equipment.

RADIATION SURVEY INSTRUMENT REQUIREMENTS

Radiation survey instruments used for area monitoring should meet certain requirements. First, these devices should be easy to carry, so that one person can operate the device in an efficient manner for a period of time. Second, survey instruments must be durable enough to withstand normal use, the routine handling that occurs during standard operating procedures. Third, area monitors must be reliable; only in such a case can radiation exposure or exposure rate in a given area be accurately assessed. Fourth, area monitoring

Table 9-2 **Summary of the Advantages and Disadvantages of Personnel Monitoring Devices**

Personnel monitoring device	Advantages	Disadvantages
Film badge	1. Lightweight, durable, easy to carry 2. Cost-efficient monitoring for large numbers of people 3. Records radiation exposure accumulated at a low rate over a long period of time 4. Provides a permanent, legally acceptable record of personnel exposure 5. Detects and records small and large exposures in a consistent, reliable manner 6. Instrument performance is usually not affected by outside influences such as heat and humidity fluctuations and non-extreme mechanical shock 7. Filters contained in the badge make it possible to estimate the direction from which the radiation came 8. Filters can indicate whether exposure was due to excessive amounts of scattered radiation as opposed to a single exposure from the primary beam 9. Control badge can indicate if a group of badges were exposed in transit to and/or from an institution 10. Can be used to monitor x-, gamma, and all but very low energy beta radiation in a reliable manner 11. Can discriminate between type of radiation and energy of x-, gamma, and beta radiation	1. Records only the exposure received in the body area in which it is worn 2. Not effective as a monitoring device if not worn 3. Temperature and humidity can cause film in the badge to fog over long periods of time, causing inaccurate exposure reading 4. Decreased film sensitivity above and below 50 keV 5. Exposure cannot be determined on day of occurrence 6. Limited in accuracy to + or − 20%

Table 9-2 **Summary of the Advantages and Disadvantages of Personnel Monitoring Devices—cont'd**

Personnel monitoring device	Advantages	Disadvantages
Pocket ionization chamber	1. Small, compact units, easy to carry, convenient to use 2. Reasonably accurate and sensitive 3. Can be used as monitors for procedures that last relatively short periods of time 4. Self-reading chambers provide an immediate exposure readout for radiation workers in high exposure areas	1. Fairly expensive, hence not cost-effective for large numbers of persons 2. Readings must be carefully obtained or they may be lost 3. To avoid inaccurate reading, dosimeter must be read each day it is used 4. Unit can discharge if subjected to some type of mechanical shock and give a false high reading 5. No permanent, legal record of exposure is provided 6. Records only the exposure received in the body area in which it is worn
Thermoluminescent dosimeter	1. Crystals contained in TLD interact with ionizing radiation as human tissue does; hence, TLD determines dose more accurately 2. Not affected by humidity, pressure, or normal temperature changes 3. Can be worn up to 3 months 4. After reading has been obtained, TLD crystals can be reused, making the device somewhat cost-effective	1. Greater initial cost than film badge service 2. Readouts must be carefully obtained or results can be lost 3. Readout process destroys information stored in TLD, which prevents the "read" TLD from serving as a permanent, legal record of exposure 4. Calibrated dosimeters must be prepared and read with each group of TLDs as they are processed 5. Records only the exposure received in the body area in which it is worn 6. Not effective as a monitoring device if not worn

devices should interact with ionizing radiation in a manner similar to that in which human tissue reacts; this permits dose to be determined more accurately. Fifth, a radiation survey instrument should be able to detect all types of ionizing radiation; such a quality increases the usefulness of an area monitoring device. Sixth, the energy of the radiation should not affect the response of the detector, and the direction of the incident radiation should not affect the performance of the unit; such characteristics ensure consistency in individual unit operation. Seventh, survey equipment should be cost-effective; the initial cost and subsequent maintenance charges should be as low as possible.

TYPES OF GAS-FILLED RADIATION SURVEY INSTRUMENTS

As mentioned, there are three types of gas-filled radiation survey instruments: the ionization chamber-type survey meter (cutie pie), the proportional counter, and the Geiger-Müller (G-M) detector.

Ionization chamber-type survey meter (cutie pie)

The ionization chamber-type survey meter or "cutie pie" (Fig. 9-10) is a rate meter device (measures exposure rate) used for area surveys. This device measures x- or gamma radiation and, if equipped with a suitable window, it can also record beta radiation.

The ionization chamber-type survey meter or "cutie pie" can measure radiation intensity ranging from 1 mR/hr to several thousand roentgen per hour. This device can be used to monitor diagnostic x-ray installations when exposure times of a second or more are chosen and to measure fluoroscopic dose rate, exposure to patients containing therapeutic doses of radioactive materials, exposure in radioisotope storage facilities, and the dose received outside protective barriers.

The advantage of using the cutie pie is that it can measure a wide range of radiation exposure within a few seconds. The delicate construction and relatively large size of the unit may be considered as something of a disadvantage. Another disadvantage is that the unit requires adequate warm-up time or its meter will drift and produce an inaccurate reading. This device cannot be used to measure exposures produced by typical diagnostic procedures because the exposure times are too short to permit the meter to respond. Instead, it is most commonly used to measure the exposure rates (mR/hr) at various distances from a patient who has received radioactive materials for diagnostic or therapeutic purposes.

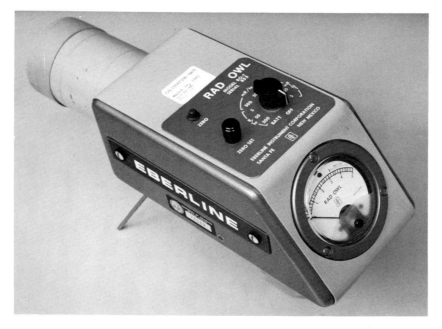

Fig. 9-10   Ionization chamber-type survey meter or "cutie-pie." (Courtesy Eberline Instruments, Santa Fe, N.M.)

Proportional counter

Proportional counters serve no useful purpose in diagnostic radiology. They are generally used in a laboratory setting to detect alpha and beta radiation and small amounts of other types of low-level radioactive contamination. The proportional counter can discriminate between alpha and beta particles; however, because alpha radiation travels only a short distance in air, the operator of the proportional counter must hold the unit's probe close to the surface of the object being surveyed to obtain an accurate reading of the alpha radiation being emitted by the object.

Geiger-Müller (G-M) detector

Geiger-Müller detectors (Fig. 9-11) serve as the primary radiation survey instrument for area monitoring in nuclear medicine facilities. The unit detects individual radioactive particles (e.g., electrons emitted from certain radioactive nuclei) or photons. Hence, it can easily detect any area contaminated by radioactive material. Because rapid monitoring can be accomplished with the G-M detector, the unit can be used to locate a lost radioactive source or to detect radioactive contamination.

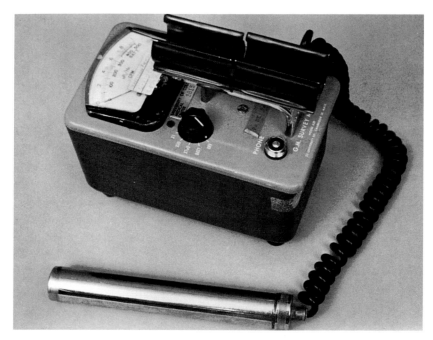

Fig. 9-11   Geiger-Müller detector.
(Courtesy Baird Corporation, Nuclear Instruments Division, Bedford, Mass.)

The G-M detector has an audible sound system (an audio amplifier and speaker), which alerts the operator to the presence of ionizing radiation. Metal encloses the counter's gas-filled tube, which is the unit's sensitive ionization chamber. When the shield covering the detector's sensitive chamber is open, beta, x-, and gamma radiation can be detected by the probe mechanism. Meter readings are usually obtained in counts per minute, which can be converted to milliroentgen per hour under some conditions. Because G-M tubes are inclined to lose their calibration, the instrument generally has a "check source" of weak uranium located somewhere on its external surface.

The meter reading of a G-M detector depends on the energy of the incident photons. This means that photons of different energies cause the instrument to respond differently, which is a disadvantage in diagnostic radiology usage. Also, the G-M detector jams when placed in a high-intensity radiation area. Because the detector's meter can deflect off scale or register zero as a consequence of entering a high-intensity radiation area, a false reading may be obtained.

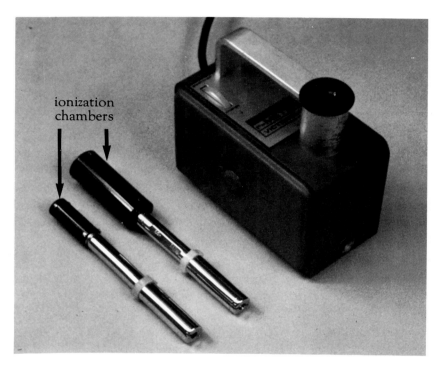

Fig. 9-12　Victoreen condenser R-meter with ionization chambers. (Courtesy Victoreen, Inc., Cleveland, Ohio)

CALIBRATION INSTRUMENTS

Gas-filled survey instruments can be used to calibrate x-ray equipment. An example of a widely used calibration instrument is the Victoreen condenser R-meter.

Victoreen condenser R-meter

The Victoreen condenser R-meter (Fig. 9-12) measures radiation by recording the total exposure received during a given period of time. The sensitivity of the unit's ionization chambers is relatively independent of the energy of the incident photon, which means that the unit is adaptable to a wide range of exposures. However, an ionization chamber suitable for the appropriate exposure range must be selected. Other types of ionization chambers are used in combination with electrometers, devices for measuring the tiny electric currents produced in the chamber when ions are liberated by radiation exposure.

SUMMARY

In this chapter the subject of radiation monitoring was introduced. The reader should now be able to identify and explain the operating principles of the various personnel and area monitoring devices and instruments.

REVIEW QUESTIONS

1. Which of the following chemicals function as the sensing material in a thermoluminescent dosimeter?
   a. calcium tungstate
   b. sodium iodide
   c. lithium fluoride
   d. barium sulphate

2. Three of the following items are basic components of the film badge; which one is *not*?
   a. radiographic film packet
   b. plastic film holder
   c. charged electrodes
   d. assortment of metal filters

3. Which of the following personnel monitoring devices looks like an ordinary fountain pen externally?
   a. pocket dosimeter
   b. film badge
   c. thermoluminescent dosimeter
   d. none of the above

4. Of the following, which are advantages of using the film badge as a personnel monitoring device?
   1. economical cost
   2. provides a permanent, legal record of personnel exposure
   3. can be used to monitor x-, gamma, and all but very low energy beta radiation
   a. 1 only
   b. 2 only
   c. 3 only
   d. 1, 2, and 3

5. Which of the following statements is *not* true?
   a. personnel monitoring becomes necessary whenever radiation workers are likely to run the risk of receiving one fourth or more of the annual dose equivalent limit
   b. personnel monitoring devices protect the radiographer or other diagnostic radiology personnel from exposure to ionizing radiation

   c. a personnel monitoring device records only the exposure received in the body area in which it is worn

   d. personnel monitoring devices measure the quantity of ionizing radiation to which they have been exposed over a period of time

6. When performing a fluoroscopic procedure, special radiographic procedures, or a mobile radiographic examination, where should nonpregnant occupationally exposed persons wear a personnel monitoring device?
   a. outside of the protective apron at hip level
   b. under the protective apron at hip level
   c. under the protective apron at the level of the sternal angle
   d. outside of the protective apron at collar level

7. The metal filters contained in the film badge are generally composed of:
   a. aluminum or copper
   b. aluminum or lead
   c. zinc or copper
   d. lead or zinc

8. When radiation interacts with the radiographic film contained in the film badge, the film after development:
   a. turns green
   b. darkens in proportion to the exposure
   c. remains unchanged in terms of density
   d. lightens in proportion to the exposure

9. The suggested maximum period of time that a film badge should be worn as a personnel monitoring device is:
   a. 1 week
   b. 2 weeks
   c. 1 month
   d. 3 months

10. Which one of the following personnel monitoring devices allows a radiation worker to determine exposure received immediately upon completion of a specific radiologic procedure?
   a. film badge
   b. self-reading pocket dosimeter
   c. non–self-reading pocket dosimeter
   d. thermoluminescent dosimeter

11. Film badges are *most* sensitive to a photon energy of:
   a. 200 keV
   b. 100 keV
   c. 50 keV
   d. 25 keV

12. When the negatively and positively charged electrodes in the pocket ionization chamber are exposed to ionizing radiation, the mechanism:
    a. charges in direct proportion to the amount of radiation to which it has been exposed
    b. discharges in direct proportion to the amount of radiation to which it has been exposed
    c. heats the central electrode
    d. heats the outer electrode

13. Before a pocket dosimeter is used to record radiation exposure, the quartz fiber indicator of the reading scale must indicate:
    a. zero
    b. 100 mR
    c. 150 mR
    d. 200 mR

14. Non–self-reading pocket ionization chambers are used:
    a. in high exposure areas when immediate readout is necessary
    b. for a period of 1 week before a readout is obtained
    c. for a period of 1 month before a readout is obtained
    d. in low exposure areas when an immediate exposure readout is not necessary

15. Of the following, which are disadvantages of using pocket ionization chambers as personnel monitoring devices?
    1. mechanical shock causes pocket chambers to discharge
    2. a permanent record of personnel exposure cannot be obtained with a pocket dosimeter
    3. false high readings may be obtained if the pocket dosimeter is not read each day
    a. 1 only
    b. 2 only
    c. 3 only
    d. 1, 2, and 3

16. Which of the following devices is used to measure the visible light emitted by the sensing material contained in the TLD after exposure to ionizing radiation and heating?
    a. x-ray tube
    b. densitometer
    c. photomultiplier tube
    d. sensitometer

17. When the sensing crystals contained in the TLD are exposed to ionizing radiation, the:
    a. protons in the crystalline lattice structure absorb energy and are excited to higher energy levels

b. neutrons in the crystalline lattice structure absorb energy and are excited to higher energy levels
c. electrons in the crystalline lattice structure absorb energy and are excited to higher energy levels
d. freed electrons are trapped at a lower energy level

18. Of the following, which are disadvantages of using thermoluminescent dosimeters as personnel monitoring devices?
  1. only one readout may be obtained
  2. readout or results can be lost if the readout procedure is not carefully conducted
  3. greater initial cost than film badge service
a. 1 only
b. 2 only
c. 3 only
d. 1, 2, and 3

19. The *maximum* period of time that a TLD may be worn as a personnel monitoring device is:
a. 1 hour
b. 1 week
c. 1 month
d. 3 months

20. Exposures from 2.58×10^{-6} C/kg to 5.2×10^{-5} C/kg (10 to 200 mR) can be recorded by using the following monitoring device(s):
  1. film badge
  2. thermoluminescent dosimeter
  3. pocket ionization chamber
a. 1 only
b. 2 only
c. 3 only
d. 1, 2, and 3

21. Which of the following personnel monitoring devices possesses the *most* mechanical integrity?
a. non–self-reading pocket ionization chambers
b. thermoluminescent dosimeters
c. self-reading pocket ionization chambers
d. film badges

22. A densitometer is used to measure the:
a. density on the processed film from a film badge
b. light emitted from the sensing material of the TLD after exposure
c. freed electrons
d. discharged electricity

23. Of the following types of personnel monitoring devices, which device is *least* sensitive to ionizing radiation?
    a. film badge
    b. thermoluminescent dosimeter
    c. self-reading pocket dosimeter
    d. non–self-reading pocket dosimeter

24. In the characteristic curve in Fig. 9-5, if the density of the dosimetry film is determined to be 1.0, the film badge has been exposed to:
    a. 1 mSv (100 mR)
    b. 0.5 mSv (50 mR)
    c. 0.15 mSv (15 mR)
    d. 0.1 mSv (10 mR)

25. The image densities cast by the filters in the film badge permit the:
    a. percentage of visible light emission to be determined
    b. film to be reused
    c. energy of the radiation to be estimated
    d. electrical discharge to be determined

26. Radiation survey instruments measure the:
    a. total quantity of electrical charge resulting from the ionization of the gas
    b. rate at which an electrical charge is produced
    c. a or b
    d. none of the above

27. The detection system of a radiation survey instrument:
    a. measures radiation intensity
    b. indicates the presence of radiation
    c. counts uncharged particles
    d. a and b

28. Which of the following instruments is used to calibrate x-ray equipment?
    a. proportional counter
    b. Geiger-Müller detector
    c. ionization chamber-type survey meter
    d. Victoreen condenser R-meter

29. Which of the following requirements should radiation survey instruments meet?
    1. instruments must be reliable by accurately recording exposure or exposure rate
    2. instruments must be durable enough to withstand normal use
    3. instruments should interact with ionizing radiation in a manner similar to the way in which human tissue interacts
    a. 1 only
    b. 2 only

    c. 3 only
    d. 1, 2, and 3

30. Which of the following instruments should be used in an x-ray installation to assess fluoroscopic dose rate?
    a. Victoreen condenser R-meter
    b. Geiger-Müller detector
    c. ionization chamber-type survey meter
    d. proportional counter

31. Which of the following instruments should be used to locate a lost radioactive source or detect radioactive contamination?
    a. Geiger-Müller detector
    b. proportional counter
    c. ionization chamber-type survey meter
    d. Victoreen condenser R-meter

32. Which of the following instruments should be used in a laboratory setting to detect alpha and beta radiation and small amounts of other types of low-level radioactive contamination?
    a. ionization chamber-type survey meter
    b. proportional counter
    c. Geiger-Müller detector
    d. Victoreen condenser R-meter

33. Which of the following instruments is called a cutie pie?
    a. Geiger-Müller detector
    b. Victoreen condenser R-meter
    c. ionization chamber-type survey meter
    d. proportional counter

34. What do ionization chamber-type survey meters, proportional counters, Geiger-Müller detectors, and Victoreen condenser R-meters have in common?
    a. these instruments all measure x-radiation only
    b. these instruments can all be used to calibrate x-ray equipment
    c. these instruments can all be used to measure the dose received outside protective barriers
    d. each of these units contains a gas-filled chamber

35. Which component of the Geiger-Müller detector alerts the operator to the presence of ionizing radiation?
    a. the shield covering the detector's sensitive chamber
    b. an audio amplifier and speaker
    c. the metal that encloses the counter's gas-filled tube
    d. the meter scale

36. Which of the following instruments generally has a check source of weak uranium located somewhere on its external surface?
    a. Victoreen condenser R-meter
    b. proportional counter
    c. Geiger-Müller detector
    d. ionization chamber-type survey meter

37. If a radiographer leaves his or her film badge in a closed car where it is exposed to sunlight for a considerable period of time, the dosimetry film in the badge will:
    a. become fogged due to increased temperature and humidity causing a false high reading
    b. decrease in sensitivity and not provide an accurate reading
    c. turn bright orange and melt
    d. not be affected by increased temperature and humidity and will provide an accurate reading

38. Select the *most* cost-effective personnel monitoring device for continual monitoring of a large number of radiography team members employed in a busy hospital Radiology Department.
    a. thermoluminescent dosimeter
    b. film badge
    c. self-reading pocket dosimeter
    d. non–self-reading pocket dosimeter

39. When performing a routine radiographic procedure, it is acceptable for a radiographer to wear a film badge monitoring device attached to the:
    1. clothing on the front of the body at chest level
    2. clothing on the front of the body at waist level
    3. wristwatch band
    a. 1 only
    b. 2 only
    c. 3 only
    d. 1 and 2 only

40. During which of the following radiologic procedures should a radiographer always wear his or her film badge on the front of the body at collar level?
    a. while assisting during fluoroscopy
    b. while radiographing a chest
    c. while radiographing an extremity
    d. while radiographing an abdomen

Bibliography

Ballinger PW: *Merrill's atlas of radiographic positions and radiologic procedures,* ed 5, vol 1, St Louis, 1982, Mosby–Year Book.

Bushong S: *Radiologic science for technologists: physics, biology, and protection,* ed 2, St Louis, 1980, Mosby–Year Book.

Bushong SC: In Ballinger PW: *Merrill's atlas of radiographic positions and radiologic procedures,* ed 7, vol 1, St Louis, 1991, Mosby–Year Book, p 18.

Bushong SC: *Radiologic science for technologists: physics, biology, and protection,* ed 5, St Louis, 1993, Mosby–Year Book.

Frankel R: *Radiation protection for radiologic technologists,* New York, 1976, McGraw-Hill.

Moscovitch M et al: A TLD system based on gas heating with linear time-temperature profile, *Radiation Protection Dosimetry* 34:361, 1990.

Moscovitch M et al: Mixed field personnel dosimetry using a nearly tissue-equivalent multi-element thermoluminescence dosimeter, *Radiation Protection Dosimetry* 34:145, 1990.

National Council on Radiation Protection and Measurements (NCRP): Report #91, *Recommendations on limits for exposure to ionizing radiation,* Bethesda, MD, 1987, NCRP Publications.

Noz ME, Maguire Jr GQ: *Radiation protection in the radiologic and health sciences,* Philadelphia, 1979, Lea & Febiger.

Noz ME, Maguire Jr GQ: *Radiation protection in radiologic and health sciences,* ed 2, Philadelphia, 1985, Lea & Febiger.

Scheele RV, Wakley J: *Elements of radiation protection,* Springfield, IL, 1975, Charles C Thomas.

Selman J: *The fundamentals of x-ray and radium physics,* ed 6, Springfield, IL, 1978, Charles C Thomas.

Travis EL: *Primer of medical radiobiology,* ed 2, Chicago, 1989, Year Book Medical Publishers.

Glossary

absolute risk   establishes a number of cancers in a specific group of people within a period of 1 year for a given level of absorbed dose (i.e., the above average number of cancer cases in 1 million [10^6] humans exposed to 1 rem)

absorbed dose   the amount of energy transferred from ionizing radiation to an irradiated object per unit mass. This absorbed energy is responsible for whatever biological damage occurs as a result of the tissues being exposed to x-radiation.

absorbed dose equivalent   the product obtained by multiplying the absorbed dose (AD) times the quality factor (QF). This quantity considers the biological effects of various types of radiation on humans.

absorbed dose equivalent limits   established guidelines for occupational and non-occupational radiation exposure

absorption   transference of energy from an x-ray beam to the atoms or molecules of the matter through which it passes

acid-base balance   state of equilibrium or stability between acids and bases

acids   hydrogen-containing compounds that can attack and dissolve metal (e.g., HNO_3, nitric acid)

acute   something that begins suddenly and runs a short but rather severe course (e.g., an acute disease)

acute effects   (*see* early effects)

acute radiation syndrome   radiation sickness that occurs in humans after whole-body absorbed doses of 1Gy (100 rad) or more of ionizing radiation delivered over a short period of time

added filtration   sheets of aluminum (or its equivalent) of appropriate thickness interposed outside of the glass window of the x-ray tube housing

adenine (A)   one of two purine bases found in both DNA and RNA.

adenosine triphosphate (ATP)   high-energy phosphate compound essential for sustaining life

agreement states   individual states of the United States that have entered into agreement with the Nuclear Regulatory Commission (NRC) to assume the responsibility for enforcing radiation protection regulations through their health departments

ALARA Concept   precept which states that "radiation exposures should be kept As Low As Reasonably Achievable"

alkali   a member of a group of elements in the periodic table that includes lithium, sodium, potassium, etc.

alkaline earth   a member of a group of elements in the periodic table that includes calcium, magnesium, strontium, etc.

alkalis   (*see* bases)

alpha particle   a particulate form of radiation. This particle is positively charged because it comprises two protons and two neutrons. Alpha particles are ejected by certain radioactive elements.

aluminum (Al)   the metal most frequently selected as filter material because it effectively removes low energy (soft) x-rays from a polyenergetic x-ray beam

American College of Radiology (ACR)   major professional organization of radiologists in the United States

amino acids   the structural units of protein

ampere   the S.I. unit of electric charge. One ampere represents the flow of electrons amounting to a charge of one coulomb crossing unit area per second.

anaphase   the phase of mitosis during which each two chromatids repel each other and migrate along the mitotic spindle to opposite sides of the cell

anemia   a condition characterized by a lack of vitality and caused by a decrease in the number of red blood cells in the circulating blood

anion   a negatively charged ion

annihilation radiation   two 0.511 keV gamma rays emitted in opposite directions. It occurs as a result of the interaction of a positron and an electron. This type of radiation is emitted from patients who have been injected with a radiopharmaceutical that contains atoms that decay by the process of positron decay.

anode   the positively charged target in the x-ray tube

antibodies   materials developed by the body in response to the presence of foreign antigens such as bacteria or a flu virus. They provide a primary defense mechanism against such antigens.

antimatter   matter composed of the counterparts of ordinary matter which does not exist freely in the universe and is unstable in the presence of ordinary matter

aperture diaphragm   a beam limitation device that consists of a flat piece of lead with a hole of a designated size and shape cut in its center

aplastic anemia   anemia resulting from bone marrow failure

artificial radiation   (*see* man-made radiation)

atom   the smallest portion of an element that has all of its chemical properties

Atomic Energy Commission (AEC)   (*see* Nuclear Regulatory Commission [NRC])

atomic number   the number of protons contained within the nucleus of an atom

attenuation   with respect to x-rays, this term refers to any process that decreases the intensity of the primary photon beam that was directed toward some destination

audible sound system   an audio amplifier and speaker. Geiger-Müller detectors contain an audible sound system.

axon   nerve cell process that extends out from the cell body and conducts impulses away from the cell body

back scatter   photons that have interacted with the atoms of an object and consequently are deflected in a backward direction (toward the x-ray tube)

bases   alkali or alkaline earth OH compounds that can neutralize acids, e.g., $Mg(OH)_2$, otherwise known as milk of magnesia

beam limitation device   a device that limits the parameters of the useful beam to a designated size and shape before it enters the area of clinical interest

becquerel   the SI unit of radioactivity. It is equal to one disintegration per second.

beta particles   high-speed electrons or positrons

binding energy   force that holds an atom together

biological damage   damage to living tissue

bone marrow syndrome   (*see* hematopoietic syndrome)

brems radiation   (*see* bremsstrahlung)

bremsstrahlung   ionizing electromagnetic radiation that is nonuniform in energy and wavelength and that is produced when a bombarding beam of electrons in an x-ray tube undergoes deceleration by interaction with the nuclei of the x-ray tube target atoms

Bucky slot shielding device   a protective device of at least 0.25 mm lead equivalent that automatically covers the Bucky slot opening during fluoroscopic examinations when the Bucky tray is positioned at the foot end of the table. This device protects the radiographer and/or the radiologist from radiation exposure at the gonadal level.

Bureau of Radiological Health (BRH)   (*see* Center for Devices and Radiological Health)

c-arm fluoroscope   a portable device for producing real-time (motion) images of a patient. The opposite ends of the "c"-shaped support arm hold the x-ray tube and the image intensifier.

carbohydrates   Compounds composed entirely of carbon, hydrogen, and oxygen. There are always twice as many atoms of hydrogen as of oxygen. Carbohydrates are involved in the chief energy releasing processes in animals and plants. Sugars and starch are examples of carbohydrates.

carbon   nonmetallic element that is the basic constituent of all organic matter

carcinogenesis   the production or origin of cancer

catalyst   agent which affects the speed of a chemical reaction without being altered itself

catalytic failure   the inability to influence the speed of a required chemical reaction; for example, during protein synthesis

cataractogenesis   the production or origin of cataracts

cataracts   a clouding of the eye lens which obstructs the passage of light

cathode   the negatively charged source of the high speed electrons in an X-ray tube

cation   a positively charged ion

cell division the multiplication process whereby one cell divides to form two or more cells

cell membrane a very frail structure encasing and surrounding the cell

cell metabolism chemical reactions which modify foods for cellular use

cells the basic units of all living matter

Center for Devices and Radiological Health (CDRH) known before 1982 as the Bureau of Radiological Health (BRH), it is responsible for conducting an on-going electronic product radiation control program

centigray one one-hundredth of a gray (1/100 Gy)

central nervous system syndrome a form of acute radiation syndrome that results from radiation doses of 50 Gy (5000 rad) or more of ionizing radiation and results in failure of the central nervous system, which causes death anywhere within a few hours to several days (two or three) after exposure

centrioles a pair of small, hollow, cylindrical structures located adjacent to the nucleus, which are believed to play some part in the formation of the mitotic spindle during cell division

centromere a clear region on a chromosome where its two—or four—arms join

centrosomes structures located in the center of the cell near the nucleus that contain the centrioles

characteristic photon a quantum or quantity of radiant energy given off by the parent atom when an electron from an outer shell drops down to fill an inner shell vacancy after the atom has interacted with an x-ray photon and lost an inner shell electron as a result. The energy of a characteristic photon is equivalent to the difference in energy level between the two electron shells.

characteristic radiation radiation released as a result of the photoelectric effect that consists of photons whose energies are representative of the electron energy level structure of the atom interacted with. Characteristic radiation composes about 10% of primary radiation, between 80 and 100 kVp.

chromatid a highly coiled strand; one of the two duplicate portions of DNA that appear during cell division

chromosome aberrations chromosome changes

chromosome breakage the breaking of one or both of the sugar-phosphate chains of a DNA molecule, which can be caused by exposure of the molecule to ionizing radiation

chromosomes small, rod-shaped bodies that contain the genes

chronic something that continues for a long time (e.g., a chronic disease)

cinefluorography the process of recording fluoroscopic images on 16 or 35 mm film

classical scattering (*see* coherent scattering)

clear lead transparent lead-plastic material that has been impregnated with approximately 30% lead by weight

cleaved chromosome broken chromosome

coherent scattering the process wherein a low-energy photon (less than 100 keV) interacts with an atom as a whole and the atom responds by releasing the excess energy it has received in the form of a scattered photon that has the same wavelength and energy as the original, incident photon but which emerges from the atom moving in a direction slightly different from that of the incident photon. This process is also known as Rayleigh scattering, classical scattering, elastic scattering, simple scattering, Thompson scattering, or unmodified scattering.

compensating filter   a material inserted between the x-ray source and the patient to modify the quality (penetrating power, spectrum) of the beam across the field of view

Compton scattered electron   a high-speed electron dislodged from the outer shell of an atom of the irradiated object as a result of interacting with an incoming x-ray photon

Compton scattering   an interaction between an incoming x-ray photon and a loosely bound outer shell electron of an atom of the irradiated object in which the photon surrenders a portion of its kinetic energy to dislodge the electron from its outer shell orbit and then continues on its way but in a new direction. This process accounts for most of the scattered radiation produced during diagnostic procedures.

Computed tomography   process of creating a cross-sectional tomographic plane (slice) of any part of the body. The image is reconstructed by a computer using x-ray absorption measurements collected at multiple points about the periphery of the part being scanned.*

cone   a circular metal tube that attaches to the x-ray tube housing or variable rectangular collimator to limit the beam to a predetermined size and shape

congenital abnormalities   defects existing at birth that are not inherited but rather acquired during development in utero

control badge   film badge that the monitoring company provides with each batch of badges it supplies to determine whether the badges have been exposed to radiation while in transit to or from the institution

controlled area   a hospital area occupied by workers who have been trained in radiation safety procedures and who wear radiation monitoring devices

cosmic radiation (cosmic rays)   very high speed particles, mainly protons, passing through the universe, that are generated as a result of extreme reactions within stars

coulomb (C)   SI unit of electric charge equal to 1 ampere-second (the quantity of electricity transferred by a current of 1 ampere in 1 second)

coulomb per kilogram (C/kg)   SI unit of radiation exposure

1 coulomb per kilogram (C/kg) of air   equals 1 SI unit of exposure or

$$1/(2.58 \times 10^{-4}) \text{ R} = 3.88 \times 10^3 \text{ R}$$

covalent bond   this refers to a chemical union between atoms that arise as a result of a sharing of one or more pairs of electrons

---

*Johnson KC, Rowberg AH: In Ballinger PW: *Merrill's atlas of radiographic positions and radiologic procedures,* ed 7, vol 3, St Louis, 1991, Mosby–Year Book, p 250.

cross-over process occurring during meiosis wherein the chromatids exchange some chromosomal material (genes)

cumulative effect an effect that increases with additional exposure to ionizing radiation

cumulative timing device a required device that times the x-ray exposure and sounds an audible alarm after the fluoroscope has been activated for 5 minutes

curie the standard unit of radioactivity in use before the SI system of units was established. One curie is equal to 3.7×10^{10} disintegrations per second.

cutie pie a nickname for an ionization chamber-type survey meter

cyclotrons machines that produce high-energy particles such as protons

cytoplasm the protoplasm that exists outside of the cell's nucleus

cytoplasmic organelles little structures present in the cytoplasm of the cell

cytosine (C) one of two pyrimidine bases found in both DNA and RNA.

daughter cell a cell resulting from division of an individual parent cell

dead-man type fluoroscopic exposure switch a fluoroscopic exposure switch (operated by foot pressure) that requires continuous pressure applied by the operator to keep it closed and the fluoroscopic tube emitting x-radiation. This means that the exposure terminates if the person operating such a switch becomes incapacitated.

deep dose defined, for example, by Landauer, Inc., Glenwood, Illinois, as the absorbed dose equivalent from all types of radiation at a depth of 1 cm in soft tissue. This number is regarded as the absorbed dose equivalent to the whole body.

dendrites nerve cell processes that extend outward from the cell body and conduct impulses toward the cell body

densitometer an instrument that measures the amount of radiation and the energy of the radiation to which a film badge has been exposed

deoxyribonucleic acid (DNA) a type of nucleic acid that carries the genetic information necessary for cell replication and directs the building of proteins

deoxyribose a five-carbon sugar molecule

diagnostic-type protective tube housing the lead-lined metal housing enclosing the x-ray tube that protects both the radiographer and the patient from leakage radiation by restricting the emission of x-rays to the area of the useful or primary beam (those x-rays emitted through the x-ray tube window or port)

dicentric chromosomes chromosomes having two centromeres

diffusion the motion of liquid, gas, or solid particles from an area of relatively high concentration to an area of lower concentration

direct effect the effect of ionizing particles interacting directly with (transferring their energy to) biologic macromolecules such as DNA, RNA, ATP, proteins or enzymes: the chemical bonds of these macromolecules break and they become abnormal structures

DNA synthesis the building up of DNA macromolecules

dominant mutation a genetic mutation that will probably be expressed in offspring

dose the amount of radiant energy absorbed by an irradiated object per unit mass

doubling dose   the dose of radiation that causes the number of spontaneous mutations occurring in a given generation to increase to two times the original number (i.e., to double)

dry air   air without humidity

dry and moist desquamation   shedding of the outer layer of skin

early effects   effects of ionizing radiation that appear within minutes, hours, days, or weeks of the time of exposure; also called acute effects

effective absorbed dose equivalent limit   conceptually, refers to upper boundary dose of ionizing radiation that a person can absorb during the course of a year, or in a single exposure in any given year, with a negligible risk of sustaining bodily injury or genetic damage as a result of the exposure

effective absorbed dose equivalent limits system   a method to equate the various risks of cancer and genetic effects to the tissue or organ exposed to radiation

effective atomic number   a composite atomic number for the many different chemical elements composing a material

effective communication   communication between the patient and the radiographer in which verbal and nonverbal messages are understood as intended

elastic scattering   (*see* coherent scattering)

electrical potential difference (voltage difference)   the change in electrical potential energy per unit electrical charge experienced by a charged particle as it moves from one position to another. The unit of electrical potential difference is called a volt.

electrical potential energy   the electrical energy acquired by a charged particle as a result of its position relative to other charged particles. The unit of electrical potential energy is the joule.

electrolytes   (*see* salts)

electromagnetic radiation   composed of interacting, varying electric and magnetic fields that propagate through space at the speed of light. It originates as a result of energy changes that occur within an atom or that are brought about as a result of interaction between an atom and some incident particle. Examples of electromagnetic radiation are radio waves, microwaves, visible light, ultraviolet rays, x-rays, and gamma rays.

electrometer   a device used to measure electrical charge

electron volt (eV)   a unit of energy equivalent to the quantity of kinetic energy an electron acquires as it is driven by a potential difference of 1 volt

electrons   negatively charged atomic particles

element   a substance made up of atoms all of which have the same atomic number and hence the same chemical properties

emaciation   the state of being extremely thin

embryological effects   damage to an organism that occurs as a result of exposure of the organism to ionizing radiation during its embryonic stage of development

endoplasmic reticulum   a vast, irregular network of tubules and vesicles spreading in all directions throughout the cytoplasm

energy   the ability to do work

entrance exposure   quantity of radiation, given in roentgens, incident upon an object. Backscatter radiation is excluded.

enzymatic proteins   proteins that control the cell's various physiological activities by functioning as catalysts

epilation   loss of hair

epithelial tissue   tissue that lines and covers body tissue the cells comprising which are highly radiosensitive

erg   a unit of energy and work

erythroblasts   red blood stem cells

erythrocytes   red blood cells

excitation   the addition of energy to a system, transforming it from a calm or low energy state to an excited or higher energy state

exposure   amount of ionizing radiation to which an object, such as a human body, may be subjected. The traditional unit of exposure is the roentgen (R). The SI unit is the coulomb per kilogram (C/kg). Exposure may also be defined as the total electric charge of one sign that x- and gamma-ray photons with energies up to 3 MeV generate in air only per unit mass of air.

exposure linearity   consistency in radiation intensity stated in milliroentgens per milliampere-seconds (mR/mAs) when changing from one milliampere station to another with a variance of not more than 10%

exposure reproducibility   consistency in output of radiation intensity from an individual exposure to other subsequent exposures

fats   compounds composed of carbon, hydrogen, and oxygen with the ratio of hydrogen to oxygen being very much greater than 2 to 1, the ratio which exists in carbohydrates. Fats are a rich energy source yielding gram for gram over twice as much energy as carbohydrates.

fatty acids   when the sugar glucose is broken down in the body during respiration, fats are among the generated intermediate products. When some of these fats combine with an acidic group of atoms (e.g., the carboxyl group: COOH), an acid is formed. It is called a fatty acid. An example is CH_3COOH, which is commonly known as acetic acid. Fatty acids are constituents of amino acids from which proteins are built.

fetus   a developing human in utero

fiber   a protracted, threadlike structure

fibril   a minute fiber or strand frequently a part of a compound fiber

film badge   the most widely used and economical type of personnel monitoring device, it records radiation exposure accumulated at a low rate over a long period of time

filtration   elements that are part of or added to the x-ray tube to reduce exposure to the patient's skin and superficial tissue by absorbing most of the lower energy photons from the heterogeneous beam, thereby increasing the mean energy of the beam

fission   the splitting of the nuclei of atoms whereby some mass is converted into energy

fixed radiographic equipment   radiologic equipment that is installed in and cannot be moved from a specific place in a radiologic facility

flat contact shield   uncontoured lead strip placed directly over the patient's reproductive organs to provide protection from exposure to ionizing radiation

focal spot   the area on the anode of the x-ray tube from which the x-rays appear to emanate

forward scatter   photons that have interacted with the atoms of an object and consequently are deflected in a forward direction (toward the radiographic film). (*See* small angle scatter.)

free air ionization chamber   an instrument used in a calibration laboratory to obtain a precise measurement of x-radiation exposure

free radicals   very reactive chemical molecules with unpaired electrons in the valence or outermost shell

frequency   the number of vibrations or waves per second (crests or cycles per second)

gadolinium   a rare-earth phosphor used in rare-earth intensifying screens

gamma rays   short-wavelength, high-energy electromagnetic waves emitted by the nuclei of radioactive substances. Although in general they are shorter in wavelength and have a different point of origin, their other characteristics are identical to those of diagnostic x-rays.

gastrointestinal (GI) syndrome   a form of acute radiation syndrome that appears in humans at a threshold dose of 6 Gy (600 rad) and peaks after a dose of 10 Gy (1000 rad)

Geiger-Müller (G-M) detector   a device that detects individual radioactive particles (e.g., electrons emitted from certain radioactive nuclei) or photons and that serves as the primary radiation survey instrument for area monitoring in nuclear medicine facilities

genes   the basic units of heredity

genetic cells (germ cells)   cells of the human body associated with reproduction

genetic damage   radiation damage to generations yet unborn

genetically significant dose   average annual gonadal absorbed dose equivalent to members of the population who are of child-bearing age. The number of children who may be expected to be conceived by members of the population is taken into account.

germ cells   reproductive cells

glycerine   a sweet, colorless, odorless, syrupy liquid obtained from fats that are soluble in water. It is often used as a moistening agent.

Golgi apparatus   tiny sacs located near the cell nucleus; the Golgi apparatus synthesizes glycoproteins and transports enzymes and hormones through the cell membrane

gonadal shielding   devices used during radiologic procedures to protect the reproductive organs from exposure to the useful beam when they are in or within close proximity (about 5 cm) of a properly collimated beam

gonads   male and female reproductive organs

gram   a unit of mass of the metric system. An object near the earth's surface that has a mass of 454 grams will weigh 1 pound.

granule   a small particle such as the insoluble nonmembranous particles found in cytoplasm

granulocyte   a type of leukocyte that fights bacteria

gray (Gy)   SI unit of absorbed dose. It is equal to 1 J of energy absorbed from any type of ionizing radiation in 1 kg of any irradiated object

guanine (G)   one of two purine bases found in both DNA and RNA

half-life   statistical quantity equal to the amount of time associated with a 50% decrease in the radioactivity of a sample containing a very large number of radioactive atoms

half value layer (HVL)   the thickness of a designated absorber (customarily a metal, e.g., aluminum) required to decrease the intensity of the primary beam by 50% of its initial value

hematopoietic syndrome (bone marrow syndrome)   a form of the acute radiation syndrome that occurs when humans are exposed to whole-body doses of ionizing radiation ranging from 1 to 10 Gy (100 to 1000 rad) and in which the reduction of the number of blood cells in the circulating blood results in a loss of the body's ability to clot blood and fight infection

hemoglobin   a protein; the oxygen-carrying pigment of the red blood cells (erythrocytes)

hemorrhage   abnormal escape of blood; heavy bleeding

hibakusha   Japanese atomic bomb survivors

highly differentiated cells   mature or more specialized cells

homeostasis   a state of equilibrium between the different elements of an organism or a tendency toward such a state; the ability of the body to return to and maintain normal functioning despite the changes to which it has been subjected

hormones   chemical secretions manufactured by various endocrine glands and carried by the bloodstream to influence activities of other parts. They regulate body functions such as growth and development.

hydrocephaly   abnormal fluid in the brain

hydrogen peroxide   a cellular poison that can result from the radiolysis of water

hydroperoxyl radical   a substance toxic to the cell that can result from the radiolysis of water

hyperbaric oxygen   high-pressure oxygen sometimes used in radiotherapy treatment of certain types of cancerous tumors to increase their radiosensitivity

hypoxic cells   cells that lack an adequate amount of oxygen

image intensification fluoroscopy   use of an image intensifier to increase the brightness of the real-time image produced on a fluorescent screen during fluoroscopy. Virtually all modern fluoroscopy is image intensification fluoroscopy.

image intensifier   a device that increases the brightness of an image. An image is produced on a fluorescent screen by x-rays at the input end (input phosphor). The bright image at the output end (output phosphor) is viewed by a television camera, film, or other recording device.

image receptor   radiographic film or phosphorescent screen

incident photon   incoming photon

incoherent scattering   (*see* Compton scattering)

indirect effect   destructive chemical changes in body molecules that result when a specific molecule such as DNA is acted upon by free radicals previously produced from the interaction of radiation with water molecules

inelastic scatter   the interaction of an incident photon with a loosely bound outer shell electron of the target atom in which the photon surrenders some of its kinetic energy to free the electron from its orbit and then continues on its way but in a new direction

inherent filtration   the glass envelope encasing the x-ray tube, the insulating oil surrounding the tube, and the glass window in the tube housing

inorganic compounds   compounds that do not contain carbon. The inorganic compounds found in the human body occur in nature independent of living things.

instant cell death   immediate death of the cell resulting from a dose of about 1000 Gy (100,000 rad) absorbed in a period of seconds or minutes

intensifying screens   devices that increase the brightness of the image produced by the action of x-rays upon a phosphor

intensity (of radiation)   quantity or amount (of radiation) crossing unit area per unit time

intermittent fluoroscopy   periodic activation of the fluoroscopic tube by the radiologist rather than long continuous activation

International System of Units (SI)   one standard system of units adopted by all countries and used in all branches of science

interphase   the period of cell growth that occurs before actual cell division

interphase death   death of a cell before the cell attempts division, which can result from exposure of the cell to radiation doses of less than 100 rad

interslice scatter   radiation that scatters from the CT slice being made into the adjacent slices

inverse square falloff of radiation intensity with distance   a consequence of this decrease in radiation intensity as the square of the distance from the radiation source is that when a small source-skin distance is employed, patient entrance exposure is significantly greater than the exit exposure. This results in the entrance surface receiving an unnecessary high exposure. When the source-to-object distance is increased, a more uniform distribution of exposure throughout the patient is maintained.

inverse square law   the intensity of the radiation at a location is inversely proportional to the square of its distance from the source of radiation

involuntary motion motion caused by muscles not under voluntary control (e.g., digestive organs)

ionization the conversion of atoms to ions

ionization chamber a device that measures the amount of electrical charge due to the presence of all the ions of one sign produced during the irradiation of a specific volume of air

ionization chamber-type survey meter (cutie pie) both a rate meter device (measures radiation exposure rate) normally used for area surveys and an integrating meter that will measure the cumulative exposure at a position for a selected time interval

ionize to remove electrons from

ionizing radiation radiation that upon passing through matter produces positively and negatively charged particles (ions)

ion pair two oppositely charged particles

ions positively and negatively charged particles

isotope an atom that contains a different number of neutrons but the same number of protons in its nucleus as a reference atom. Radioactive isotopes of atoms that make up biological materials may be used in medical imaging nuclear medicine studies.

joule (a unit of energy) the work done on energy expended when a force of 1 Newton acts on an object along a distance of 1 meter

key molecule (*see* master molecule)

kiloelectron volt (keV) a unit used to measure the kinetic energy of an individual electron in the high-speed electron stream within the x-ray tube and which is equivalent to 1000 electron volts (1 keV = 1000 eV). This unit is also used to measure the energies of x-rays.

kilogram (kg) 1000 grams

kilovolt (kV) electrical potential equal to 1000 volts

kinetic energy energy of motion

lanthanum a rare-earth phosphor used in rare-earth intensifying screens

late effects nongenetic effects that appear after a period of months or years after exposure to ionizing radiation

latent period the period after the prodromal stage of the acute radiation syndrome during which there are no visible effects or symptoms of radiation exposure

Law of Bergonié and Tribondeau "The radiosensitivity of cells is directly proportional to their reproductive activity and inversely proportional to their degree of differentiation."

LD 50/30 the whole-body dose of radiation that can be lethal to 50% of the exposed population within 30 days

LD 50/60 the whole-body dose of radiation that can be lethal to 50% of the exposed population within 60 days

lead-equivalent thickness of radiation-absorbing material that produces an attenuation equivalent to that which would be accomplished by a specified amount of lead

leukemia   a neoplastic overproduction of white blood cells

leukemogenesis   the production or origin of leukemia

leukocytes   white blood cells

linear energy transfer (LET)   the average energy deposited per unit path length to a medium by ionizing radiation as it passes through that medium

linear, nonthreshold dose-response relationship   a relationship between dose and response which, in terms of radiation dose and biological response, means that the chance of sustaining biological damage and the amount of biological damage sustained as a result of exposure to ionizing radiation are directly proportional to the magnitude of the exposure and that even the most miniscule dose of radiation has the potential to cause some damage

lipids   water-insoluble organic macromolecules that consist only of carbon, hydrogen, and oxygen. Among other functions, lipids store energy for the body for long periods of time.

long scale of radiographic contrast   radiographic contrast in which there are many shades of gray. A wide range of exposures will produce a wide range of shades of gray when a long scale image receptor or display is used.

low-level radiation   "an absorbed dose of 10 rem or less delivered over a short period of time" or "a larger dose delivered over a long period of time, for instance, 50 rem in 10 years"*

lymphocyte   a type of white blood cell that plays an active role in producing immunity for the body by producing antibodies to combat disease. Lymphocytes are the most radiosensitive blood cells in the human body.

lysosomes   small pealike sacs containing digestive enzymes

macromolecule   large molecule built up from smaller chemical structures

manifest illness   the stage of the acute radiation syndrome during which symptoms become visible

man-made radiation   artificially produced radiation such as radionuclides generated in atomic reactors or by use of cyclotrons

mAs   (*see* milliampere-seconds)

master molecule (key molecule)   a molecule vital to the survival of the cell. It maintains normal cell function.

matter   the constituent material of which all things are made

matter-antimatter annihilation reaction   the destructive interaction between matter and antimatter (matter composed of the counterparts of normal matter). In pair production, the combining of a positron with an electron it encounters resulting in the destruction of the electron, the disappearance of the positron, and the transformation of the positron and electron masses into energy in the form of two photons of 0.51 MeV each, moving in opposite directions. In this process, mass is converted into energy.

maximum permissible dose (MPD)   term used previously to indicate the maximum absorbed dose equivalent of ionizing radiation that an occupationally ex-

---

*Ritenour ER: In Hendee WR, editor: *Health effects of low-level radiation*, Norwalk, CT, 1984, Appleton-Century-Crofts, p 13.

posed person could absorb without sustaining appreciable bodily injury as a result of the exposure

mean energy   the average energy of an x-ray beam

mean marrow dose (MMD)   "that dose of radiation averaged over the entire active bone marrow"*

megakaryocytes   platelet stem cells

meiosis   the process of germ (genetic) cell division, which reduces the chromosomes in each daughter cell to half the number of chromosomes in the parent cell

mesons   penetrating, unstable, subatomic particles that are components of cosmic radiation (e.g., pions)

metaphase   that phase of cell division during which the mitotic spindle is completed

milliampere-seconds (mAs)   the product of x-ray electron tube current and the amount of time in seconds that the x-ray is on

milligray (mGy)   one one-thousandth of a gray (1/1000 Gy)

millirad (mrad)   one one-thousandth of a rad (1/1000 rad)

millirem (mrem)   one one-thousandth of a rem (1/1000 rem)

millisievert (mSv)   one one-thousandth of a sievert (1/1000 Sv)

mitochondria   large bean-shaped structures containing highly organized enzymes in their inner membrane, which function as "powerhouses" of the cell

mitosis   the process of somatic cell division wherein a parent cell divides to form two daughter cells identical to the parent cell

mitotic death (genetic death)   cell death occurring after one or more divisions after irradiation

mitotic delay   the failure of a cell to start dividing on time

mobile radiographic equipment   manually portable radiologic equipment

modified scattering   (*see* Compton scattering)

molecular change   an alteration in the basic structure of a molecule caused by some type of destructive process such as exposure to ionizing radiation

molecular lesions   (*see* point lesions)

molecule   the smallest unit of a specific substance composed of one or more atoms

molten   melted or liquefied by heat

mutagens   agents that can increase the frequency of occurrence of mutations, such as elevated temperatures, ionizing radiations, viruses, and chemicals

mutation frequency   the number of spontaneous or mutagen-caused mutations that occur in a given generation

mutations   changes in genes

myeloblasts   white blood stem cells

natural background radiation   radiation from natural sources, including radioactive materials in the earth, cosmic radiation from outer space, and radionuclides deposited in the human body

negatron   an ordinary electron; it carries a negative charge

---

*Bushong SC: *Radiologic science for technologists: physics, biology, and protection,* ed 4, St Louis, 1988, Mosby–Year Book, p 577.

neutron   an electrically neutral particle, one of the fundamental constituents of the atom and, like the proton, located within the nucleus of the atom. The mass of the neutron is just slightly greater than that of the proton.

neutrophils   a type of leukocyte that plays a role in fighting infection

newton   unit of force in the meter-kilogram-second system of physical units. One newton corresponds to approximately one quarter of a pound.

nitrogen   a tasteless, odorless, colorless gaseous chemical element found free in the air. Since nitrogen is an integral part of protein and nucleic acids and thus found in every living cell, it is important biologically.

nitrogenous bases   organic bases that contain the element nitrogen

nonagreement states   individual states in the United States in which both the state Department of Environmental Protection and the Nuclear Regulatory Commission (NRC) enforce radiation protection regulations

nonoccupational exposure   radiation exposure received by members of the general population who are not employed as radiation workers

nonoccupational persons   any persons not employed as radiation workers

non–image-intensified fluoroscopy   a procedure that employs a fluoroscopic screen made of zinc cadmium sulfide that produces a fluoroscopic image of the area of clinical interest of a very low brightness level. This technique is considered outmoded and has been superseded by image-intensified fluoroscopy.

non–self-reading pocket dosimeter   a pocket ionization chamber that requires a special accessory electrometer to read the device and is used for personnel monitoring in low radiation exposure areas when immediate readout is not necessary

nonspecific life span shortening   life span shortening that results from premature yet not peculiar diseases. Radiation-induced life span shortening is nonspecific.

nonstochastic effects   biological effects of ionizing radiation that demonstrate the existence of a threshold and the severity of the biological damage increases as a consequence of increased absorbed dose

nonverbal messages   unconscious actions or body language

nuclear medicine procedure   the administration, either orally or intravenously, of a radioactive isotope for the purpose of conducting a diagnostic study of a body area. The isotope is associated with a chemical compound that preferentially concentrates in the body area of interest.

nuclear reactor   a mechanism for creating and continuing a controlled nuclear chain reaction in a fissionable fuel for the production of energy or supplementary fissionable material

Nuclear Regulatory Commission (NRC) (formerly known as The Atomic Energy Commission [AEC])   federal agency that has the power to enforce radiation protection standards established by an Act of Congress or other law-making body

nucleic acids   large, complex macromolecules made up of nucleotides

nucleotides   units formed from a nitrogenous base such as adenine, guanine, cytosine or thymine, a five-carbon sugar molecule, deoxyribose, and a phosphate molecule. A group of nucleotides make up a nucleic acid.

nucleus   the center of the cell; a spherical mass of protoplasm containing the genetic material (DNA), which is stored in its molecular structure. The nucleus also contains a rounded body called the nucleolus, which holds a large amount of RNA.

occupancy factor (T)   a factor used to indicate the fraction of time that an area in the immediate vicinity of an x-ray room is likely to be occupied by a given individual

occupational exposure   radiation exposure received by radiation workers in the course of exercising their professional responsibilities

occupational persons   individuals employed as radiation workers

off-focus radiation (stem radiation)   x-rays emitted from parts of the tube other than the focal spot

oogonium   female germ cell

organic acids   organic compounds containing the carboxyl (COOH) group, e.g. acetic acid (the distinctive component of vinegar) has the chemical formula CH_3COOH

organic compounds   all carbon compounds, those found in nature and those produced artificially

organic damage   genetic or somatic changes in the organism such as mutations, cataracts, and leukemia, which result from sufficient radiation-induced damage at the cellular level

organogenesis   period of gestation from the second to the eighth week after conception during which the nerve cells in the brain and spinal cord of the fetus develop and the fetus is most susceptible to radiation-induced congenital abnormalities

organ weighing factor (W_T)   a factor that "indicates the ratio of the risk of stochastic effects attributable to irradiation of a given organ or tissue (T) to the total risk when the whole body is uniformly irradiated"*

osmotic pressure   the force created when a semipermeable membrane separates two solutions of different concentration

osteogenic sarcoma   bone cancer

osteoporosis   decalcification of the bone

oxidation   most simply, the combining of a substance with oxygen. The oxidation of iron leads to iron oxide, commonly known as rust. The definition of oxidation, however, has been broadened to include reactions in which electrons are lost by an atom.

pair production   interaction between an incoming photon of at least 1.022 MeV and an atom of the irradiated object in which the photon approaches and strongly interacts with the nucleus of the atom of the irradiated material and disappears. In the process the energy of the incoming photon is transformed into two new particles, a negatron and a positron, after which these particles exit from the atom.

particulate radiation   in distinction to x- and gamma rays, examples are: electrons, protons, neutrons, alpha particles (nuclei of helium), and so forth

---

*National Council on Radiation Protection and Measurements (NCRP): Report #91, *Recommendations on limits for exposure to ionizing radiation,* Bethesda, MD, 1987, NCRP Publications, p. 52.

peak voltage   maximum voltage directed across an x-ray tube

peptic bond   chemical bond connecting two amino acids

permeable   penetrable

photoelectric absorption   an interaction between an x-ray photon and an inner shell electron in which the photon surrenders all of its kinetic energy to the electron and ceases to exist and the atom responds by ejecting the electron from its inner shell. Photoelectric absorption is the process most responsible for the contrast between bone and soft tissue in diagnostic radiographs.

photoelectron   the electron ejected from its inner shell orbit during the process of photoelectric absorption

photon   a particle associated with electromagnetic radiation that has neither mass nor electric charge

picocurie   a very small quantity of radioactivity equivalent to one trillionth (10^{-12}) of a curie

platelets   circular or oval discs found in the blood of all vertebrates. Platelets initiate blood clotting and prevent hemorrhage.

pocket ionization chamber (pocket dosimeter)   a personnel monitoring device that contains a positively charged electrode and a negatively charged electrode; when these electrodes are exposed to ionizing radiation, the air around the positively charged electrode is ionized and discharges the mechanism in direct proportion to the amount of radiation to which it has been exposed.

point lesions (molecular lesions)   injured areas in molecules caused by the breaking of a single chemical bond

point mutations   genetic mutations in which the chromosome is not broken but the DNA within it is damaged

positive beam limitation (PBL)   a feature of current radiographic collimators that automatically adjusts the collimators so that the radiation field size matches the film size

positron   an unstable, positively charged electron, which is a form of antimatter

potential difference   the difference in electrical potential or voltage between two points in a circuit

precursor cells   (*see* stem cells)

primary beam   (*see* useful beam)

primary protective barrier   a barrier located perpendicular to the line of travel of the primary x-ray beam to afford protection from the primary beam

primary radiation   radiation that emerges from the x-ray tube target (the anode), which consists of brems radiation and characteristic radiation

prodrome   the first stage of the acute radiation syndrome, which occurs within hours after radiation exposure

prophase   the phase of cell division during which the nucleus and the chromosomes enlarge and the DNA begins to take structural form

proportional counter   a radiation survey instrument usually used in a laboratory setting to detect alpha and beta radiation and small amounts of other types of low-level radioactive contamination

protective apparel items of clothing (i.e., aprons, gloves) that attenuate ionizing radiation to provide some degree of radiation protection for the wearer

protective barrier any medium of adequate composition and thickness that functions to absorb primary and/or secondary radiation, thereby reducing exposure of persons located on the other side of the barrier

protein amino acids that link together in various patterns and combinations. They contain carbon, hydrogen, nitrogen, oxygen, and occasionally other elements such as sulfur.

protein synthesis the making of new proteins

proton one of the three main constituents of an atom, the other two being electrons and neutrons. The proton carries a positive electrical charge equal in magnitude to that of an electron. The proton, which is located within the central core or nucleus of the atom, has a mass in excess of 1800 times that of an electron. The combination of one proton and one electron constitutes the simplest atom.

protoplasm the building material of all living things, consisting of inorganic substances such as water and mineral salts and organic substances, including proteins, carbohydrates, lipids, and nucleic acids

purines a class of nitrogenous bases found in DNA or RNA. These bases include adenine (A) and guanine (G).

pyrimidines a class of nitrogenous bases found in DNA or RNA. These bases include cytosine (C), thymine (T), or uracil (U).

quality factor (QF) a modifying factor used in the calculation of the dose equivalent to determine the ability of a dose of any kind of ionizing radiation to cause biological damage

quantum mottle faint blotches in the recorded radiographic image produced by an intrinsic fluctuation in the incident photon intensity. This effect is more noticeable when using very high, rare earth systems.

rad ("*r*adiation-*a*bsorbed-*d*ose") unit used to measure the amount of radiant energy transferred to an irradiated object by any type of ionizing radiation. One rad is equivalent to an energy transfer of 100 erg per gram.

radiant energy energy that moves in the form of a wave and is transmitted by radiations such as x-rays and gamma rays

radiation transfer of energy that results either because of a change occurring naturally within an atom (*see* radiation decay) or a process caused by the interaction of a particle with an atom

radiation biology the branch of biology concerned with the effects of ionizing radiations on living systems

Radiation Control for Health and Safety Act of 1968 law passed by Congress (Public Law 90-602) to protect the public from the hazards of unnecessary radiation exposure resulting from electronic products such as microwave ovens, color televisions, and diagnostic x-ray equipment

radiation decay a naturally occurring process whereby an unstable atomic nucleus relieves its instability through the emission of one or more energetic particles

radiation hormesis effect a beneficial consequence of radiation for populations continuously exposed to moderately high levels of radiation

radiation monitoring device a device worn by diagnostic radiology personnel to indicate occupational exposure by measuring the quantity of radiation to which it has been exposed over a period of time

radiation permeability the ability of a structure to be penetrated by radiation

radiation protection tools and techniques employed by radiation workers to protect patients and personnel from exposure to ionizing radiation

radiation safety officer a qualified individual designated by an institution to ensure that internationally accepted guidelines for radiation protection are followed by the institution. The radiation safety officer is responsible for maintaining radiation monitoring records for all personnel.

radiation survey instruments area monitoring devices that detect and/or measure radiation

radiation therapy treatment use of x- or gamma rays, usually with energies much greater than those employed for diagnostic purposes, to destroy the cells composing a tumor while sparing the surrounding nontumor tissues

radicals groups of atoms that remain together during a chemical change behaving almost like a single atom. Atoms in a radical are held together by covalent bond.

radioactive nuclides (radionuclides) unstable atomic species that change naturally into other atomic species by altering their nuclear structure. They give off ionizing radiation during their disintegration (radioactive decay) process.

radiogenic malignancies cancerous neoplasms induced by exposure to ionizing radiation

radiographer a person qualified through formal education and certification to practice medical radiography and provide related patient care

radiographic beam (light beam coincidence) means that both physical size (length and width) and alignment between the radiographic beam and the localizing light beam must correspond to within 2% of the source-image distance (SID)

radiographic contrast differences in density level between the radiographic images of objects in a radiograph

radiographic grid a device (made of parallel radiopaque lead strips alternated with radioparent strips of aluminum, plastic, or wood) placed between the patient and the film to remove scattered x-ray photons that emerge from the object being radiographed before they reach the film. Use of a grid improves image quality.

radiologist a qualified physician who specializes in diagnosis and treatment through the use of radiant energy

radiolucent transparent to radiation; a material that allows radiation to pass through

radiolysis of water interaction of radiation with water

radionuclide any atom that emits radiation

radiosensitive capable of being damaged or destroyed by ionizing radiation

radon   radioactive gas that decays with a half-life of 3.8 days by way of alpha particles emission

Rayleigh scattering   (*see* coherent scattering)

recessive mutation   a genetic mutation that will probably not be expressed for a number of generations because both parents must possess the same mutation. If only one parent possesses the mutation, it will not be expressed.

recoil electron   (*see* Compton scattered electron)

relative biological effectiveness (RBE)   relative capability of radiations with various LETs to produce a particular biological reaction. Simply defined, it is the dose of a reference radiation quality (conventionally, this has been chosen to be 250 kVp x-ray), stated in gray, that is necessary to produce the same biological reaction in a given experiment that is produced by a dose of the test radiation, also stated in gray

relative risk   assumes exposure to radiation will end in a steady percentage increase of cancers over the normal risk of malignancy occurring in people of all ages

rem ("*rad-equivalent-man*")   traditional unit of absorbed dose equivalent; 1 rem is the absorbed dose of any type of ionizing radiation that produces the same biological effect as 1 rad of x-radiation and is equivalent to 1/100 J/kg

remnant radiation   all of the x-ray photons that reach their destination (the film) after passing through the object being radiographed

repair enzymes   enzymes that can mend damaged molecules

repeat analysis program   procedure that helps a Radiology Department determine the number of repeat radiographs and reasons for producing unacceptable radiographs, thereby identifying existing problems and conditions

repeat radiograph   any radiograph that must be performed more than once because of some human or mechanical error in the process of producing the initial radiograph. Radiation exposure for the patient and the radiation worker increases when a radiograph must be repeated.

reproductive cells   male and female germ cells

reproductive death   a cell's loss of its ability to reproduce resulting from exposure of the cell to a moderate dose of ionizing radiation (100 to 1000 rad)

retina   the rod- and cone-containing area of the eye; the retina receives the image formed by the lens

ribonucleic acid (RNA)   a type of nucleic acid that carries the genetic information from the DNA in the cell nucleus to the ribosomes located in the cytoplasm

ribosomes   small, spherical cytoplasmic organelles that attach to the endoplasmic reticulum. They are the cell's "protein factories."

risk   the possibility of inducing a radiogenic cancer or genetic defects after irradiation

roentgen (R)   internationally accepted unit for measurement of exposure to x- and gamma radiation. One roentgen is the photon exposure that produces under standard conditions of pressure and temperature a total positive or negative ion charge of 2.58×10^{-4} coulombs per kilogram of dry air.

rung   a step in the DNA ladder-like structure composed of a pair of nitrogenous bases

safe industries   industries that have "an associated annual fatality accident rate of 1 or less per 10,000 workers, i.e., an average annual risk of 10^{-4}."* Safe industries include manufacturing, trade, service, and government.

salts (electrolytes)   chemical compounds that result from the action of an acid and a base upon each other

scattered radiation   all of the radiation that arises from the interactions of an x-ray beam with the atoms of an object in the path of the beam

scattering   the process wherein x-ray photons undergo a change in direction after interacting with the atoms of an object

secondary protective barrier   a barrier that affords protection from secondary radiation (leakage and scattered radiation) only

secondary radiation   the radiation that results from the interaction between primary radiation and the atoms of the irradiated object and the off-focus or leakage radiation that penetrates the x-ray tube protective housing. Secondary radiation consists of scattered radiation and characteristic radiation.

self-reading pocket dosimeter   a pocket ionization chamber that contains a built-in electrometer and provides an immediate exposure readout for radiation workers who work in high exposure areas

semipermeable membrane   a film that permits the passage of a pure solvent such as water but does not allow materials dissolved by the solvent to pass through

shadow shield   a shield of radiopaque material suspended from above the radiographic beam-defining system to cast a shadow in the primary beam over the patient's reproductive organs

shallow dose   defined, for example, by Landauer, Inc., Glenwood, Illinois, as "the absorbed dose equivalent from all radiations at approximately 0.007 cm depth in soft tissue." This dose is considered by Landauer as the "equivalent to the dose to the skin of the whole body."

shaped contact shield   a cup-shaped radiopaque shield that encloses the scrotum and penis to protect the male reproductive organs from exposure to ionizing radiation

short-term somatic effects (early or acute effects)   somatic effects that appear within minutes, hours, days, or weeks of the time of radiation exposure

side scatter   photons that interact with the atoms of an object and consequently are deflected to the side

sievert (Sv)   SI unit of absorbed dose equivalent. One sievert equals 1 J/kg (for x-radiation, QF = 1).

simple scattering   (*see* classical scattering)

skin dose   the absorbed radiation dose, stated in gray or rads, delivered to the most superficial layers of the skin as a result of a radiation exposure. Back-scatter radiation contribution is included.

---

*National Council on Radiation Protection and Measurements (NCRP): Report #91, *Recommendations on limits for exposure to ionizing radiation,* Bethesda, MD, 1987, NCRP Publications, p 8.

skin erythema dose   the dose of radiation (usually about 200 rad, or 2 Gy) that causes diffused redness over an area of skin after irradiation

small angle scatter   photons that pass through the object being radiographed, interact with the atoms of the object, and are deflected only at a small enough angle so that they reach the film, thereby degrading the radiographic image by producing small amounts of radiographic fog.

somatic cells   all of the cells in the human body with the exception of the germ cells

somatic effects   biological damage sustained by living organisms such as human beings as a consequence of exposure to ionizing radiation

source-image distance (SID)   the distance from the anode focal spot to the radiographic film

spermatogonium   the male germ cell

spontaneous mutations   mutations in genes and DNA that occur at random and without a known cause as a natural phenomenon

stem cells   immature or precursor cells

stochastic effects   nonthreshold, randomly occurring biological effects of ionizing radiation in which the probability of occurrence of the effects rather than the severity is proportional to the dose. Examples of stochastic effects are cancer and genetic effects.

structural proteins   those proteins from which the body acquires its shape and form

super lethal radiation dose   a deadly dose of radiation, which for humans is any whole body dose greater than 6 Gy (600 rad) of ionizing radiation. All individuals in a population would be dead within 30 days after such a dose.

target theory   the theory that the cell will die if inactivation of the master molecule occurs as a result of exposure to ionizing radiation

telophase   the phase of mitosis during which cell division is completed with the formation of two new daughter cells, each of which contains exactly the same genetic material as the parent cell. Telophase in meiosis involves not only division of the parent cell into two daughter cells but also division of these daughter cells into two granddaughter cells each. Because this second division does not involve DNA replication, the result of these two successive divisions is the formation of four granddaughter cells, each of which contains only half the genetic material of the original parent cell.

10-day rule   a rule based on the low degree of probability that a woman would be pregnant during the first 10 days after the onset of menstruation. The rule suggests that abdominal x-rays of fertile women be postponed until sometime during the first 10 days after the onset of the next menstruation if the results of the examination are not of importance in connection with an immediate illness

terrestrial radiation   radiation resulting from radioactive minerals found in natural deposits within the earth

thermal neutron   nominally classified as a neutron whose kinetic energy is approximately less than or equal to 1 eV. Typically, these are neutrons whose kinetic energy has been significantly degraded as a result of multiple energy loss collisions.

thermoluminescent dosimeter (TLD) badge   a personnel monitoring device that most often contains a crystalline form (powder or chips) of lithium fluoride as its sensing material. When the device is placed in a TLD analyzer and heated, the crystals emit visible light in proportion to the amount of radiation to which the TLD badge was exposed.

Thompson scattering   (*see* coherent scattering)

threshold   the point at which a response or reaction to an increasing stimulation first occurs. Threshold may also be defined as a dose below which a person has a negligible chance of sustaining specific biological damage.

thrombocytes   (*see* platelets)

thymine (T)   a pyrimidine base found only in DNA

thymus gland   an organ of the lymphatic system, located in the mediastinal cavity anterior to and above the heart. It plays a critical role in the body's defense against infection.

thyroid gland   a gland located in the neck just below the larynx. The hormone produced by this gland helps to regulate the body's metabolic rate and the process of growth.

total filtration   inherent filtration plus added filtration

tubule   a small tube

tungsten   a metal with a high melting point (greater than 3400° C) and high atomic number ($z = 74$). The anode in the x-ray tube is usually made primarily of this metal.

umbra   (*see* useful beam)

uncontrolled area   area in which members of the "general public" (i.e., individuals who are not trained to work with radiation) may be found

undifferentiated cells   immature or nonspecialized cells

unit   a fixed amount of some property or characteristic (e.g., distance-meter, time-second, energy-joule, etc.) used as a measure for which other amounts of that property or characteristic can be described

unmodified scattering   (*see* coherent scattering)

unnecessary exposure   any radiation exposure that does not benefit a person in terms of diagnostic information obtained or any radiation exposure that does not enhance the quality of the study

unnecessary radiologic procedure   radiologic examination for which there is no sufficient justification to subject a patient to the minimal risk of absorbed radiation dose that will result from the procedure

uracil (U)   a pyrimidine base found only in RNA. It replaces thymine (T) as the nitrogenous base in ribonucleic acid.

use factor (U) (beam direction factor)   the proportional amount of time during which the x-ray beam is energized or directed toward a particular barrier

useful beam   primary beam or umbra

variable rectangular collimator   a box-shaped device containing the radiographic beam-defining system; the device most often used to define the size and shape of the radiographic beam

vesicle   a small cavity or sac containing liquid

Victoreen condenser R-meter   a gas-filled radiation survey instrument used to calibrate x-ray equipment

visual acuity   ability to discriminate small images

volt (V)   SI unit of electric potential and potential difference

voltage   electric potential at a point or position relative to ground potential

voluntary motion   motion controlled by will (i.e., skeletal muscle)

wavelength   distance between two consecutive crests or troughs in a wave

working level month (WLM)   quantitatively is an exposure for 170 hours to radon and its daughter products at a concentration of 100 pCi/L. The occupational limit for miners is 4 WLM/yr, which corresponds to a dose equivalent of approximately 15 rem (0.15 Sv) per year.

workload (W)   the maximum voltage and milliamperage (mA) of the x-ray generator and the amount of x-ray activity (the number of x-ray examinations performed per week) (i.e., the amount of radiation produced per week). Workload is measured in milliampere-minutes per week. A typical value is 1000 mA-min/week in a busy radiographic room.

x-rays   electromagnetic radiation that emerges from the anode of an x-ray tube after bombardment of this target by high-speed electrons in a highly evacuated glass tube

yttrium   a rare-earth phosphor used in rare-earth intensifying screens

Appendix A

Answers to Review Questions

Chapter 1
1. c
2. b
3. c
4. a
5. d
6. b
7. b
8. d
9. b
10. d
11. b
12. d
13. a
14. a
15. c
16. c
17. d
18. c
19. d
20. b

Chapter 2
1. b
2. d
3. c
4. a

5. b
6. b
7. a
8. a
9. b
10. c
11. c
12. c
13. a
14. d
15. a
16. a
17. b
18. d
19. b
20. b
21. d
22. b
23. b
24. c

Chapter 3
1. c
2. b
3. d
4. b
5. a

6. d
7. b
8. c
9. d
10. a
11. b
12. d
13. d
14. b
15. d
16. c
17. a
18. a
19. d
20. d
21. d
22. c
23. a
24. c
25. c

Chapter 4
1. b
2. c
3. a
4. d
5. d

6. d
7. c
8. b
9. a
10. a
11. b
12. b
13. c
14. d
15. a
16. c

Chapter 5
1. c
2. c
3. b
4. b
5. d
6. b
7. b
8. d
9. b
10. d

Chapter 6
1. b
2. a
3. b
4. c
5. a
6. d
7. c
8. b
9. b
10. b
11. a
12. b
13. a
14. c
15. d
16. d

17. a
18. d
19. d
20. b
21. d
22. c
23. c
24. b
25. c
26. d
27. d
28. a
29. d
30. d
31. d
32. d
33. c
34. d
35. b
36. d
37. b
38. d
39. c
40. a

Chapter 7
1. d
2. a
3. b
4. b
5. b
6. d
7. c
8. c
9. b
10. d
11. a
12. b
13. d
14. d
15. c

16. c
17. d
18. b
19. b
20. a
21. b
22. a
23. c
24. d
25. b
26. b
27. c
28. d
29. a
30. d
31. c
32. a
33. d
34. b
35. b
36. c
37. a
38. d
39. a
40. d

Chapter 8
1. b
2. a
3. c
4. d
5. d
6. b
7. b
8. c
9. a
10. a
11. d
12. c
13. c
14. b

15. b

16. d

17. c

18. d

19. c

20. b

21. d

22. a

23. d

24. d

25. d

26. b

27. d

28. c

29. c

30. a

Chapter 9

1. c

2. c

3. a

4. d

5. b

6. d

7. a

8. b

9. c

10. b

11. c

12. b

13. a

14. d

15. d

16. c

17. c

18. d

19. d

20. d

21. d

22. a

23. a

24. b

25. c

26. c

27. b

28. d

29. d

30. c

31. a

32. b

33. c

34. d

35. b

36. c

37. a

38. b

39. d

40. a

Appendix B

Metric System Equivalents for Length

Metric System Equivalents for Length

Length	Symbol	Power of ten fractional form	Power of ten decimal form	Scientific notation
terameter	T	1,000,000,000,000	1,000,000,000,000	10^{12} (m)
gigameter	G	1,000,000,000	1,000,000,000	10^{9} (m)
megameter	M	1,000,000	1,000,000	10^{6} (m)
kilometer	k	1,000	1,000	10^{3} (m)
hectometer	h	100	100	10^{2} (m)
dekameter	da	10	10	10^{1} (m)
meter	m	1	1	10^{0} (m)
decimeter	d	1/10	0.1	10^{-1} (m)
centimeter	cm	1/100	0.01	10^{-2} (m)
millimeter	mm	1/1,000	0.001	10^{-3} (m)
micrometer	μm	1/1,000,000	0.000001	10^{-6} (m)
nanometer	nm	1/1,000,000,000	0.000000001	10^{-9} (m)
picometer	pm	1/1,000,000,000,000	0.000000000001	10^{-12} (m)

Appendix C

Consumer-Patient Radiation Health and Safety Act of 1981

[Consumer-Patient Radiation Health and Safety Act of 1981.]

SUBTITLE I—CONSUMER-PATIENT RADIATION HEALTH AND SAFETY ACT OF 1981

Short title

[42 USC 10001] note.

Sec. 975. This subtitle may be cited as the "Consumer-Patient Radiation Health and Safety Act of 1981."

Statement of findings

[42 USC 10001.]

Sec. 976. The Congress finds that—

(1) it is in the interest of public health and safety to minimize unnecessary exposure to potentially hazardous radiation due to medical and dental radiologic procedures;

(2) it is in the interest of public health and safety to have a continuing supply of adequately educated persons and appropriate accreditation and certification programs administered by State governments;

(3) the protection of the public health and safety from unnecessary exposure to potentially hazardous radiation due to medical and dental radiologic procedures and the assurance of efficacious procedures are the responsibility of State and Federal governments;

(4) persons who administer radiologic procedures, including procedures at Federal facilities, should be required to demonstrate competence by reason of education, training, and experience; and

(5) the administration of radiologic procedures and the effect on individuals of such procedures have a substantial and direct effect upon United States interstate commerce.

Statement of purpose

[42 USC 10002.]

Sec. 977.   It is the purpose of this subtitle to—

(1) provide for the establishment of minimum standards by the Federal Government for the accreditation of education programs for persons who administer radiologic procedures and for the certification of such persons; and

(2) insure that medical and dental radiologic procedures are consistent with rigorous safety precautions and standards.

Definitions

[42 USC 10003.]

Sec. 978.   Unless otherwise expressly provided, for purposes of this subtitle, the term—

(1) "radiation" means ionizing and nonionizing radiation in amounts beyond normal background levels from sources such as medical and dental radiologic procedures;

(2) "radiologic procedure" means any procedure or article intended for use in—

   (A) the diagnosis of disease or other medical or dental conditions in humans (including diagnostic X-rays or nuclear medicine procedures); or

   (B) the cure, mitigation, treatment, or prevention of disease in humans; that achieves its intended purpose through the emission of radiation;

(3) "radiologic equipment" means any radiation electronic product which emits or detects radiation and which is used or intended for use to—

   (A) diagnose disease or other medical or dental conditions (including diagnostic X-ray equipment); or

   (B) cure, mitigate, treat, or prevent disease in humans; that achieves its intended purpose through the emission or detection of radiation;

(4) "practitioner" means any licensed doctor of medicine, osteopathy, dentistry, podiatry, or chiropractic, who prescribes radiologic procedures for other persons;

(5) "persons who administer radiologic procedures" means any person, other than a practitioner, who intentionally administers radiation to other persons for medical purposes, and includes medical radiologic technologists (including dental hygienists and assistants), radiation therapy technologists, and nuclear medicine technologists;

(6) "Secretary" means the Secretary of Health and Human Services; and

(7) "State" means the several States, the District of Columbia, the Commonwealth of Puerto Rico, the Commonwealth of the Northern Mariana Islands, the Virgin Islands, Guam, American Samoa, and the Trust Territory of the Pacific Islands.

Promulgation of standards

[Regulation. 42 USC 10004.]

Sec. 979.   (a) Within twelve months after the date of enactment of this Act, the Secretary, in consultation with the Radiation Policy Council, the Administrator of Veterans' Affairs, the Administrator of the Environmental Protection Agency, appropriate agencies of the States, and appropriate professional organizations, shall by regulation promulgate minimum standards for the accreditation of educational programs to train individuals to perform radiologic procedures. Such standards shall distinguish between programs for the education of (1) medical radiologic technologists (including radiographers), (2) dental auxiliaries (including dental hygienists and assistants), (3) radiation therapy technologists, (4) nuclear medicine technologists, and (5) such other kinds of health auxiliaries who administer radiologic procedures as the Secretary determines appropriate. Such standards shall not be applicable to educational programs for practitioners.

[Regulation.]

(b) Within twelve months after the date of enactment of this Act, the Secretary, in consultation with the Radiation Policy Council, the Administrator of Veterans' Affairs, the Administrator of the Environmental Protection Agency, interested agencies of the States, and appropriate professional organizations, shall by regulation promulgate minimum standards for the certification of persons who administer radiologic procedures. Such standards shall distinguish between certification of (1) medical radiologic technologists (including radiographers), (2) dental auxiliaries (including dental hygienists and assistants), (3) radiation therapy technologists, (4) nuclear medicine technologists, and (5) such other kinds of health auxiliaries who administer radiologic procedures as the Secretary determines appropriate. Such standards shall include minimum certification criteria for individuals with regard to accredited education, practical experience, successful passage of required examinations, and such other criteria as the Secretary shall deem necessary for the adequate qualification of individuals to administer radiologic procedures. Such standards shall not apply to practitioners.

Model Statute

[42 USC 10005.]

Sec. 980. In order to encourage the administration of accreditation and certification programs by the States, the Secretary shall prepare and transmit to the States a model statute for radiologic procedure safety. Such model statute shall provide that—

(1) it shall be unlawful in a State for individuals to perform radiologic procedures unless such individuals are certified by the State to perform such procedures; and

(2) any educational requirements for certification of individuals to perform radiologic procedures shall be limited to educational programs accredited by the State.

Compliance

[42 USC 10006.]

Sec. 981. (a) The Secretary shall take all actions consistent with law to effectuate the purposes of this subtitle.

(b) A State may utilize an accreditation or certification program administered by a private entity if—

(1) such State delegates the administration of the State accreditation or certification program to such private entity;

(2) such program is approved by the State; and

(3) such program is consistent with the minimum Federal standards promulgated under this subtitle for such program.

(c) Absent compliance by the States with the provisions of this subtitle within three years after the date of enactment of this Act, the Secretary shall report to the Congress recommendations for legislative changes considered necessary to assure the States' compliance with this subtitle.

[Report to Congress.]

(d) The Secretary shall be responsible for continued monitoring of compliance by the States with the applicable provisions of this subtitle and shall report to the Senate and the House of Representatives by January 1, 1982, and January 1 of each succeeding year the status of the States' compliance with the purposes of this subtitle.

(e) Notwithstanding any other provision of this section, in the case of a State which has, prior to the effective date of standards and guidelines promulgated pursuant to this subtitle, established standards for the accreditation of educational programs and certification of radiologic technologists, such State shall be deemed to be in compliance with the conditions of this section unless the Secretary determines, after notice and hearing, that such State standards do not meet the minimum standards prescribed by the Secretary or are inconsistent with the purposes of this subtitle.

Federal radiation guidelines

[42 USC 10007.]

Sec. 982. The Secretary shall, in conjunction with the Radiation Policy Council, the Administrator of Veterans' Affairs, the Administrator of the Environmental Protection Agency, appropriate agencies of the States, and appropriate professional organizations, promulgate Federal radiation guidelines with respect to radiologic procedures. Such guidelines shall—

(1) determine the level of radiation exposure due to radiologic procedures which is unnecessary and specify the techniques, procedures, and methods to minimize such unnecessary exposure;

(2) provide for the elimination of the need for retakes of diagnostic radiologic procedures;

(3) provide for the elimination of unproductive screening programs;

(4) provide for the optimum diagnostic information with minimum radiologic exposure; and

(5) include the therapeutic application of radiation to individuals in the treatment of disease, including nuclear medicine applications.

Applicability to federal agencies

[42 USC 10008.]

Sec. 983. (a) Except as provided in subsection (b), each department, agency, and instrumentality of the executive branch of the Federal Government shall comply with standards promulgated pursuant to this subtitle.

[Regulations.]

[38 USC 101 *et seq.*]

(b)(1) The Administrator of Veterans' Affairs, through the Chief Medical Director of the Veterans' Administration, shall, to the maximum extent feasible consistent with the responsibilities of such Administrator and Chief Medical Director under subtitle 38, United States Code, prescribe regulations making the standards promulgated pursuant to this subtitle applicable to the provision of radiologic procedures in facilities over which the Administrator has jurisdiction. In prescribing and implementing regulations pursuant to this subsection, the Administrator shall consult with the Secretary in order to achieve the maximum possible coordination of the regulations, standards, and guidelines, and the implementation thereof, which the Secretary and the Administrator prescribe under this subtitle.

[Report to congressional committees.]

(2) Not later than 180 days after standards are promulgated by the Secretary pursuant to this subtitle, the Administrator of Veterans' Affairs shall submit to the appropriate committees of Congress a full report with respect to the regulations (including guidelines, policies, and procedures thereunder) prescribed pursuant to paragraph (1) of this subsection. Such report shall include—

(A) an explanation of any inconsistency between standards made applicable by such regulations and the standards promulgated by the Secretary pursuant to this subtitle;

(B) an account of the extent, substance, and results of consultations with the Secretary respecting the prescription and implementation of regulations by the Administrator; and

(C) such recommendations for legislation and administrative action as the Administrator determines are necessary and desirable.

[Publication in Federal Register.]

(3) The Administrator of Veterans' Affairs shall publish the report required by paragraph (2) in the Federal Register.

Index

Page numbers followed by *f* indicate figures, by *t* indicate tables, by *n* indicate footnotes.